SPORTS
INJURIES
AND
EMERGENCIES

W9-AWQ-651

SPORTS INJURIES AND EMERGENCIES

A Quick-Response Manual

Editor

Aaron Rubin, MD

Program Director
Kaiser Permanente Sports Medicine
Fellowship–Fontana
Team Physician
Rubidoux High School
University of California, Riverside
Riverside, California

McGraw-Hill
Medical Publishing Division

New York   Chicago   San Francisco   Lisbon   London   Madrid
Mexico City   Milan   New Delhi   San Juan   Seoul
Singapore   Sydney   Toronto

The McGraw·Hill Companies

SPORTS INJURIES AND EMERGENCIES: A Quick-Response Manual

1234567890   DOCDOC   098765432

ISBN 0-07-139610-1

This book was set in Times Medium by Matrix Publishing Services.
The editors were Darlene Barela Cooke, Michelle Watt, and Lester A. Sheinis.
The production supervisor was Richard C. Ruzycka.
The cover designer was Janice Bielawa.
The indexer was Alexandra Nickerson.
The illustrator was William N. Winn.
RR Donnelley was printer and binder.

This book is printed on acid-free paper.

Inside Back Cover: Reprinted from *Emergent Management of Trauma,* 2d edition, by Thomas A. Scaletta and Jeffrey J. Schaider, New York: McGraw-Hill, 2001, with permission.

Library of Congress Cataloging-in-Publication Data
Sports injuries and emergencies : a quick-response manual / edited by
  Aaron Rubin.
      p. ; cm.
    Includes bibliographical references and index.
    ISBN 0-07-139610-1
      1. Sports injuries—Handbooks, manuals, etc. I. Rubin, Aaron.
    [DNLM: 1. Athletic Injuries—diagnosis—Handbooks. QT 29 S7637
    2003]
    RD97 .S6884 2003
    617.1′027—dc21
                                                        2002030911

CPT codes, descriptions, and material only are Copyright © 2001 American Medical Association. All Rights Reserved. No fee schedules, basic units, relative values, or related listings are included in CPT. The AMA assumes no liability for the data contained herein. Applicable FARS/DFARS restrictions apply to government use.

*Dedicated to my wife, Paula, my children, Kristen and Ryan, and
my parents and sister for providing my foundation.
To my teachers and colleagues for building the framework.
And to my fellows, residents, students, and athletes for continuing
to add the details.
The best way to learn is to teach.*

Contents

PART 4   GENERAL TOPICS

PART 5   APPENDIXES

Contributors

Special Consultant: Orthopedic Section
David Anderson, MD
Chief, Orthopedic Surgery
Director Orthopedic Sports Medicine
Kaiser Permanente Medicine Fellowship Program
Fontana, California

Tony Alamo, MD
Athletic Commissioner State of Nevada (Boxing)
Past Chairman Medical Advisory Board to Boxing Commission
Past Ring Physician (Boxing)
Tactical Physician Metropolitan Police (SWAT Division Las Vegas)
Chief of Staff Sunrise Adult and Pediatric Hospital
Diplomat American Board of Internal Medicine
Las Vegas, Nevada
Chapter 33

Evan S. Bass, MD
Sports Medicine Fellowship Director and Clinical Faculty
Harbor-UCLA Family Medicine Residency Program
Primary Care Sports Medicine, Kaiser Permanente
Harbor City, California
Chapters 36, 51

Brian Birnie
LaFollette, Johnson, DeHaas, Fesler, Silberberg, & Ames
Los Angeles, California
Chapter 57

Mark P. Bouchard, MD
Assistant Director
Maine Medical Center Sports Medicine Program
Assistant Professor
Department of Family Medicine
University of Vermont School of Medicine
Portland, Maine
Chapter 14

Kevin J. Broderick, MD
Sports Medicine Fellow 2001–2002
Maine Medical Center Sports Medicine Fellowship Program
Team Physician, North Reading High School, 2001–2002
Family Medicine Associates
Middleton, Massachusetts
Chapter 28

C. Mark Chassay, MD
Team Physician, Intercollegiate Athletics
The University of Texas at Austin
Austin, Texas
Chapter 49

John Cheng, MD
Family Medicine and Sports Medicine
Aliso Viejo, California
Chapter 40

Robert Corb, PhD
University of California, Riverside
Riverside, California
Chapter 58

Brian A. Davis, MD, FABPMR, FACSM
Co-Director of Sports Medicine and Director of Spine Care
Assistant Professor, Department of Physical Medicine & Rehabilitation
Assistant Professor, Department of Anesthesiology & Pain Management
University of California, Davis Medical Center
California State Ringside Physician
Physician to USA Boxing, Track and Field, Swimming and Tae
  Kwon Do
Sacramento, California
Chapter 33

William W. Dexter, MD, FACSM
Director
Maine Medical Center Sports Medicine Program
Associate Professor
Department of Family Medicine
University of Vermont School of Medicine and University of Maine
  Division of Sports Medicine
Team Physician
Portland Pirates (AHL)
University of Southern Maine
Portland, Maine
Chapter 15

T. Ted Funahashi, MD
Kaiser Permanente
Chief, Department of Orthopedic Surgery
Assistant Area Medical Director, Orange County
Coordinating Chief of Orthopedic Surgery, Southern California
Associate Clinical Professor of Orthopedic Surgery
UC Irvine Medical School
Irvine, California
Chapter 26

Jeff T. Grange, MD
Medical Director, California Speedway
Medical Director, San Bernardino Sheriff's Air Rescue Team
Assistant Professor, Emergency Medicine
Loma Linda School of Medicine
Loma Linda, California
Chapters 41, 55

David L. Haller, MD
Partner, Physician Southern California Permanente Medical Group
Team Physician
University of California, Irvine
Saddleback Community College
Garden Grove High School
San Juan Capistrano, California
Chapter 7

Kimberly G. Harmon, MD
Clinical Assistant Professor Department of Family Practice
Clinical Assistant Professor Department of Orthopaedics and
    Sports Medicine
Team Physician
University of Washington
Seattle, Washington
Chapters 37, 53

Benjamin A. Hasan, MD
Family Practice and Sports Medicine
Associate Director
Resurrection Family Practice Residency
Resurrection Medical Center
Team Physician
North Park University
Chicago, Illinois
Chapter 13

Sandra J. Hoffmann, MD, FACSM, FACP
New River Medical Associates
Hilton Head, South Carolina
Chapter 9

Ken Honsik, MD
Family and Sports Medicine
Faculty
Kaiser Permanente Sports Medicine Fellowship
Program
Fontana, California
Chapters 11, 16, 19, 54

Mark R. Hutchinson, MD
Associate Professor of Orthopaedics and Sports Medicine
University of Illinois at Chicago
Chicago, Illinois
Chapter 18

Carrie Jaworski, MD
Family Practice and Sports Medicine
Associate Director
Resurrection Family Practice
Residency
Team Physician
North Park University
Chicago, Illinois
Chapters 3, 4, 5, 39

Robert J. Johnson, MD
Director, Primary Care Sports Medicine
Department of Family Practice
Hennepin County Medical Center
Associate Professor, Department of Family Practice and Community
    Medicine
University of Minnesota
Minneapolis, Minnesota
Chapter 56

Todd Jorgenson, MD
Family Practice and Sports Medicine
Allina Medical Clinic, Woodlake
Minneapolis, Minnesota
Chapter 47

Joseph P. Luftman, MD
Attending Physician
Kaiser Permanente Medical Center
Department of Family Practice
Associate Director Sports Medicine Fellowship Program
Assistant Clinical Professor, UCLA Department of Family Practice
Los Angeles, California
Chapter 35

Gregory B. Maletis, MD
Assistant Chief of Orthopedics
Kaiser Permanente Baldwin Park
Associate Clinical Professor of Orthopedics
USC/Keck School of Medicine
Baldwin Park, California
Chapters 26, 38

D. Scott Marr, MD
Assistant Program Director, Maine Medical Center
Sports Medicine Fellowship Program
Assistant Program Director, Maine Medical Center
Family Practice Residency
Assistant Clinical Professor, Department of Family Medicine, University
  of Vermont School of Medicine
Portland, Maine
Chapter 27

John Martinez, MD
Sports Medicine Fellow
Kaiser Permanente Sports Medicine Fellowship
Program 2001–2002
Graybill Medical Group Inc.
Escondido, California
Chapters 32, 34, 52

Julie Max, ATC
Head Athletic Trainer
California State University Fullerton
Fullerton, California
Chapter 60

Timothy R. McCurry, MD
Program Director
Resurrection Family Practice Residency Program
Clinical Assistant Professor
Department of Family Medicine
Loyola University, Chicago/Stritch School of Medicine
Chicago, Illinois
Chapter 44

Chris McGilmer, MD
Kaiser Permanente Sports Medicine Fellowship
Program 2001–2002
Staff Physician
Kaiser Permanente
Panorama City, California
Chapters 25, 29

Bernadette Pendergraph, MD
Primary Care Sports Medicine Faculty
Harbor-UCLA Medical Center
Torrance, California
Chapters 36, 51

Chad A. Roghair, MD
Associate Team Physician
Lead Urgent Care Physician
University of California, Berkeley
Berkeley, California
Chapter 8

Joseph P. Romeo, MD, MS
President, California Day Spa and Cosmetic Surgery
Reconstructive Head and Neck Surgery
Turlock, California
Chapter 10

Sam J. Romeo, MD
CEO
Romeo Medical Clinic, Inc.
Clinical Faculty of the University of California
Davis School of Medicine
Team Physician, California State University, Stanislaus
Team Physician, Pitman High School
Turlock, California
Chapter 10

Denise M. Romero
Medical Student
University of California, San Francisco
San Francisco, California
Chapter 31

Aaron Rubin, MD
Program Director
Kaiser Permanente Sports Medicine Fellowship–Fontana
Team Physician
Rubidoux High School
University of California, Riverside
Riverside, California
Chapters 1, 43, 59, 63

Marc R. Safran, MD
Codirector, Sports Medicine
Associate Professor
Department of Orthopaedic Surgery
University of California, San Francisco
San Francisco, California
Chapters 23, 24, 31, 50

Robert E. Sallis, MD
Codirector
Kaiser Permanente Sports Medicine Fellowship–Fontana
Team Physician, Pomona College
Rancho Cucamonga, California
Chapter 6

Jim Schiller
Paramedic
Ontario Fire Department
Ontario, California
Chapters 61, 62

Lauren M. Simon, MD, MPH
Associate Professor, Department of Family Medicine
Director, Primary Care Sports Medicine
Loma Linda University School of Medicine
Team Physician, University of California-Riverside
Team Physician, University of Redlands
Race Medical Director, Redlands Bicycle Classic
Loma Linda, California
Chapters 12, 42

Sam Sunshine, MD
Family and Sports Medicine
Private Practice
Alisa Viejo, California
Chapter 48

Joseph P. Tansey MD
Resident Physician
University of Illinois at Chicago Hospital
Chicago, Illinois
Chapter 18

R. Tucker Thole, MD
Washoe Family Care–Vista
University of Nevada-Reno Team Physician
Reno, Nevada
Chapters 17, 45

Ray Tufts, ATC
Athletic Trainer, San Jose Sharks
San Jose, California
Chapter 38

Daniel V. Vigil, MD
Sports Medicine Fellowship Director
Kaiser Permanente
Los Angeles Medical Center
Center for Medical Education
Los Angeles, California
Chapter 46

Quincy Wang, MD
Family and Sports Medicine
Kaiser Permanente Long Beach
Long Beach, California
Chapters 2, 20, 22, 30

Frank Winton, MD
Sports Medicine Fellow
Kaiser Permanente Sports Medicine Fellowship
Program 2001–2002
Family Medicine and Sports Medicine
Graybill Medical Group Inc.
Fallbrook, California
Chapter 21

Preface

Our fellowship program organizes care for many local high school, college, and public events. We designed a training program to teach sideline behavior and treatment. As we reviewed the many fine sports medicine publications to find information to teach our residents, fellows, and attending physicians, we noted a lack of material directly related to the immediate, sideline care of the athlete.

We had to teach them how to practice medicine with little more than the equipment they could carry in their pockets. They had to be taught how to protect themselves from the changing elements, errant footballs, players charging off the field, and the occasional overexcited coach. This became the basis for this book.

The sports medicine provider always had to consider injury to player and spectator. Whether there was a team designated to care for spectators in a large arena or an individual physician at a high school game called to evaluate an injury in the stands, there was a need to have knowledge and planning.

This book is divided into five sections. The first section covers the basic approaches to the athlete and primary care issues. The second section covers specific orthopedic and musculoskeletal problems. The third section covers sports-specific concerns. The fourth section, General Topics, review important topics for the sideline medical provider. The Appendixes (the fifth section) are designed to be copied and customized for your individual needs.

I have asked experienced sports medicine physicians to provide expertise in these chapters but also to provide personal insight into the intricacies of managing acute injuries of athletes. I enlisted the aid of an attorney to discuss legal issues, a sports psychologist for the psychology of injury, an athletic trainer regarding equipment needs, and a fire captain/paramedic trained in emergency equipment and the incident command system.

And due to the aftermath of 9/11, more attention is turned to potential for disasters to occur at sporting events. We included chapters on the Incident Command System, Spectator Care, and the equipment and supplies utilized by emergency medical systems.

Remember the athletes of all ages and ability. Use this text to provide care and caring for them. Get out on the field and volunteer; your presence will be appreciated.

SPORTS
INJURIES
AND
EMERGENCIES

Part 1

Primary Concerns

1

Preparation

Aaron Rubin

Overview

- Any athletic event can lead to injury
- Both athletes and spectators are subject to medical problems
- Appropriate care can minimize long-term disability
- Care depends on the training of the medical providers and equipment availability

Training

- Medical providers should be adequately trained
  - Basic life support or equivalent training
  - Basic first aid
- Physician should have special training in sports medicine
  - Advanced cardiac life support or equivalent
  - Specialized training in care of the athlete by fellowship, residency, preceptorship, sports medicine meetings, and continuing medical education

Team Approach

- Physician should be leader of sports medicine team
  - Be readily available for care of athletes prior to game and make sure that all have been cared for at end of contest
  - Aid the athletic trainer in coordinating medical care
  - Make transport, care, and return-to-play decisions during contest
- Athletic trainer
  - Medical team member with most contact with the athletes
  - Arranges for preparticipation screening
  - Keeps injury records on athletes
  - Arranges for proper equipment
  - Coordinates medical care
  - Establishes and maintains disaster plan
  - Maintains medical control in absence of the team physician

- Coach
  - Generally has the most contact with the athletes
  - Must make sure that each athlete is properly trained for activity
  - Must see that safety equipment (helmets, shoulder pads, etc.) are properly fitted and maintained
  - Makes sure that the practice and playing venues are safe
  - Must have at least basic first aid training to offer in the absence of medical personnel
  - Must be well versed on the disaster plan for the facilities
  - Must ensure maximal safety of training exercises
- Facilities director or athletic director
  - Establishes budget for equipment and operating costs
  - Makes sure facilities are well maintained
  - Coordinates with security personnel
  - Assures access to facilities by emergency personnel
  - Maintains liaison with press
- Paramedics
  - Work with team medical personnel
  - Stabilize and transport injured athletes
  - Maintain communications with hospitals, communications centers, and other emergency personnel
- Police/security
  - Keep access to facilities and injured athlete open
  - Maintain communications
  - Provide security for medical personnel, athletes, families
  - Prevent injury to spectators and others by unruly fans

Equipment

- Medical supplies
  - Physician's medical bag (see Chap. 59)
  - Trainer's kit (see Chap. 60)
  - Emergency medical (see Chap. 61)
- Communication
  - Cellular phones
    - Ubiquitous
    - Generally one-to-one communications
    - Relative low in cost
    - Fairly highly secured communications
    - May be unreliable in certain areas
    - May have limited standby and talk time
  - Family Radio System/Citizen's Band Radio
    - Inexpensive
    - May "broadcast" to several users
    - Poor security
    - Limited range
  - "Ham" radio
    - More expense and training involved

- Long distance coverage
- "Police/emergency" frequency radios
  - Require special training, licensing. and equipment
  - High expense
  - High reliability in most areas

Bibliography

Mellion MB, Walsh WM, Shelton GL (eds): *The Team Physician's Handbook,* 2d ed. Philadelphia: Hanley & Belfus, 1997.

Safran MR, McKeag DP, VanCamp SP: *Manual of Sports Medicine.* Philadelphia: Lippincott-Raven, 1998.

2

Approach to the Downed Athlete

Quincy Wang

Assume the Worst

- Every downed athlete should be approached as having a life- or limb-threatening injury until proven otherwise
- Survey the scene and make sure it is safe to approach the downed athlete

Three Levels of Injury Priority

- First priority—injuries that pose an immediate threat to life
  - Airway obstruction (see Chap. 3)
  - Respiratory failure (see Chap. 4)
  - Cardiac arrest (see Chap. 5)
  - Uncontrolled hemorrhage
- Second priority—urgent injuries that are potential threats to life or limb
  - Head trauma (see Chap. 6)
  - Neck and spinal cord injuries (see Chap. 20)
  - Visceral injuries—ruptured spleen or bowel (see Chap. 14)
  - Seizures
  - Severe musculoskeletal trauma with neurovascular compromise
- Third priority—non-life-threatening injury, fortunately the most common type
  - Mild musculoskeletal injuries, sprain/strains
  - Lacerations and contusions (see Chap. 16)

Downed Athlete Survey

- When evaluating the downed athlete, survey the athlete with the three levels of injury priority in mind
- Primary survey—airway, breathing, circulation (ABCs)
  - Responsiveness—see whether the athlete is conscious

- Check for open airway; open if closed
- Check for breathing and prepare for ventilation
- Check for pulse/circulation
- Activate EMS if any one of the above is absent and begin CPR if necessary
- Secondary survey
  - If the athlete is conscious, obtain a brief history of the injury from the athlete
  - Ask whether there is any neck pain.
  - If there is neck pain or if the athlete is unconscious, **assume a cervical spine injury**. **DO NOT** move the athlete. **DO** stabilize the head and neck. (**DO NOT** remove the helmet, chin straps, or shoulder pads when treating a football player.)
  - Ask the athlete if there is any numbness, burning, or tingling down the arms or legs
  - Palpate the neck gently, feeling for point tenderness of the spinous processes and paraspinal musculature of the cervical spine
  - Perform a brief head-to-toe evaluation. Observe for gross deformities and acute hemorrhage. Palpate the arms, chest, abdomen, pelvis, and legs, noting any tenderness, numbness, swelling, or bone crepitus.
  - Determine gross motor function by asking athlete, if he or she is able, to move the fingers and toes, hands and feet, then arms and legs
  - Activate EMS for loss of consciousness, cervical spine injury, or other injury that poses a threat to life or limb (i.e., open fracture, uncontrolled hemorrhage, respiratory/cardiac arrest)
- Tertiary survey—by far the most common survey performed
  - Usually involves a musculoskeletal injury, laceration, or contusion
  - Perform a brief on-the-field examination of the injury
- Remove the athlete from the field of play
  - If there is no cervical spine or head injury, allow the athlete to sit up
  - Allow the athlete to stand, with assistance if needed
  - Allow the athlete to ambulate off the field of play to the medical station under his or her own power or with assistance
  - Perform a complete examination at the medical station. Afterwards, a decision must be made for return to play, removal from the contest, or transport to a medical facility.

Return to Play—General Principles

- Musculoskeletal injuries
  - The severity of the injury determines whether the athlete can return to play
  - Often, a short period of rest is all that is needed for the athlete to recover sufficiently to return safely to the game
  - For minor injuries, taping, stretching/massaging, padding the injury, or icing may be of benefit prior to return to play

- For return to play, the athlete must demonstrate on the sideline to the team physician that he can competently perform all the skills needed for that particular sport
- The athlete must be able to run, jump, squat, throw, kick, block, catch, or demonstrate any other appropriate skill at full speed and strength without pain
- The athlete can be cleared to play if the team physician determines that he or she can safely return with a low risk of reinjury or causing new injury to others while contributing to team performance
- Observation of play and reassessment must continue periodically for the remainder of the competition. Return of injury symptoms and diminished performance should warrant permanent removal from the contest.
- Neurologic/spinal cord/c-spine injuries
  - Neurologic injuries to the brain and spinal cord and/or cervical spine injuries warrant removal from the contest
  - Any loss of consciousness, persistent numbness, or weakness of the extremities mandates withdrawal from further competition
  - Athletes with concussion symptoms that have completely resolved after 15 min of rest with no return after provocative sideline testing can return to the game. Immediate removal from the game should occur if the concussion symptoms return (i.e., headache, nausea, memory problems).

Bibliography

Ewald M, Moeller JL: Urgent and emergent situations in sports medicine coverage. *Clin Fam Pract* 1(1):21–35, 1999.

Johnson RJ: Evaluating the injured athlete, in Safran MR, McKeag DB, Van Camp SP (eds): *Manual of Sports Medicine*. Philadelphia: Lippincott-Raven, 1998, pp 33–36.

Rubin AL, Sallis RE: Management of on-the-field emergencies, in Safran MR, McKeag DB, Van Camp SP (eds): *Manual of Sports Medicine*. Philadelphia: Lippincott-Raven, 1998, pp 43–53.

3

Airway

Carrie Jaworski

PATHOLOGY

- The sudden collapse of an athlete can result in an airway emergency
- The numerous causes leading to collapse and airway compromise include:
  - Status asthmaticus, anaphylaxis, seizure, cardiac arrythmias, heat exhaustion/heat stroke, hypoglycemia
  - Foreign-body obstruction
    - Mouthpiece, teeth, vomitus, blood
- Airway compromise is most often secondary to the tongue falling back in the throat
- Direct and indirect trauma can also interfere with an athlete's airway
  - Soft tissue trauma to neck
  - Laryngeal or facial fractures
    - Bilateral anterior mandibular fractures cause loss of anterior support of the tongue
    - Maxillary (Le Fort) fractures can cause rapid soft tissue swelling and airway obstruction (see Chap. 10)
  - Indirect traumas such as cervical spine and head injuries can affect airway patency

DIAGNOSTIC KEYS

- Ability to speak without hoarseness or stridor indicates a patent airway
- Reassess regularly for changes in status
- Assume cervical spine injury in the unconscious athlete (see Chap. 20)

EXAMINATION / EVALUATION

- Remember that establishing an airway is the first priority in the ABCs (airway, breathing, circulation) of emergency medical care
- A face-down athlete requires "log-rolling" to allow for airway access
  - Cervical spine immobilization is necessary

- Proper technique and regular practice are required (see Chaps. 2 and 20)
- Face mask removal through the use of a "Trainer's Angel" or equivalent is also necessary in an athlete wearing a helmet/face mask
  - Cervical spine immobilization and regular practice, as above, are required
- Proper positioning is necessary to allow for evaluation
- The head-tilt, chin-lift (Fig. 3.1), or jaw-thrust maneuver (Fig. 3.2) can be used to elevate the tongue out of the airway
- Jaw thrust without head tilt is the preferred method in suspected cervical spine injuries
  - Place the third, fourth, and fifth fingers of each hand under the angle of the athlete's mandible
  - Push the mandible upward while maintaining cervical stabilization
- "Look, listen, and feel" for signs of breathing
  - Observe for chest rise and fall
  - Listen and feel by placing your ear close to athlete's mouth and nose
- If there are no signs of breathing, reposition the athlete after looking for signs of foreign-body obstruction
  - If there is no risk of injury to the cervical spine, it is acceptable to turn the athlete on his or her side to clear foreign-body obstruction

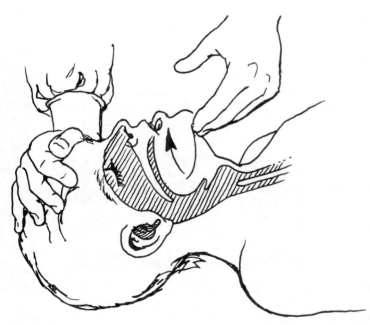

Figure 3.1 Chin lift.

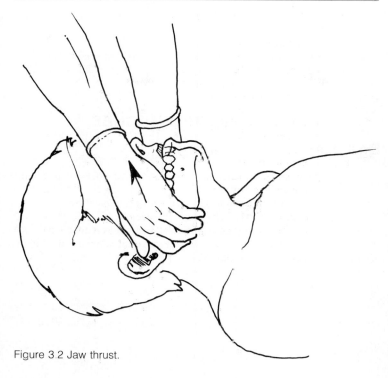

Figure 3.2 Jaw thrust.

- You can use a finger sweep with proper precautions (gloves) in an adult
- Use the Heimlich maneuver as indicated

EMERGENT TREATMENT

- Establishment of a patent airway is the only acceptable treatment
- Activate Emergency Medical Service (EMS) immediately
- Proper positioning may be all that is required
  - Maintain airway with an oropharyngeal airway (OPA) in the unconscious athlete
    - Can aid rescuer in ventilation and airway maintenance
    - Appropriate size is distance from incisors to tragus
    - Insert using tongue blade and slide posteriorly along tongue
    - If no tongue blade is available, reverse OPA so concave portion faces palate and rotate 180 degrees as it reaches back of tongue; avoid in small children
    - Can elicit gag reflex and possibly vomiting in conscious victim
- A nasopharyngeal airway can be used to maintain the airway in a semiconscious athlete

- Contraindicated in basilar skull fractures; therefore avoid in head-injured athletes
- Same sizing as OPA
- Use vasoconstricting drops, if available, in nostril prior to insertion to reduce bleeding risk
- Insert with bevel toward septum

ADVANCED TECHNIQUES

Endotracheal Intubation

- When done properly, method considered most effective in establishing airway
- Requires extensive training and continuous reinforcement
- May be difficult in an athletic setting, especially if cervical spine injury is suspected—requires in-line stabilization (**not traction**)
- Have patient preoxygenated with bag-valve-mask device and 100% oxygen while equipment is prepared
- Endotracheal tube (ETT) sizing:
  - Adult male: 8.0 mm
  - Adult female: 7.0 mm
  - Child: (age in years +16)/4 or size of child's little finger
- "BURP" (backward, upward, and rightward pressure) larynx to visualize glottis
- Pass ETT between cords once glottis is seen
- Depth of insertion: stop when the "19–23 cm" indicator marks are at the anterior teeth in adults or (internal diameter $\times$ 3) at the incisors in children
- Can cause harm in inexperienced hands:
  - Esophageal intubation
  - Trauma to oropharynx
  - Prolonged time to ventilation
- Alternative methods—including nasotracheal intubation, manual digital intubation, and rapid sequence inductions (RSI)—are best left to extensively trained practitioners

Laryngeal Mask Airway (LMA) (Fig. 3.3)

- The LMA is a reusable airway device approved by the American Heart Association (AHA) as an alternative airway during Advanced Cardiac Life Support (ACLS)
- Requires blind insertion into the pharynx until resistance is felt at the hypopharynx
- Distal cuff is then inflated, which seals the larynx and leaves the distal end above the glottis to provide a stable airway
- Advantages
  - Requires minimal instruction
  - Eliminates need to master laryngoscopy

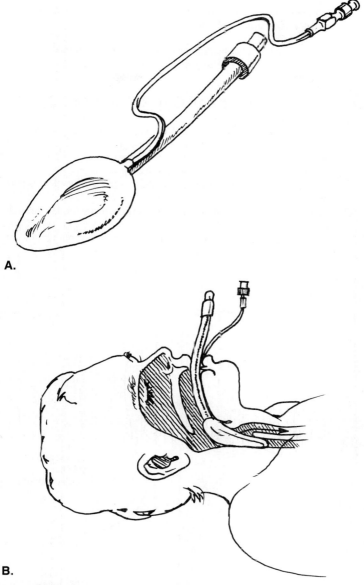

A.

B.

Figure 3.3 Laryngeal mask. *A.* Laryngeal mask airway. *B.* Proper insertion of laryngeal mask airway.

- Rapid insertion times
- Ventilation volumes equivalent to endotracheal tube, better than bag-valve-mask ventilation
- Disadvantages
  - Does not provide absolute protection against aspiration
  - Still requires practice and reinforcement

Esophageal-Tracheal Combitube (ETC)

- The ETC (Kendall, Mansfield, MA) (Fig. 3.4) is a single-use, double-lumen airway comprising a tracheal tube joined to an esophageal obturator
- Approved by AHA for use in ACLS setting
- Blind insertion usually results in esophageal placement (98–99 percent)
- Inflate both cuffs, assume esophageal insertion, and ventilate through esophageal obturator side (blue lumen)
- If tube is in esophagus, air enters trachea through vents on side of obturator

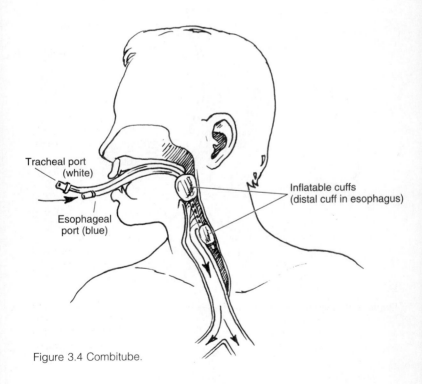

Figure 3.4 Combitube.

- If no chest rise, assume tube is in trachea and change ventilations to white tracheal tube lumen
- Advantages
  - Blind insertion
  - Protects against aspiration
  - Ventilates better than face mask and equivalent to endotracheal tube
- Disadvantages
  - More complicated confirmation of placement than LMA
  - Risk of esophageal trauma
  - Requires training and reinforcement
- Contraindications
  - Esophageal disease
  - Caustic ingestion
  - Active gag reflex
  - Standard size ETC is contraindicated in athletes less than 5 ft tall
  - Small adult model contraindicated in athletes less than 4 ft or more than 5.5 ft tall

Confirmation of Airway Placement

- The ETT, LMA, and ETC all require confirmation of placement
  - **Primary confirmation** is done clinically
    - Lungs with bilateral breath sounds (best heard in each axilla)
    - Chest wall movement
    - Absence of stomach gurgling
  - **Secondary confirmation** required through use of end-tidal CO_2 detector or esophageal detector devices
    - **End-tidal CO_2 detector** measures exhaled CO_2 from lungs
      - Qualitative, quantitative, and continuous models are available
      - Measure after six breaths to wash out any CO_2 in the esophagus
      - Can get incorrect readings in low perfusion states (cardiac arrest)
    - **Esophageal detector devices** work via a suction force at the end of the tube by either withdrawing on a large syringe or applying a compressed aspiration bulb
      - Only effective in endotracheal intubation or ETC use
      - Suction will pull the esophageal mucosa against the tube and prevent reexpansion if improperly placed in esophagus
      - Potential for error in morbid obesity, status asthmaticus, tracheomalacia, or late stages of pregnancy
      - Easy to construct for sideline bag using 60-mL catheter-tip syringe connected to an adapter with a 15-mm internal diameter (catalog # 48312, Hudson Oxygen Company) with a length of semirigid tubing in between (uncuffed 6-mm endotracheal tube)

SURGICAL AIRWAYS

- If airway cannot be secured by conventional means, a surgical airway is indicated
- Laryngeal fracture or edema, massive facial injuries, and obstruction can necessitate a surgical airway

Percutaneous Needle Cricothyrotomy (PNC)

- Method of choice in athletes age 10 and under
- Locate cricothyroid membrane (CTM) by palpating down from the notch of the thyroid cartilage
- Prepare area with skin antiseptic as time allows
- Insert a 14-gauge intravenous catheter needle through the membrane while stabilizing the larynx
- Aspiration should yield a free flow of air
- Angle needle caudally 45 degrees and advance the catheter over the needle into the trachea
- Remove the needle and begin ventilation using appropriate oxygen delivery device (jet ventilator, high-pressure oxygen extension tubing, or resuscitation bag with proper adapter attachment)
- Contraindicated when there is complete upper airway obstruction that cannot be corrected due to risk of barotrauma from trapped air
- Commercial cricothyrotomy kits are available

Surgical Cricothyrotomy

- Preferred method in those over 10 years of age (Fig. 3.5)
  - Locate the CTM as above
  - Prepare skin as time allows
  - Stabilize the larynx with your nondominant hand
  - Longitudinal incision 2 to 3 cm along midline of and down to the CTM using a scalpel with a #10 or #11 blade
  - Retract skin edges and make a transverse incision across the CTM
  - Maintain incision opening with finger placement, hemostat, nasal speculum, tracheal hook, or end of scalpel until airway is placed
  - Insert a tracheostomy tube or 5- to 6-mm endotracheal tube (3 mm in a child) and secure
  - Ventilate—attach bag-valve device
  - Commercially prepared kits are available to aid in the procedure
  - Lifestat is an example—trocar and cannula with universal adapter that allows ventilation via rescue breaths, bag-valve devices, or a ventilator

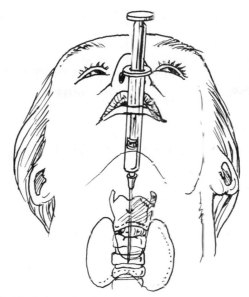

Figure 3.5 Surgical airway landmarks.

Complications of Surgical Airways (Table 3.1)

- Can be minimized with proper training and practice
- Emergency tracheostomy is best left to the hospital setting

Table 3.1 Complications of Surgical Airways

Percutaneous needle cricothyrotomy
1. Inadequate ventilations causing hypoxia or death
2. Aspiration
3. Hematoma
4. Subcutaneous or mediastinal emphysema
5. Esophageal laceration
6. Posterior tracheal wall perforation
7. Thyroid perforation

Surgical cricothyrotomy
1. Asphyxia
2. Aspiration
3. Creation of false passage into the tissues
4. Subglottic stenosis or edema
5. Laryngeal stenosis
6. Laceration of the esophagus or trachea
7. Mediastinal emphysema
8. Vocal cord paralysis
9. Hoarseness
10. Hemorrhage or hematoma
11. Cellulitis

DEFINITIVE TREATMENT/FOLLOW-UP

- Proceed to assess remainder of ABCDEs (airway, breathing, circulation, disability, environment, examination)
- Transport athlete to hospital for definitive treatment of underlying pathology
- Return to play is based on cause of airway compromise and use clinical judgment

COMPLICATIONS

- Anoxic injury
- Death

Bibliography

Advanced Trauma Life Support Program for Doctors. Chicago: American College of Surgeons, 1997, pp 1–504.

Chameides L, Hazinski MF (eds): *Pediatric Advanced Life Support.* Dallas: American Heart Association, 1997.

Cummins RO (ed): *ACLS Provider Manual.* Dallas: American Heart Association, 2001.

Doerges V, Sauer C, Ocker H, et al: Airway management during cardiopulmonary resuscitation—a comparative study of bag-valve-mask, laryngeal mask airway and Combitube in a bench model. *Resuscitation* 41:63–69, 1999.

Guidelines 2000 for cardiopulmonary resuscitation and emergency cardiac care. *Circulation* 102(suppl I):I-95–I-104, 2000.

Jaworski C: Advances in emergent airway management. *Curr Sports Med Rep* 1:133–140, 2002.

Norris RL, Peterson J: Airway management for the sports physician. Part 1: Basic techniques. *Phys Sportsmed* 29:23–29, 2001.

Norris RL, Peterson J: Airway management for the sports physician. Part 2: Advanced techniques. *Phys Sportsmed* 29:15–28, 2001.

Tintinalli JE, Kelen GD, Stapczynski JS (eds): *Emergency Medicine: A Comprehensive Study Guide,* 5th ed. New York: McGraw-Hill, 2000.

4

Breathing

Carrie Jaworski

Introduction

The second step in the airway, breathing, circulation (ABCs) of resuscitation, breathing, goes hand in hand with the airway issues outlined in Chap. 3. Any breathing difficulties encountered must be addressed in a rapid and efficient manner to prevent serious, life-threatening sequelae.

Pathology

- Many times, proper positioning to elevate the tongue out of the airway is all that is required to enable an injured athlete to resume spontaneous breathing (see Chap. 3)
- Respiratory effort can also be compromised by several life-threatening etiologies:
  - Status asthmaticus
  - Anaphylactic reactions
    - Acute allergic reaction leading to respiratory difficulty
    - Reaction to insect bite/bee sting, most common reason in athletic setting
  - Pneumothorax
    - Escape of air into the pleural space, resulting in lung collapse/compression and respiratory compromise
    - Secondary to trauma versus spontaneous event
      - Traumatic pneumothorax is usually caused by blunt trauma to chest with or without rib fracture
      - Spontaneous pneumothorax can be precipitated by physical activity; it is seen frequently in tall, thin young males
      - Tension pneumothorax results when accumulated inspired air cannot escape with expiration
    - Direct and indirect trauma can also impair breathing, as discussed in related chapters

Diagnostic Keys

- History of asthma
- History of previous reactions to bites
- Chest trauma

Examination

- Look, listen, and feel for signs of breathing, as described previously
- In asthma and anaphylaxis, labored breathing may be present
  - Nasal flaring, accessory muscle use, retractions
  - Cyanosis
  - Erythema at site of insect bite or diffuse urticaria
- Pneumothorax
  - Pleuritic chest pain, dyspnea, cough in simple pneumothorax
  - Tracheal deviation, cyanosis, neck vein distention, hemodynamic compromise = tension pneumothorax
  - Unilateral absence of breath sounds
  - Hypertympany of affected side
  - Tachypnea

Emergent Treatment

- Anaphylaxis, asthma, and pneumothorax (see Chaps. 7, 8, and 13)
- Activate Emergency Medical Service (EMS) if not already done
- Once airway is established, a lack of spontaneous respirations requires initiation of artificial ventilations
- **Mouth-to-mouth resuscitation**: Not recommended unless mask or shield is unavailable
- **Barrier devices** should be carried by all health care providers:
  - Face shield
    - Easily portable
    - Does not protect against aspiration or victim's exhaled gases
  - Mouth-to-pocket mask
    - One-way valve to protect against victim's exhaled air
    - Some models allow for supplemental oxygen, 10–15 L/min
    - Use long, slow breaths over at least 2 s
    - Some studies demonstrate superiority to bag-valve-mask technique
    - Easier to use than bag-valve-mask device, especially in one-rescuer situations
  - **Bag-valve-mask technique**: best option if done properly
    - Two rescuers recommended—one to hold mask, one to bag
    - Ventilate at least 2 s for each bag ventilation
    - Sellick maneuver—third rescuer can apply cricoid pressure to prevent aspiration of gastric contents and/or gastric inflation with positive-pressure ventilation

- Difficult to do in single-rescuer situations
- Use oropharyngeal airway in patients who can tolerate insertion without gagging
- Definitive airway control as described in Chap. 3

Definitive Treatment/Follow-up/ Return to Play

- Proceed to assess circulation (Chap. 5)
- Transport to hospital for definitive care of underlying pathology
- Return to play (RTP) or is based on cause of breathing difficulty and clinical judgment

Complications

- Anoxic injury
- Death

Bibliography

Advanced Trauma Life Support Program for Doctors. Chicago: American College of Surgeons, 1997, pp 1–504.

Chameides L, Hazinski MF (eds): *Pediatric Advanced Life Support.* Dallas: American Heart Association, 1997.

Cummins RO (ed): *ACLS Provider Manual.* Dallas: American Heart Association, 2001.

Guidelines 2000 for cardiopulmonary resuscitation and emergency cardiac care. *Circulation* 102(suppl I):I-95–I-104, 2000.

Norris RL, Peterson J: Airway management for the sports physician. Part 1: Basic techniques. *Phys Sportsmed* 29:23–29, 2001.

Norris RL, Peterson J: Airway management for the sports physician. Part 2: Advanced techniques. *Phys Sportsmed* 29:15–28, 2001.

Tintinalli JE, Kelen GD, Stapczynski JS (eds): *Emergency Medicine: A Comprehensive Study Guide,* 5th ed. New York: McGraw-Hill, 2000.

5

Circulation

Carrie Jaworski

INTRODUCTION

The next critical step in stabilizing an athlete is assessing perfusion of vital organs. The sports medicine team must be prepared to perform basic life support (BLS), including chest compressions and rapid defibrillation as indicated. Team physicians should also be trained in advanced cardiac life support (ACLS) and consider certification in advanced trauma and life support (ATLS).

PATHOLOGY

- In the athletic setting, the most frequent causes of perfusion problems include:
  - Hypovolemia—loss of blood leading to decreased preload and therefore decreased cardiac output
  - Dysrhythmias—usually ventricular fibrillation with underlying cardiovascular disease
  - Myocardial infarction
- Other causes include electrocution from lightning strikes and commotio cordis
- Victim is more likely to be a spectator, coach, or official

DIAGNOSTIC KEYS

- Determine whether pulse is present
- Often difficult to obtain blood pressure (BP) in athletic setting
- Estimate BP by measuring pulse:
  - Palpable carotid pulse indicates systolic BP of at least 60 mmHg
  - Palpable radial pulse indicates systolic BP of at least 80 mmHg
- Weak pulse indicates shock
  - Rapid identification of the cause of shock is paramount
  - Hypovolemic shock—hemorrhage, fluid losses, dehydration

- Cardiogenic shock—myocardial infarction, pulmonary embolus, pericardial tamponade, tension pneumothorax, cardiomyopathy
- Vasogenic shock—sepsis, anaphylaxis, pharmacologic overdose
- Neurogenic shock—spinal cord injury
- No pulse: assume ventricular fibrillation

EXAMINATION

- Look for areas of trauma/hemorrhage and apply pressure as indicated
- Patients in shock may be suffering from:
  - Hypovolemic shock—cool, clammy, or mottled extremities; tachycardic; tachypneic; flat neck veins; pallor; and decreased peripheral pulses
  - Cardiogenic shock—distended neck veins, rales, diaphoresis, narrowed pulse pressure, and cool, clammy, sweaty extremities
  - Vasogenic shock—flushing, widened pulse pressure, urticaria, and throat tightness/hoarseness if anaphylactic
  - Neurogenic shock—flaccid paralysis and hypotension with bradycardia
- Monitor cardiac rate and rhythm

EMERGENT TREATMENT

- Activate Emergency Medical Service (EMS)
- Follow cardiopulmonary resuscitation (CPR) guidelines (see Appendix)

Cardiac Arrest

- Most commonly ventricular fibrillation (VF) or pulseless ventricular tachycardia (VT)
- Chest compressions until defibrillator available
  - Two rescuers: 15 compressions to 2 breaths
  - Single rescuer and pediatrics: 5-to-1 ratio
  - Depth of compression: ~2 in. in adult, ~1 to 1.5 in. in child 1 to 8 years of age
- Early defibrillation is of utmost importance
  - Chances of resuscitation decrease 7–10 percent for each minute that elapses
  - Most will survive if defibrillation occurs in less than 3 min
  - Few will survive if delay is greater than 16 min. despite CPR
- **Automatic external defibrillators (AEDs)**—serve as an excellent alternative to standard defibrillators in an athletic setting/mass participation events
  - Ease of use—limited training required
  - Less cumbersome—portable and lightweight
  - Less costly than a standard defibrillator

- "Shock-advisory" type most commonly used. It alerts user, by voice command, to push well-marked button to deliver shock as indicated.
- Four universal steps of AED operation:
    - Power on, attach electrode pads to patient's chest, analyze rhythm, shock (if indicated)
- See Chap. 65 for specific algorithm on use in CPR
- Contraindicated in children less than 8 years of age
- **ACLS** (see Appendix for algorithm) (Chap. 64)
    - Protocols beyond defibrillation unlikely to be used at most athletic venues. However, they should be available at any mass-participation event.
    - Medications typically administered en route to hospital by EMS
    - Epinephrine 1 mg IV push every 3 to 5 min is standard as next line of treatment after three attempts at defibrillation in VF/pulseless VT
    - 40 U of vasopressin administered intravenously (one dose only) can also be used
    - Amiodarone, lidocaine, magnesium, procainamide, and sodium bicarbonate can also be considered
    - Resume attempts to defibrillate after each medication or after each minute of CPR

Shock

- Contain areas of hemorrhage
- Insert two large-bore (16-gauge or larger) peripheral intravenous lines
- Administer intravenous crystalloid fluids rapidly—normal saline or lactated Ringer's solution
- 3:1 rule—for each 1 unit volume of blood loss, give 3 volumes crystalloid
- Fluids not recommended if cardiogenic shock suspected—use inotropes instead
- Monitor cardiac rate and rhythm
- Administer supplemental oxygen
- Apply medical antishock trousers (MAST) (contraindicated in acute pulmonary edema)

Intravenous Access

- Large-bore needle
- Aseptic technique insofar as possible
- Choose technique most experienced with to decrease complication rate
- Peripheral venipuncture is procedure of choice during CPR
- Femoral line may be necessary for rapid fluid replacement and is often easier in emergency situations

- Medial to femoral artery
- If pulseless, vein is found at junction of medial and middle third of inguinal ligament
- Venous cutdown—use "minicutdown" approach to avoid sacrificing vessel
  - Saphenous vein most often used
  - Can find anterior to medial malleolus or 5 cm below inguinal ligament at junction of medial and middle third of thigh with patient supine
  - Incision perpendicular to vein
  - Expose vein and elevate with hemostat
  - Insert over-the-needle catheter into vein under direct visualization
  - Can occlude distal vessel temporarily to control bleeding
  - Close skin after successfully placed

DEFINITIVE TREATMENT/ RETURN TO PLAY

- Stabilize as above and transfer to hospital
- Treatment of underlying cause of perfusion deficits
- Dictated by underlying pathology and clinical judgment

Bibliography

Advanced Trauma Life Support Program for Doctors. Chicago: American College of Surgeons, 1997, pp 1–504.

Cantwell JD: Automatic external defibrillators in the sports arena: The right place, the right time. *Phys Sportsmed* 26(12):33, 1998.

Chameides L, Hazinski MF (eds): *Pediatric Advanced Life Support.* Dallas: American Heart Association, 1997.

Cummins RO (ed): *ACLS Provider Manual.* Dallas: American Heart Association, 2001.

Guidelines 2000 for cardiopulmonary resuscitation and emergency cardiac care. *Circulation* 102(suppl I):I-95–I-104, 2000.

Rubin AL: Automated external defibrillators: Selection and use. *Phys Sportsmed* 8(3):112–114, 2000.

Tintinalli JE, Kelen GD, Stapczynski JS (eds): *Emergency Medicine: A Comprehensive Study Guide,* 5th ed. New York: McGraw-Hill, 2000.

6

Head Injuries in the Athlete

Robert E. Sallis

INTRODUCTION

- Head injuries are frequently seen in a variety of sports. Along with neck injuries, they are the most common cause of catastrophic sports injuries.
- Sports with the highest incidence of head injuries are football, boxing, ice hockey, rugby, skiing, gymnastics, aquatic sports, martial arts, biking, motor sports
- Sideline physicians must be prepared to respond quickly and appropriately to the head-injured athlete to avoid a tragic outcome

THE EFFECTS OF HEAD INJURY

- **Cerebral concussion**—the most common consequence of a head injury in sports (see below)
- **Cerebral contusion**—implies "bruising" of the brain. Best seen with MRI
  - Symptoms—usually persistent headache or neurologic deficit, possibly also seizures
  - Treatment—symptomatic. Usually does not require surgery
- **Intracerebral hematoma**—bleeding into brain substance itself. Can be seen on CT or MRI scan
  - Symptoms—similar to contusion but often more severe. May progress rapidly to death
  - Treatment—may require surgical evacuation to reduce intracranial pressure if the hematoma is large
- **Epidural hematoma**—from an arterial bleed between the skull and the dura of the brain. Often associated with a temporal skull fracture. Can be seen with CT scan or MRI.
  - Symptoms—often initial short loss of consciousness followed by lucid interval associated with increasing headache and progressive deterioration in level of consciousness (usually within 1–2 h)
  - Treatment—prompt surgical evacuation may prevent permanent neurologic injury

- **Subdural hematoma**—from a venous bleed between the brain surface and the dura. Often associated with injury to the brain tissue. Can be seen with CT or MRI scan.
  - Symptoms—depend on type
    - Acute—usually unconscious with focal neurologic findings. Usually indicate significant brain injury.
    - Subacute or chronic—often mild symptoms of headache along with mild mental, motor, or sensory signs. Develops over 24 h to 2 weeks or more.
  - Treatment—surgical evacuation can lead to full recovery in subacute/chronic cases. Much poorer results with acute cases.

CEREBRAL CONCUSSION

Definition

A temporary disturbance of brain function that occurs without structural change in the brain.

Incidence

- Over 250,000 concussions each year in football alone (likely more)
- High school football players have about a 20 percent risk of concussions every year of play

Consequences

- Athletes with one concussion have a fourfold greater risk of sustaining repeated concussions
- Repeated concussions appear to impart a cumulative effect. They tend to produce symptoms of increasing severity and curation.

EFFECTS OF REPEATED CONCUSSIONS

- **Postconcussive syndrome**—persistent symptoms occurring after concussion
  - Headache and dizziness are typically the most prominent symptoms, often associated with nausea and vomiting
  - Other symptoms include tiredness, difficulty concentrating, memory disturbances, irritability, anxiety, blurred vision, problems sleeping, etc
  - Etiology is uncertain—psychological factors may play a role. Need to rule out structural injury with CT or MRI scan.
  - Treatment is symptomatic, as symptoms tend to spontaneously abate with time

- Dementia pugilistica (punch-drunk syndrome)—chronic brain damage resulting from repeated head trauma. Described in boxers.
  - Symptoms of personality disturbances, organic mental syndrome, dysarthria, and cerebellar or Parkinson's-like disturbance
  - Correlates with the number of fights and length of career. Most common in slugging-type, heavyweight, and second-rate boxers.
  - While not described in other sports, it has been shown that repeated concussions in football players do lead to abnormal neuropsychological tests, indicating some degree of brain damage
- **Second-impact syndrome (SIS)**—massive and often fatal brain swelling occurring after a head injury
  - First described in 1984 by Saunders and Harbaugh. Between 1980 and 1991, there were only 17 probable cases of SIS identified in U.S. football players.
  - Occurs in athletes who are still symptomatic after a recent minor head injury and then sustain a second minor head injury
  - Injury leads to autoregulatory dysfunction of the cerebral vasculature → cerebral congestion → intracranial hypertension → temporal lobe or cerebellar herniation → death
  - A common feature of all reported cases is persistent symptoms after the first minor head injury (e.g., headaches, dizziness, or visual, motor, or sensory changes)
  - The second blow may be quite minor and the athlete may appear stunned but usually does not lose consciousness. The athlete generally remains on his or her feet for 15 s to a minute or so and may leave the field without assistance.
  - After 15 s to a few minutes, the athlete quite precipitously collapses to the ground semicomatose, with rapidly dilating pupils and imminent respiratory failure
- On-field treatment requires rapid intubation, hyperventilation (to decrease CO_2, which causes vasoconstriction), and intravenous administration of an osmotic diuretic (usually 20% mannitol). This must be followed by immediate hospital transport. Surgery is generally not helpful and treatment is supportive.
- **Prevention is the key treatment for SIS.** Athletes who remain symptomatic after a head injury must not participate in contact or collision sports until all symptoms have cleared.

PROGRESSION OF SYMPTOMS IN CONCUSSIONS

- Concussion symptoms indicate the severity of the concussion. This forms the basis for concussion classifications schemes.
  - Confusion
  - Confusion + post-traumatic amnesia (PTA)
  - Confusion + PTA + retrograde amnesia (RGA)
  - Coma → confusion + PTA + RGA
  - Coma → persistent vegetative state
  - Coma → death

CLASSIFICATION OF CEREBRAL CONCUSSION

Colorado Medical Society Guidelines

- Grade 1 (mild)—confusion without amnesia. No loss of consciousness (LOC).
- Grade 2 (moderate)—confusion *with* amnesia. No LOC.
- Grade 3 (severe)—any LOC

American Academy of Neurology (AAN) Guidelines

- Grade 1—transient confusion. No LOC. Symptoms resolve in less than 15 min.
- Grade 2—transient confusion. No LOC. Symptoms last more than 15 min.
- Grade 3—any LOC, either brief (seconds) or prolonged (minutes)

GUIDELINES FOR RETURN TO PLAY (ADAPTED FROM COLORADO AND AAN GUIDELINES)

Grade 1 Concussion

- First grade 1 concussion—remove athlete from contest. Observe every 5 min for the development of amnesia or postconcussive symptoms, both at rest and with exertion. Athlete may return if no amnesia or other symptoms appear after 20 min.
- Second grade 1 concussion—if in the same game, athlete should be eliminated from that game and should sit out play for 1 week symptom-free

Grade 2 Concussion

- First grade 2 concussion—remove athlete from contest with no return that day. Observe for signs of evolving intracranial pathology (see patient handout). May return to play after 1 week symptom-free.
- Second grade 2 concussion—hold athlete out for 2 weeks symptom-free

Grade 3 Concussion

- If athlete remains unconscious, assume cervical spine fracture and place on spine board. Transport to nearest hospital for evaluation. Strongly consider CT or MRI scan. Admit to hospital if signs of pathology are detected.

- First grade 3 concussion—if brief (seconds), hold athlete out for 1 week symptom-free. If prolonged (minutes), hold athlete out for 2 weeks.
- Second grade 3 concussion—hold athlete out for 1 month symptom-free at minimum (possibly longer)

Further Considerations

- Consider getting a CT or MRI scan if headache or associated symptoms worsen or persist longer than a few days with any concussion
- Athletes with persisting symptoms should be restricted from any physical activity. Once symptoms clear, they may resume *noncontact* physical activity until the time when guidelines permit a return to contact sports.
- Terminate season for any abnormality on CT or MRI consistent with brain swelling, contusion, bleeding, or other intracranial pathology

SIDELINE EVALUATION FOR ATHLETES WITH HEAD INJURIES

The sideline evaluation of a head-injured athlete should include an assessment of the following.

Mental Status Testing

- Orientation—time, person, place, and situation (circumstances of injury)
- Concentration—serial sevens, months of year in reverse order
- Memory—names of teams in prior contests, principal, president, three words and three objects at 0 and 5 min

Neurologic Tests

- Pupils—symmetry and reaction to light
- Coordination—finger-nose-finger and tandem gait
- Sensation—fingers to nose (eyes closed) and Romberg test

Exertional Provocative Tests

- Do 40-yd sprint, five pushups, and five knee bends
- Any associated symptoms should preclude a return to play (e.g., headache, dizziness, nausea, unsteadiness, blurred or double vision, photophobia, emotional lability, or mental status changes)

Bibliography

Erlanger DM, Kutner KC, Barth JT, et al: Neuropsychology of sports-related head injury: Dementia pugilistica to postconcussion syndrome. *Clin Neuropsychol* 13(2):193–209, 1999.

Kelly JP, Rosenberg JH: Diagnosis and management of concussion in sports. *Neurology* 48:575–580, 1997.

McCrory PR, Berkovic SF: Second impact syndrome. *Neurology* 50:677–683, 1998.

Practice parameter: The management of concussion in sports (summary statement): Report of the Quality Standards Subcommittee. *Neurology* 48:581–585, 1997.

Sallis RE, Jones K: Prevalence of headache in football players. *Med Sci Sports Exerc* 32(11):1820–1824, 2000.

The Sports Medicine Committee, Colorado Medical Society. Guidelines for the management of concussion in sports Denver, CO: Colorado Medical Society; May, 1990. revised May, 1991.

7

Anaphylaxis

David L. Haller

Mechanism of Injury/Pathology

- Anaphylaxis is a severe, systemic allergic reaction caused by the release of histamine and other mediators
- Anaphylaxis cascade:
  - Exposure to an allergen results in binding of that allergen to IgE antibodies on mast cells
  - Degranulation of mast cells causes the release of histamine and other mediators of anaphylaxis, resulting in the following:
    - Increased vascular permeability, producing angioedema, hives, and laryngeal edema
    - Vasodilatation, resulting in flushing and warmth
    - Bronchial constriction and smooth muscle contraction, responsible for the symptoms of dyspnea, wheezing, and chest tightness
    - Recruitment of other inflammatory cells
    - Severe reactions possibly resulting in hypotension, vascular collapse, and death
- Common causes of anaphylactic reactions:
  - Foods—shellfish, soybeans, nuts, wheat, milk, eggs, monosodium glutamate, nitrates, and other food additives
  - Drugs—aspirin and nonsteroidal anti-inflammatory drugs, sulfa, and penicillin
  - Insects—Hymenoptera stings, insect parts
  - Other—latex, molds, pollen extracts and contrast dye
  - Ingestion of offending foods or drugs in combination with exercise or exercise in and of itself

Diagnostic Keys

- History of anaphylaxis
- Large (10- to 25-mm) urticarial rash or angioedema
- Respiratory symptoms
- Shock

Examination/Evaluation

- Symptoms typically appear within a few minutes after contact with allergen
- The following history should be obtained when assessing an athlete having an anaphylactic reaction:
  - General—feeling of doom, light-headedness, flushing, chills, or sweating
  - Pulmonary—chest tightness, hoarseness, wheezing, or shortness of breath
  - Skin—rash or swelling
  - Gastrointestinal—nausea, vomiting, abdominal cramps, or diarrhea
  - Recent food and medication history
  - Past medical history of a rash or anaphylaxis with exercise (personal and family history)
- Particular attention should be paid to the following on the physical examination:
  - General—airway, breathing, circulation (ABCs), vital signs, presence of respiratory distress, and level of consciousness
  - Skin—angioedema, especially of the head, neck, and face; hives, usually 10–25 mm in length
  - Pulmonary—stridor or wheeze

Differential Diagnosis

- Cholinergic urticaria
  - Cholinergic urticaria is a physical allergy manifest by small, 2- to 5-mm papules
  - Vascular collapse is unusual, but pulmonary symptoms may occur
  - Lesions usually resolve within 20 min
  - Occurs in response to heat, stress, and exercise
  - A passive body-warming test can reproducibly cause these lesions
- Other causes of collapse in the differential of an athlete in shock:
  - Pulmonary embolism, tension pneumothorax, status asthmaticus, airway obstruction
  - Myocardial infarction, cardiac arrhythmias
  - Dehydration, heat stroke, vasovagal syncope
  - Can usually be distinguished from anaphylaxis by the presence of hives or angioedema with cardiopulmonary symptoms.

Tests

- No laboratory or radiographic tests are helpful in making the diagnosis of anaphylaxis
- Tests may be helpful in ruling out other conditions if there is doubt as to the diagnosis
- Allergist may recommend radio allergosorbent test (RAST), skin, or food allergen testing to identify the agent responsible for anaphylaxis

Treatment

- Activate your emergency plan (see Chap. 63)
    - Airway must be secured (see Chap. 3)
    - Oxygen will be helpful if available and pulmonary symptoms are present
    - Intravenous fluids if hypotension is present
    - Elevating the legs can improve venous return if the athlete is hypotensive
    - If an insect bite or sting is responsible, a tourniquet may slow the uptake of the toxin into the remainder of the body
        - If used, tourniquet should be released after epinephrine is given to avoid limb injury
        - Ice may also help delay uptake of toxin into the body
- Epinephrine
    - The drug of choice in treating anaphylaxis
    - Mechanism
        - Increases peripheral resistance and cardiac output
        - Reduces permeability of blood vessels
        - Dilates bronchioles
    - Dose
        - In adults, 0.3–0.5 mg, usually given as 0.3–0.5 mL of a 1:1000 dilution SC or IM
        - The pediatric dose is 0.01 mg/kg in children up to 30 kg
        - Epinephrine injections may have to be repeated as often as every 15 min for recurrent symptoms
        - The Epi-pen (0.3 mg) and Epi-pen Jr. (0.15 mg) are useful, allowing an athlete or bystander to give a standardized dose of epinephrine

Follow-up Care

- Emergency room transfer
    - Patients with significant reactions should be observed in an emergency room setting
    - Delayed reactions and recurrence of symptoms when epinephrine is metabolized are known to occur
    - Other treatments for severe allergic reactions should be strongly considered and include the following:
        - Antihistamines ($H_1 \pm H_2$), which are helpful in treating allergic reactions
        - Corticosteroids, which may protect against or lessen delayed reactions
- Allergist consultation
    - Any patient with a serious anaphylactic reaction should be referred to an allergist
    - An allergist may test to identify the agent responsible for anaphylaxis and suggest preventive strategies

- Immunotherapy is helpful for bee- and wasp-induced anaphylactic reactions but not those that are food-induced
- Prevention
  - A patient who has had a prior anaphylactic reaction should be educated on the symptoms of anaphylaxis and in the use of the Epi-pen
  - If exercise was a trigger, the patient should exercise with a partner knowledgeable in basic life support and the use of the Epi-pen
    - Exercise should cease at the first sign of anaphylaxis
    - Epinephrine administration if symptoms do not rapidly abate, followed by a physician's evaluation
  - Food and medication avoidance if implicated in triggering anaphylaxis
  - Antihistamines are partially effective in preventing anaphylaxis associated with exercise
  - Cromolyn, H_2 blockers, and tricyclic antidepressants such as doxepin have been tried but not extensively studied in their effectiveness

Complications

- Shock, airway obstruction, and death are potential complications from severe anaphylactic reactions
- Anaphylactic reactions are responsible for several hundred deaths per year

ICD-9 Codes

- 995.0 Other anaphylactic shock
- 995.6 Anaphylaxis due to food ingestion
- 989.5 Anaphylaxis due to Hymenoptera sting
- 995.1 Angioneurotic edema
- 995.2 Unspecified adverse effect of drug, medicinal, and biological substance

Bibliography

Hosey RG, Carek PJ, Goo A: Exercise-induced anaphylaxis and urticaria. *Am Fam Physician* 64:1367–1372, 2001.

Kay AB: Allergy and allergic diseases. *N Engl J Med* 344:109–113, 2001.

Salomone JA: Anaphylaxis and acute allergic reactions, in Tintinalli JE, Ruiz E, Krome RL (eds): *Emergency Medicine*. 4th ed. New York: McGraw-Hill, 1996, p 209.

Terrell T, Hough DO, Alexander R: Identifying exercise allergies: Exercise-induced anaphylaxis and cholinergic urticaria. *Phys Sportsmed* 24(11): 76–89, 1996.

8

Asthma and Exercise-Induced Bronchospasm

Chad A. Roghair

ASTHMA

- A lower airway condition characterized by increased responsiveness of airways to stimuli leading to airway obstruction

Mechanism/Pathology

- Inciting factor/stimuli: allergen, smoke, drugs, cold air, exercise
- Release of inflammatory mediators
  - Macrophages, eosinophils, mast cells, basophils
- Mast cell degranulation causes release of multiple factors such as:
  - Histamine, bradykinins, leukotrienes, prostaglandin, thromboxane A_2, plasminogen activating factor (PAF)
- Inflammatory mediator effect
  - Smooth muscle contraction
  - Mucous secretion
  - Increase vascular permeability and edema
- Bottom line—airway narrowing

EXERCISE-INDUCED BRONCHOSPASM (EIB)

- Transient increase in airway obstruction following approximately 8 min of strenuous exercise
  - Exercise at 75–85 percent of maximum heart rate will trigger bronchoconstriction in large and small airways
  - This may include moderate to severe airway obstruction within 5–8 min of cessation of exercise
  - There is a late-response inflammatory event that may occur 6–8 h following the initial obstruction and recovery

- Symptoms:
  - Wheezing
  - Dyspnea out of proportion to task
  - Cough—especially postexercise
  - Chest tightness
- Prevalence of EIB
  - Exact percentage is unknown
  - However:
    - 90 percent of chronic asthmatics demonstrate symptoms consistent with EIB
    - 7 percent of randomly sampled asymptomatic children
    - 10–50 percent of athletes, especially those in cold, dry air (cross-country skiing, skiing, hockey)
    - 67 of 597 athletes on the 1984 U.S. Olympic team, 41 of whom won medals

Diagnosis/Examinations

- History of symptoms consistent with EIB
- Trial of beta$_2$ agonist medication improves symptoms
- Exercise challenge test:
  - Exercise 6–8 min at 90 percent of maximum heart rate
  - 10 percent reduction in FEV_1 or peak expiratory flow rate is suggestive of EIB

Emergent Treatment

- Early identification and intervention are the keys to preventing disaster
  - Know the participants of the sporting event who have a history of asthma or bronchospasm
  - Observe such participants vigilantly during the event for early signs of respiratory distress, such as
    - Lagging behind other athletes, labored breathing pattern
- Early evaluation of the individual with respiratory symptoms
  - Examination performed in a controlled environment
  - Mental status changes, ability to speak in complete sentences, accessory muscle use, quality of air movement with chest auscultation
- Emergency management
  - If the individual has altered mental status or absent breath sounds, activate the EMS system, supply oxygen (if available), and attempt to administer a beta$_2$ agonist
  - If the individual is alert but audibly wheezing and unable to speak in complete sentences secondary to bronchospasm, remove athlete from competition, administer beta$_2$ agonist. Reevaluate every 15 min.
  - DO NOT leave the individual unattended
  - Monitor for abrupt changes in condition. If a peak flow meter is available, obtain a reading. If the peak flow remains less than 50

percent of the predicted value 1 h after treatment, hospitalization is indicated.

- If the individual is alert and chest auscultation demonstrates air movement throughout lung fields but with trace expiratory wheeze, administer beta$_2$ agonist and reevaluate. If improved, have the patient exercise on the sideline and reevaluate for worsening symptoms. If no change in status, the individual may return to play with careful observation.
- Any individual who experiences an asthma attack during competition must have follow-up with either the team or his or her private physician to optimize treatment

DEFINITIVE TREATMENT

- Evaluate for underlying asthma and associated triggers
- Determine frequency of episodes per week
  - If more than two significant episodes per week, consider treating for typical asthma. With frequent episodes, the patient may benefit from more aggressive prophylactic treatment.
  - Inhaled corticosteroids daily
  - Beta$_2$ agonists as needed
  - Adjunctive leukotriene inhibitors if not controlled

Nonpharmacologic Treatment

- Exercise should occur in a high-humidity environment
- Advise nose breathing to warm the air prior to contact with the lungs
- Exercise at maximum work load for more than 5 min will induce a refractory period
- Physical training does not prevent asthma but alters threshold of symptom onset
- Caution to avoid environmental pollutants and to control factors such as allergic rhinitis or infection

Pharmacologic Treatment

- Current pharmacologic treatment standards for EIB
  - Inhaled beta$_2$ agonists (albuterol)
    - Drug of choice
      - Use 30 min prior to exercise
      - Lasts up to 6 h
      - May prevent symptoms in up to 90 percent of cases
  - Long-acting beta$_2$ agonists
    - Initially show a longer protective effect
      - However, if used over time, the protective effect diminishes and medication will need to be used more frequently, increasing chance of tachyphylaxis

- Inhaled mast cell stabilizers (e.g., cromolyn)
  - Second-line medications
  - Inhibit immediate and delayed bronchoconstrictive reaction to inhaled antigens
  - Have no bronchodilator or antihistamine effect
  - If used 20 min prior to exercise can reduce symptoms in 70–85 percent of patients
  - May be most beneficial to patients who exercise repeatedly in a single day, as the dose can be repeated
  - Helpful in preventing delayed-onset symptoms
- Leukotriene-receptor antagonist (i.e., montelukast)
  - Used as adjunct to different regimens, may be helpful for patients with chronic asthma
  - Wide range of benefit; up to 25 percent will have no improvement in EIB symptoms

COMPLICATIONS AND CLINICAL PRACTICE

- EIB is probably underdiagnosed
  - Clinician should ask patients about symptoms during both sports physicals and health maintenance examinations
  - If not diagnosed and treated appropriately, asthma and bronchospasm can lead to respiratory failure and death
- If managed appropriately, treatment is highly effective
  - Initial treatment with beta$_2$ agonists 30 min prior to exercise
  - If symptoms not adequately controlled, add an inhaled mast cell stabilizer 20 min prior to activity; may be repeated if there are multiple episodes of exercise during the day
  - Leukotriene-receptor antagonist—especially for patients with chronic asthma as adjunctive therapy
  - If patient experiences frequent severe symptoms, inhaled corticosteroid

SPORTS POSING RISK FOR EXERCISE-INDUCED BRONCHOSPASM

High Risk

- High minute ventilation
  - Basketball, cycling, track, soccer
- Cool, dry air
  - Cross-country skiing, ice hockey, skiing, skating

Lower Risk

- Low minute ventilation
  - Golf, archery, goalie in soccer or hockey

- Warm, moist air
  - Surfing, kayaking, swimming

ICD-9 CODES

- 493.9 Asthma
- 493.91 Asthma with status asthmaticus
- 493.92 Asthma with acute exacerbation

Bibliography

Kobayashi R, Mellion M: Exercise-induced asthma, anaphylaxis and urticaria. *Clin Prim Care* 18:809–831, 1991.

McFadden ER, Gilbert IA: Exercise-induced asthma. *N Engl J Med* 330:1362–1367, 1994.

National Asthma Education Program, Expert Panel Report: Guidelines for the diagnosis and management of asthma. National Heart, Lung, and Blood Institute, National Institutes of Health, Bethesda, MD. *J Allergy Clin Immunol* 88:425–534, 1991.

Rupp NT, Brudno DS, Guill MF: The value of screening for risk of exercise-induced asthma in high school athlete. *Ann Allergy* 70(4): 339–342, 1993.

Shapiro SG: Management of pediatric asthma. *Immunol Allergy Clin North Am* 18:1–23, 1998.

Spahn J, Szefler S: Pharmacologic management of pediatric asthma. *Immunol Allergy Clin North Am* 1:165–179, 1998.

Thole RT, Sallis RE, Rubin AL, Smith GN: Exercise-induced bronchospasm prevalence in collegiate cross-country runners. *Med Sci Sports Exerc* 33(1c):1641–1646, 2001.

9

Chest Pain

Sandra J. Hoffmann

Overview of Chest Pain

- Differential diagnosis includes conditions of the cardiovascular, gastrointestinal, respiratory, and musculoskeletal systems
- Can be a manifestation of a serious medical condition and a precursor to impending death or disability at all ages
- In younger population, more likely benign condition unrelated to cardiovascular system
- Thorough preparticipation examination should focus on cardiovascular risk factors

Diagnostic Keys

- Aggravated by movement—musculoskeletal, cardiac
- Precipitated by activity—cardiac
- Relieved by rest—cardiac
- Responds to nitroglycerin—cardiac
- Personal or family history of coronary artery disease—cardiac
- Aggravated by eating—gastrointestinal, cardiac
- Painful breathing—pulmonary

Examination

- ABCs (airway, breathing, circulation) (see Chaps. 3, 4, and 5)
- Blood pressure measurement—bilateral, upper and lower extremities
- Chest wall palpation for tenderness and abnormal wall motion
- Auscultation for murmurs, breath sounds
- Palpation of peripheral pulses
- Inspection of neck veins
- Thoracic inspection, palpation, percussion, auscultation
- Examination of the extremities for cyanosis and edema
- Abdominal palpation for mass, tenderness

Emergent Treatment

- Treatment of ABCs
- Thorough examination
- Stabilization (if cardiac, rapid activation of EMS and transport for definitive treatment)
  - Aspirin (ASA) 81–325 mg chewed
  - Nitroglycerin (NTG) spray or 0.4 mg sublingual repeated every 5 min for three doses or until pain relieved
  - Oxygen
  - Morphine sulfate for pain control if available
  - Intravenous beta blocker (unless signs of heart failure)
    - Atenolol 5 mg over 5 min then 5 mg IV in 10 min
    - Metoprolol 5 mg IV every 2 min for three doses
  - Heparin/low-molecular-weight heparin/thrombolysis as soon as possible. Generally administered once patient reaches emergency department.
- Cardiac monitoring/defibrillation if ventricular fibrillation

Tests

- 12-lead ECG
- Chest x-ray
- Blood work
  - Complete blood cell count (CBC), thyroid, chemistry panel, lipid panel, troponin, creatine phosphokinase (CPK) with isoenzymes
- Consider
  - Echocardiogram
  - Exercise stress test
  - Holter monitor/event recorder
  - Cardiac catheterization
  - Electrophysiologic study

Definitive Treatment/Follow-up/ Return to Play

- Musculoskeletal
  - Rest, ice, compression and elevation (RICE)
- Cardiac
  - Appropriate medical management
  - Evaluation by cardiologist
  - Consideration for long-term medical or surgical management
- Respiratory
  - Resolution of symptoms
  - Temperature $<100.5°$
- Gastrointestinal
  - Antireflux measures
  - Treatment of irritable bowel syndrome

- Psychological
  - Counseling
  - Medications

Complications

- Sudden death
  - Commotio cordis (sudden cardiac death from a blow to the precordium during cardiac repolarization)
  - Structural heart disease <30 years old
  - Coronary artery disease >30 years old
- Acute myocardial infarction
- Dysrhythmias
- Aortic dissection
- Pulmonary embolism
- Pneumothorax

Bibliography

Albert CM, Mittleman MA, Chae CU, et al: Triggering of sudden death from cardiac causes by vigorous exertion. *N Engl J Med* 343:1355–1361, 2000.

Maron BJ: Cardiovascular risks to young persons on the athletic field. *Ann Intern Med* 129:379–386, 1998.

Maron BJ, Araujo CG, Thompson PD, et al: Recommendations for preparticipation screening and the assessment of cardiovascular disease in masters athletes. *Circulation* 103:327–334, 2001.

Maron BJ, Mitchell JH (eds): 26th Bethesda Conference: Recommendations for determining eligibility for competition in athletes with cardiovascular abnormalities. *J Am Coll Cardiol* 24:845–899, 1994.

Maron BJ, Thompson PD, Puffer JC, et al: Cardiovascular preparticipation screening of competitive athletes: A Statement for Health Professionals From the Sudden Death Committee (Clinical Cardiology) and Congenital Cardiac Defects Committee (Cardiovascular Disease in the Young), American Heart Association. *Circulation* 94:850–856, 1996.

10

Facial Injury

Sam J. Romeo
Joseph P. Romeo

OVERVIEW

- Because facial structures are usually exposed during participation in sports, they are susceptible to injury
- Injury patterns vary by sport, but this chapter focuses on the initial management of soft tissue injuries such as contusions and lacerations and bony injuries such as fractures (for dental injuries, see Chap. 11; for eye injuries, see Chap. 12)
- Sporting activities account for 3–29 percent of all facial injuries, approximately 10–42 percent of all facial fractures, with men accounting for approximately 60–90 percent of injuries (these numbers may vary depending on clinical setting)
- The U.S. Consumer Product Safety Commission reported in 1996 that more than half of the injuries that occurred in children under age 11 occurred in the head or neck

Mechanism of Injury

- Facial injuries result from direct impact with the following:
    - Another player's body part (head, fist, elbow, etc.)
    - Equipment (ball, puck, goalpost, handlebars, etc.)
    - The ground (wrestling mat, gym floor, etc.)
    - The environment (tree on a ski slope, outfield wall in baseball)

Examination and Evaluation

- All initial assessments should include the airway, breathing, circulation (ABCs) (see Chaps. 3, 4, and 5)
- Cervical spine precautions should be taken when necessary (see Chap. 20)
- Can patient be safely removed from area of competition (field, court, track, etc.)? If so, do so immediately.

- Because facial injuries frequently involve bleeding, apply pressure with gauze to appropriate area while obtaining the athlete's medical history

Pertinent History

- What was the mechanism of injury?
- Does the athlete have any signs or symptoms of a concussion? (See Chap 6.)
- Where is the athlete's pain located?
- Does he or she complain of blurred vision or diplopia?
- Was the athlete wearing a protective mouth guard?

Physical Examination

- Careful inspection:
  - Identify areas of ecchymosis, edema, or active bleeding
  - Inspect nasal septum and external ears for the presence of hematomas
  - Early recognition of facial asymmetry and/or structural depressions is key to clinically diagnosing facial fractures before edema distorts the overlying soft tissue
  - Look for a sunken globe suggestive of a blowout fracture
  - Note lacerations or deep abrasions overlying suspected fractures
- Palpation:
  - Palpate the bones of the face in a systematic way noting the presence of significant tenderness, crepitus, numbness, and/or contour irregularities
  - Palpate the orbital rims, nasal bones, and temporomandibular joints
  - Palpate the maxilla and mandible bimanually. Stabilize the forehead with one hand while gently pulling on the maxillary incisors with a gloved hand to demonstrate midface instability or crepitus. Directly palpate along the course of the mandible (one hand palpating intraorally) to discover instability, irregularity, or tenderness.

Evocative Examination

- Assess extraocular eye movements and cranial nerves (CN) III, IV, and VI by having patient track an examiner's finger in all four quadrants while keeping the chin in a fixed position. Ability to do so without complaints of diplopia rules out acute entrapment of extraocular eye muscles secondary to an orbital blowout fracture (see Chap. 12).
- Lacerations or fractures can injure the facial nerve (CN VII) or one of its branches, so assess facial symmetry
- Ask patient to
  - Raise his or her eyebrows—innervated by the temporal branch
  - Close eyes tightly—innervated by the zygomatic branch with some cross innervation from buccal branch

- Big smile—forehead–temporal branch, midface–buccal branch with cross innervation from zygomatic branch, corner of mouth—marginal mandibular branch
- Open mouth widely or pucker lips—innervated by marginal mandibular branch
- Ask the patient to open his or her mouth as wide as possible
  - Inability to do so, trismus, or severe pain along the lateral aspect of cheek or jaw is suggestive of a fracture of the mandible or zygoma
  - Assess oral cavity to rule out damage to the teeth and lacerations in the intraoral mucosa or tongue (see Chaps. 11 and 16)
- Ask athlete to close his or her mouth
  - A sense of malocclusion is highly suggestive of a significant fracture of the mandible, maxilla, or palate

Tests

- To determine whether there is a leak of cerebral spinal fluid from a suspected fractured cribiform plate in a stable patient, perform the "ring test" by having patient sit with neck in flexion. The test is positive if a clear fluid ring forms around a drop of nasal blood on gauze.
- Although not necessary for most nasal fractures, a plain radiograph facial series may be indicated if there is suspicion of other fractures. Include Panorex views to assess the mandible.
- Computed tomography (CT) scans are extremely sensitive and extensively used to detect bony abnormalities of the face

SOFT TISSUE INJURIES

Contusions

- Contusions are the most commonly encountered facial injuries and usually result from blunt trauma to the face

Emergent Treatment

- Aimed at minimizing the inflammatory response. Applying ice for 20 minutes on then off several times per day for the first 48 hours following initial injury and consider nonsteroidal anti-inflammatory drugs.

Definitive Treatment/Follow-up/Return to Play

- Athletes may return to play if there is no visual obstruction secondary to edema

Complications

- Uncommon, but may include a large, persistent, painful or disfiguring hematoma requiring surgical evacuation

ICD-9 Code

- 920 Contusion of face, scalp, and neck except eye(s)
- 921 Contusion of eye and adnexa

Abrasions

- Abrasions are common partial-thickness disruptions of the epidermis often resulting from blunt trauma or sudden forcible friction along the face
- The prominent structures of the face (such as nose, cheek, eyebrow, or raised chin) are more prone to abrasion-type injuries; as with all soft tissue injuries, additional underlying injury must be ruled out

Emergent Treatment

- Gently cleanse the skin of all debris (primary debridement). If the athlete is unable to tolerate this process, a 4% lidocaine solution can be topically applied or a regional block can be used. Occasionally, wounds require extensive cleaning and debridement; these patients should be referred to an emergency room, urgent care facility, or surgery center for management.
- Lubricating the wound with antibiotic ointment and then covering it with a sterile dressing encourages healing
- Athletes should be taught basic wound care

Definitive Treatment /Follow-up/ Return to Play

- Athletes may generally return at their discretion

Complications

- "Tattooing" can occur when foreign debris is left in an abrasion. This gives the skin an irregular, hyperpigmented look and can lead to a poor cosmetic outcome.
- Secondary infections of facial abrasions are rare due to the rich blood supply of the facial tissues

ICD-9 Code

- 910.0 Abrasion or friction burn without mention of infection
- 959.09 Injury of face and neck

Lacerations (See Chap. 16)

- Tongue lacerations heal extremely well and rarely require sutures. Attention should focus on hemostasis.

- Lacerations with any of the following characteristics pose a high risk for poor cosmetic or functional outcomes and should be definitively managed in an appropriately equipped and staffed emergency room/hospital/urgent care or surgery center (referral considerations—head and neck surgery, plastic surgery, ophthalmology):
  - Large tissue deficits or irregular edges requiring debridement with the possible need for a skin graft or flap placement
  - Significant disruption of the vermilion border
  - Large through-and-through lacerations of the cheek or lip that may require approximation of the underlying musculature
  - Facial nerve deficits
  - Involvement of ear or nose cartilage with poor blood supplies; these are prone to secondary infections and chondritis
  - Suspicion of an underlying fracture
  - Deep laceration possibly involving the parotid duct, which generally courses along an imaginary line from the tragus to the maxillary second molar
  - Involvement of the eyelid or lacrimal duct

Definitive Treatment/Follow-up/Return to Play

- Irrigation and conservative debridement. Close wound as soon as possible.
- Superficial laceration—athlete can return to activity immediately if wound is protected
- Deep laceration—complex closure after surrounding structures (nerves, glands, etc.) are identified
- Return to play in 7–21 days depends on deep structures involved
- Follow up in 5–7 days

Complications

- Persistent bleeding with hematoma formation, infection with possible reopening of the wound, unacceptable scar

ICD-9 Code

- 870 Open wound of ocular adnexa
- 872 Open wound of ear
- 873 Other open wound of head

NASAL INJURIES

Overview

- Due to the nose's protrusion from the face and the fact that few sports utilize protective face masks, nasal injuries are extremely common in athletics

- Injuries range from contusions to fractures and generally result from a direct or glancing blow to the nose
- Epistaxis is a common presenting symptom that is easily identified. Most cases originate from the anterior septum (Kiesselbach's plexus) and are easily visualized with a nasal speculum.

Diagnostic Keys

- Athletes who have sustained a nasal fracture frequently report having heard a "crunch" or "crack" such as the sound of biting into uncooked macaroni
- Blows to the cartilaginous complex frequently cause septal fractures and dislocations, while lateral blows often displace the nasal bones
- Nasal fractures are diagnosed clinically (imaging studies are generally not needed), which highlights the importance of recognizing a deformity prior to the rapid onset of edema

Examination/Evaluation

- See "Physical Examination," above

Emergent Treatment

- Anterior epistaxis is best controlled by slightly reclining the patient and applying direct pressure to the nasal septum for 5–10 min. Applying ice to back of neck may assist in causing reflex vasoconstriction.
- Persistent epistaxis occasionally requires nasal packing with a nasal tampon covered in topical antibiotic or a topical coagulant (such as Floseal). Neo-Synephrine or oxymetazolone may also be used to cause vasoconstriction. Persistent and/or profuse bleeding may indicate a complex nasal fracture with an injury to the ethmoid artery, requiring more invasive visualization. Posterior epistaxis is usually atraumatic and might sometimes be encountered on the sidelines.
- Focus initial treatment on hemostasis and minimizing swelling by applying ice.
- Treatment of nasal fractures includes ice, pain control, and nasal decongestants for up to 3 days. Displaced nasal fractures may be reduced immediately (within the first hour).

Definitive Treatment/Follow-up/ Return to Play

- Referral to a head and neck surgeon for reduction once swelling has decreased approximately 3–5 days later

- Can be as early as 7–14 days after date of injury if appropriate facial protection is used (custom acrylic face shields, helmets with face masks, etc.). This should be worn for the following 4 weeks during competitive play.

Complication

- If an athlete has sustained a nasal contusion or fracture, it is imperative to rule out the presence of a septal hematoma (blood beneath the septal perichondrium). It presents as a bulging bluish septal mass and requires prompt surgical drainage, nasal packing, and prophylactic antibiotics. Failure to drain can lead to infection or pressure necrosis of the underlying bone and cartilage. If this occurs, the septum can collapse, causing chronic nasal obstruction and a cosmetic appearance known as a "saddle-nose" deformity.

ICD-9 Codes

- 802 Fracture of face bones
- 802.0 Nasal bones, closed
- 802.1 Nasal bones, open

EAR INJURIES

Mechanism of Injury/Pathology

- Contusions to the external ear caused by shearing forces or blunt trauma applied to the external ear are common in sports (most notably in wrestling)

Diagnostic Keys

- Include ecchymosis, erythema, and pain
- Auricular hematomas usually present, with palpable collections of fluid that are painful and throbbing

Examination/Evaluation

- Swelling of external ear with loss of anatomic landmarks (helix, antihelix etc.) and severe pain, which may not appear consistent with the extent of injury

Emergent Treatment

- Application of ice for 20 min on/off with continuous compression can minimize the risk of developing an auricular hematoma
- Treatment consists of prompt aspiration using a 20-gauge needle or incision and drainage using sterile technique. To avoid reaccumulation of blood, compression for 5–7 days is adequate. There are several techniques for applying compression:
  - Apply fine gauze to anterior and posterior surfaces and then layers of collodion
  - Apply dental rolls or a button to the anterior and posterior surfaces of the ear and fix in place with through-and-through sutures

Tests

- Physical examination is the key to diagnosis. See "Physical Examination," above.

Definitive Treatment/Follow-up/ Return to Play

- Athletes participating in noncontact sports may return to play immediately. Ear protection such as headgear or helmet is needed for immediate return to contact sports. If sutures were placed to hold the dental rolls or buttons for compression, contact sports may be resumed approximately 24–48 h after sutures are removed.
- Prophylactic use of antibiotics such as cephalosporin is recommended for 7–10 days

Complications

- Auricular hematomas, like septal hematomas, can cause pressure necrosis of the underlying cartilage by separating the blood supply found in the perichondrium from the underlying cartilage. This may result in a severe deformity of the external ear ("cauliflower ear").

ICD-9 Code

- 380.31 Hematoma of auricle or pinna

Table 10.1 The Most Common Facial Fractures

Fracture/ICD-9	Mechanism of Injury	Characteristic Signs and Symptoms	Diagnostic Imaging	Usual Definitive Treatment	Return to Play
Mandible/ ICD-9 802.2,802	Trauma to lower face	Malocclusion, swelling and pain over fracture site	Plain film with Panorex view	1. Nondisplaced closed single fracture—conservative treatment with observation. 2. Displaced/unstable/complex/open—open reduction internal fixation.	6–8 weeks
Zygoma (tripod)/ ICD-9 802.4,802.5	Blunt trauma to cheek	Pain, swelling, ecchymosis over fracture site, numbness along infraorbital nerve (upper lip/cheek),depressed malar eminence and inferior orbital rim	CT scan	1. Nondisplaced closed fracture—conservative treatment with observation. 2. Displaced/unstable/complex/depressed fragment—open reduction internal fixation.	4 weeks
Nasal/ ICD-9 802.0,802.1	Direct or glancing blow	Heard "crack," ecchymosis, tearing, epistaxis, crepitus, asymmetry	None	1. Displaced—closed reduction 2. Comminuted—possible open reduction	1–2 weeks with face guard
Zygomatic arch/ ICD-9 802.4,802.5	Blunt trauma to cheek	Central depression/asymmetry of cheek bone, trismus caused by impingement of the arch on the coronoid process of the mandible or temporalis muscle	Submental vertex view radiograph	1. Nondisplaced closed fracture—conservative treatment with observation. 2. Displaced/unstable/complex/depressed fragment—open reduction, rarely with internal fixation.	4 weeks
Maxilla or LeFort/ ICD-9 802.4,802.5	High-velocity shearing force to midface (i.e., motor cross accident; bat, baseball, or hockey puck to face)	Elongated, distorted face, mobile maxilla with bimanual exam, malocclusion.	CT scan	1. Nondisplaced closed fracture—conservative treatment with observation. 2. Displaced/unstable/complex/depressed fragment—open reduction and internal fixation.	Wide variations depending on fracture characteristics. Minimum 4–6 weeks.
Orbital blowout/ ICD-9 802.6,802.7	Direct trauma to globe (usually a ball)	Periorbital edema, ecchymosis, subconjunctival hemorrhage, numbness along infraorbital nerve (upper lip/cheek); limitation of upward gaze resulting from entrapment of the inferior rectus and superior oblique extraocular muscles, diplopia, sunken globe	CT scan	1. No entrapment—close observation to ensure entrapment does not occur. 2. Entrapment of extraocular muscles—open reduction and internal fixation. Nondisplaced closed fracture—conservative treatment with observation.	Wide variations depending on fracture characteristics. Minimum 4–6 weeks.

FRACTURES

- Although one would expect variation depending on sports played, the mandible, zygoma, and nose account for nearly 75 percent of facial fractures
- A standard, thorough physical examination (as previously described) is designed to clinically detect all facial fractures and guide management decisions
- Early recognition is the key to appropriate management of facial fractures
- Open fractures require prompt treatment
- See Table 10.1 for characteristics of the more common facial fractures seen in athletes

Bibliography

Crow RW: Diagnosis and management of sports-related injuries to the face. *Dent Clin North Am* 35(4): 719–733, 1991.

Iida S, Koga M, Sugiura T, et al: Retrospective analysis of 1502 patients with facial fractures. *Int J Oral Maxillofac Surg* 30:286–290, 2001.

Perkins RA, Dayan SH, Sklarew EC, et al: The incidence of sports-related facial trauma in children. *Ear Nose Throat J* 8:632–638, 2000.

Stackhous T: On-site management of nasal injuries. *Phys Sports Med* 26:8, 1998.

Study of protective equipment for baseball. Washington, DC: US Consumer Product Safety Commission, 1996.

Tanaka N, Hayashi S, Amagasa T, et al: Maxillofacial fractures sustained during sports. *J Oral Maxillofac Surg* 54:715–719, 1996.

11

Dental Injuries

Ken Honsik

INTRODUCTION

Anatomy

- Root
  - Attached to tooth socket
  - Periodontal ligaments
  - Pulp
- Crown
  - Dentin—soft inner layer
  - Enamel—hard outer shell

TOOTH FRACTURE (FIG. 11.1)

Mechanism/Pathology

- Caused by direct blow to tooth or by indirect blow transmitted through jaw
- Types
  - Enamel only—chip fracture
  - Enamel and dentin—uncomplicated
  - Enamel, dentin, and pulp—complicated
  - Root fracture—complicated

Diagnostic Keys

- Pulp involvement
  - Occurs in Type III or root fractures
  - More severe injury
  - Very painful
  - Found as bleeding site or pink/red dot in middle of dentin

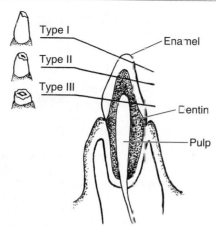

Figure 11.1 Ellis fracture classification. (From Scaletta TA, Schaider JJ: *Emergent Management of Trauma,* 2d ed. New York: McGraw-Hill, 2001. Used by permission.)

Evaluation/Examination

- Determine alertness of athlete
  - May have increased risk of aspirating tooth fragments if diminished level of consciousness
- Visually inspect entire mouth and maxillofacial region
  - Use a light source
  - May need to rinse mouth with clean water in order to inspect
  - Do not discard spit right away—may contain tooth fragments
  - Palpate all rows with a sterile glove for asymmetry and looseness
  - Search for tooth fragments
  - Athlete's mouth
  - Field/court where injury occurred
  - Athlete's clothes

Emergent Treatment

- Fragments should be found, saved, and sent with athlete to dentist
  - Handle fragments by enamel surface
  - Transport in sterile gauze soaked in normal saline
- Be cautious of aspiration in unconscious athlete
- Bleeding controlled by having athlete gently bite down on sterile gauze or clean towel. Ice may also help, but area may be extremely sensitive if root is exposed or near surface.
- Pain control if nerve root exposed
  - Place drop of cyanoacrylate to cover nerve root (not FDA-approved for this purpose)

Definitive Treatment/Follow-up/ Return to Play

- Referral to dentist
  - Fracture
  - Complicated—involving pulp: within 3 h
  - Uncomplicated—enamel/dentin: within 48 h
  - Loose tooth
  - Refer for radiographic evaluation by dentist
  - May involve simple fracture of enamel
- Athlete may continue to play if fragment is recovered and bleeding controlled
- **Athlete has 3 h to get to dentist if pulp is involved**
- Use protective mouth guard for all contact sports or any sport where loose tooth may be acquired during contest

LUXATION (DISPLACED TOOTH)

Mechanism/Pathology

- See "Tooth Fracture," above
- Types
  - Extruded—appears longer than adjacent teeth
  - Laterally displaced—extends anterior or posterior to normal row
  - Intruded—appears shorter than adjacent teeth

Diagnostic Keys

- Look for row asymmetry and inner cheek lacerations

Evaluation/Examination

- See "Tooth Fracture," above

Emergent Treatment

- Extruded and laterally displaced teeth
  - Immediately reposition on field
  - Use dry, gloved hand
  - If unable to reposition or there is severe pain, refer to dentist
- Intruded teeth
  - **DO NOT** reposition on field

Definitive treatment/Follow-up/ Return to Play

- Refer to dentist within 48 h
- Custom-fit mouth guard—athlete may return immediately
- Intruded tooth or no custom mouth guard—recommend athlete not return until dental consultation

AVULSION

Mechanism/Pathology

- See "Tooth Fracture," above
- Complete separation of tooth from socket
- Rupture of periodontal ligaments

Diagnostic Keys

- Obvious missing tooth

Evaluation/Examination

- See "Tooth Fracture," above

Emergent Treatment

- Find the tooth!!
  - Examine athlete's mouth, clothing, equipment, ground
- Clean tooth if dirty
  - Use saline or clean water
- Reimplant the tooth
  - Best option if done within 30 min
  - Decreases chance of root resorption
  - Poor outcomes after 2 h
  - Be sure to place correct side forward !
  - Do not irrigate socket
  - Palpable click is noted with proper placement
- Splint tooth to row
  - Advise use of custom mouth guard
  - Use "Silly Putty" or chewing gum (preferably sugar-free) to splint
- Storage of tooth (if unable to implant)
  - Hank's balanced salt solution
  - Milk
  - Athlete's mouth (if athlete is completely alert)
  - Normal saline

- Antibiotics
  - Penicillin if athlete is not allergic
  - Check athlete's tetanus status

Definitive Treatment/Follow-up/ Return to Play

- **Refer to dentist within 1 h**
- Tooth survival greatly decreases by 2 h after injury
- Dentist <u>must clear athlete</u> for contact sports

ALVEOLAR (SOCKET) FRACTURE

Mechanism/Pathology

- Fracture of socket of mandible or maxilla

Diagnostic Keys

- Commonly associated with gingival laceration

Evaluation/Examination

- See "Tooth Fracture," above
- Palpate along gum line
  - Step-off
  - Crepitus
  - Movement of entire segment or row when checking for loose teeth
  - Bony ledges
- Bite changes
- Radiographs required

Emergent Treatment

- If alveolar fracture suspected, do not attempt to replace avulsed teeth

Definitive Treatment/Follow-up/ Return to Play

- Immediate referral to dentist/dental surgeon
- Should be cleared by dentist

Associated Injuries

- Lip/mucosal lacerations (see Chap. 16)
- Tongue lacerations are vascular and generally heal well without intervention
- Mandibular/maxillary fractures
- Tempromandibular joint (TMJ)
  - Assess for range of motion
  - Sounds: clicks or pops
- Concussion (see Chap. 6)

Mouthguards

- Should be used in all contact sports
- Protect soft tissues
  - Custom vacuum-molded guard supplied by dentist/orthodontist are best
  - Stock and mouth-formed guards
  - Have questionable fit
  - Allow more tooth movement than custom guards

Bibliography

Dale, RA: Oral-facial emergencies, dentoalveolar trauma. *Emerg Med Clin North Am* 18(3):521–538, 2000.

Roberts WO: Field care of the injured tooth. *Phys Sports Med* 28:(1): 101–102, 2000.

Tu HK, Davis LF, Nique TA: Maxillofacial injuries, in Mellion M, Walsh M, Shelton G (eds): *The Team Physician's Handbook,* 2d ed. Philadelphia: Hanley & Belfus, 1997, p 429.

12

Eye Injury

Lauren M. Simon

OVERVIEW

- Sports are a significant source of ocular trauma
- Basketball and baseball are the sports that most frequently lead to injury
- Other high-risk sports for eye injuries are racquet sports, martial arts, soccer, and boxing
- Prompt recognition and management of ocular injuries reduces the chance of diminished visual acuity

Mechanism of Injury

- Blunt injuries
  - Objects smaller than orbital opening transmit force to the globe; larger objects transmit force to globe and surrounding tissue
- Lacerations
  - To lids, cornea, sclera, or globe, usually from projectile objects
- Associated trauma
  - Head or facial injuries may be associated with ocular injuries usually seen in collision sports.

Examination/Evaluation

- History
  - Mechanism of injury
  - Length of symptoms
  - Previous eye injury/eye disease
- Signs and symptoms
  - Pain, diminished vision, diplopia, bleeding, foreign-body sensation, flashing lights, paresthesia around orbit or nose
- Visual acuity
  - Snellen card preferable; if card not available, use print material (magazine, newspaper)

- Gross inspection
  - Evaluate eyelids, corneas, conjunctiva, anterior chamber, pupils, lens, and fundi for irregularities or hemorrhage
  - Assess for eye symmetry, ptosis of lids, proptosis of eye
  - Assess symmetry of pupillary light reflex on both corneas
  - Check visual fields by confrontation
- Direct visualization with ophthalmoscope
- Extraocular muscle function
  - Look at six cardinal fields of gaze:
    - Right and up (R. superior rectus; L. inferior oblique)
    - Right (R. lateral rectus; L. medial rectus)
    - Right and down (R. inferior rectus; L. superior oblique)
    - Left and up (L. superior rectus, R. inferior oblique)
    - Left (L. lateral rectus; R. medial rectus)
    - Left and down (L. inferior rectus; R. superior oblique)
  - Limitation of eye movement may indicate orbital soft tissue injury or extraocular muscle entrapment
- Fluorescein stain
  - To assess for abrasions or foreign bodies

CORNEAL TRAUMA

Corneal Abrasion/Corneal Foreign Body

- Disruption of surface epithelium

Signs/Symptoms

- Pain, photophobia
- Increased conjunctival tearing
- Possible decrease visual acuity

Examination

- Use topical anesthetic to decrease pain for examination
- Fluorescein stain reveals abrasion and some foreign bodies under cobalt blue light
- Rule out associated ocular injury
- Evert upper eyelid and inspect for foreign body
- Look in upper and lower conjunctival fornices

Emergency Treatment

- Irrigate with sterile saline to remove debris
- With topical anesthetic in place, remove foreign body with hypodermic needle or cotton-tipped swab
- Administer topical antibiotic (although postinjury infection is uncommon)

- Patching eye for 24 h reduces eyelid motion for pain control
- Avoid topical corticosteroids, as these may promote fungal or viral infections
- Long-term use of topical anesthetics is contraindicated (impairs corneal reepithelialization)
- Large abrasions may require cycloplegic agent to control pain

Return to Play

- Resolution of pain
- Return of visual acuity to baseline
- Usually within 24–48 h

Complication

- Recurrent epithelial erosion

Ocular Burn (Ultraviolet Keratitis)

- "Sunburn" of corneal epithelium

Signs/Symptoms

- Delayed onset 6–12 h postexposure
- Intense pain, photophobia
- Possible decrease in visual acuity
- Tearing, conjunctival hyperemia, corneal haziness
- Fluorescein stain shows punctate epithelium on cornea

Treatment

- Pain relief—cycloplegic drugs to relieve ciliary body spasms
- Systemic analgesic
- Topical antibiotics and eye patch
- Sometimes topical corticosteroids used briefly (generally under direction of ophthalmologist)
- Recovery time averages 12–36 h

Corneal Laceration

- Fluorescein stain useful to visualize laceration
- Treatment—ophthalmology referral for repair

IRIS TRAUMA

Traumatic Iridocyclitis : *blurry vision*

Mechanism of Injury

- Blunt trauma irritates iris and ciliary body
- Inflammation of anterior chamber

Signs/Symptoms

- Pain, photophobia, blurry vision

Examination

- Affected pupil constricted

Traumatic Miosis/Mydriasis

Mechanism of Injury

- Blunt trauma irritates iris and ciliary body

Examination

- Constricted pupil (miosis) or dilated pupil (mydriasis)
- Treatment is supportive; spontaneous resolution expected

LENS TRAUMA

Lens Subluxation or Dislocation

Mechanism of Injury

- Blunt trauma in anteroposterior direction
- Tearing of zonule fibers attaching the lens, subluxing or dislocating lens into anterior chamber

Signs/Symptoms

- Decreased visual acuity

Treatment

- Prompt ophthalmologic consultation for possible repair

Complications

- Glaucoma

Traumatic Cataract

Mechanism of Injury

- Blunt or penetrating trauma
- Lens becomes opacified

Treatment

- Refer to ophthalmologist

RETINAL INJURY

Retinal Detachment

- Hole or tear in retinal tissue: fluid collects between retina and retinal pigment epithelium

Mechanism of Injury

- Blunt trauma; vitreous traction; head injury
- Can occur spontaneously

Signs/Symptoms

- Flashes of light; floaters
- Curtain over eye (vision loss in peripheral vision)
- Immediate loss of vision in detached segment

Examination

- Ophthalmoscopic Examination
  - Gray-white color of retina indicating elevation of retina or edema
  - Gray-white color of retina that moves with change in eye position
  - Partially or completely absent red reflex

Treatment

- Ophthalmologic referral
- Cryosurgery, laser surgery, or surgical intervention

Complication

- If untreated can progress to total retinal detachment

SUBCONJUNCTIVAL HEMORRHAGE

- Choroid highly vascular (lying between the sclera, retina, and vitreous) can be penetrated by blunt or sharp trauma resulting in subconjunctival, subscleral, subretinal, or vitreous hemorrhage

Examination

- Blood under conjunctiva, nonpainful

Treatment

- Reassurance

ANTERIOR CHAMBER

Traumatic Hyphema

Mechanism of Injury

- Blunt trauma to globe
- Blood in anterior chamber of the eye from tear of ciliary body or iris

Signs/Symptoms

- Pain, photophobia, blurred vision
- If small hyphema may not affect visual acuity
- Somnolence may indicate associated head injury

Examination

- Crescent-shaped blood-fluid level often visible in anterior chamber

Emergency Treatment

- Immediate ophthalmologic referral
- Elevate athlete's head to 45 degrees (**DO NOT** place head-down or prone)
- Restrict physical activity. Place on bed rest
- Use protective shield over affected eye

- Control intraocular pressure
- Avoid NSAIDs to prevent more bleeding
- Give antiemetics
- May require surgical treatment

Complications

- Recurrent bleeding can occur, usually within 4 days of injury
- Can result in glaucoma or hypopyon (white cells and protein in the anterior chamber)
- Sickle cell patients can have complications of sludging
- Can lead to permanent loss of vision

ORBITAL INJURY

Orbital Fracture

Mechanism of Injury

- Blunt trauma

Examination/Evaluation

- Ecchymosis, lid swelling, hemorrhage within orbit, proptosis
- Fracture of orbital rim usually causes no decrease in function
- Medial fracture of ethmoid bone associated with subcutaneous emphysema of eyelids
- Fracture near optic canal can damage optic nerve, with resultant loss of vision

Blowout Orbital Fracture

- Type of orbital fracture
  - Blunt trauma compresses orbital tissue, increasing pressure into orbit
  - Orbit "blows out" at weakest point, the floor
  - Orbital contents protrude into maxillary sinus
  - Symptoms similar to those of other orbital fractures plus blowout fracture triad:
    - Diplopia
    - Obscured maxillary sinus cavity on x-ray
    - Hypesthesia of face (ipsilateral side of nose and lower lid)
  - Infraorbital branch of trigeminal nerve may be damaged
  - Orbital contents may get trapped in maxillary antrum trapping inferior rectus, inferior oblique muscles
  - Impairs upward gaze, causing diplopia

Tests

- Clinical examination
- X-ray: Waters' view—shows opacified maxillary antrum
- CT scan delineates orbital floor fracture

Treatment

- Surgical repair if there is herniation of orbital contents

Globe Contusion

Ruptured Globe

Mechanism of Injury

- Blunt trauma or indirect forces increase intraocular pressure acutely, causing rupture of globe

Examination/Evaluation

- Do not press on the eye
- Decreased visual acuity, lack of light perception
- Pain, hyphema, vitreous hemorrhage
- Distortion/displacement of pupil
- Loss of fundal red reflex

Emergency Treatment

- Cover eye with hard ocular shield
- Keep patient upright or supine, not prone
- Transport to ophthalmologist for repair

Vitreous Hemorrhage

- Vitreous detachment when retina or superficial retinal vessels are torn

Signs/Symptoms

- Painless loss of vision, floaters or waterfalls (stream of blood)

Treatment

- Athlete must sit in head-up position for 24 h
- Avoid NSAIDs
- Refer to ophthalmologist

LID LACERATIONS

Mechanism of Injury

- Blunt trauma, sharp objects
- Rupture of protective eye equipment

Examination/Evaluation

- Swelling, hemorrhage, anatomic malalignment of lids
- Subtle lacerations, hard to visualize; compare side to side
- Globe injuries may be associated
- Medial eyelid laceration may involve nasolacrimal duct system, impairing tear drainage
- Upper lid laceration may involve levator muscle, resulting in ptosis

Treatment

- Refer to ophthalmologist
- Lacerations involving eyelid margin, levator, canthal tendons, or lacrimal duct system require ophthalmologist to repair
- Full-thickness lacerations require separate-layer closure
- Nonophthalmologist may repair small, nonmarginal lacerations except those listed above

EQUIPMENT

- Ophthalmoscope with blue light, fluorescein strips
- Penlight/flashlight
- Visual acuity card
- Topical ophthalmic anesthetic
- Eye shield, eye patch, tape

PREVENTION

- Protective eyewear use. Polycarbonate lenses preferred
- Purpose: impact-alleviating properties of frame and lens
- American National Standards Institute (ANSI)
- American Society for Testing and Materials (ASTM) Sports Standards
- Listing available of standard eye protection for specific sports

ICD-9 CODES

- 361.0 Retinal detachment with retinal defect
- 364.00 Acute and subacute iridocyclitis, unspecified

- 772.8 Subconjunctival hemorrhage
- 918.1 Corneal abrasion
- 918.9 Other and unspecified superficial injuries of eye
- 921.3 Traumatic hyphema

Bibliography

Christensen GR: Eye injuries in sports: Evaluation, management, and prevention, in Mellion MB, Walsh WM, Shelton GL (eds): *The Team Physician's Handbook,* 2d ed. Philadelphia: Hanley & Belfus, 1997, pp 407–425.

Rubin A, Cheng J: Facial trauma. *Clin Fam Pract* 2(3):565–580, 2000.

Witherspoon CD, Kuhn F, Morris R: Epidemiology of general and sports eye injuries. *Ophthalmol Clin North Am* 12(3):333–343, 1999.

Woods TA: Protective eyewear. *Ophthalmol Clin North Am* 12(3):381–406, 1999.

13

Chest Trauma

Benjamin A. Hasan

RIB FRACTURES

Mechanism of Injury/Pathology

- Blunt trauma
- Falls
- Projectiles
- One or multiple ribs may fracture
- Fractures most often nondisplaced or minimally displaced
- Significant displacement possible
- Comminution possible but also less common
- There may be associated pulmonary contusion, pneumothorax from fractured end of rib nicking the pleura, hemothorax from bleeding onto the pleural space

Diagnostic Keys

- Pain over the rib(s)
- Pain with respiration and other chest wall motion

Examination

- Significant tenderness is the most important clinical finding
- Auscultation is important
  - Abnormal lung sounds initially can be key to finding a pneumothorax or hemothorax
  - Continue auscultation in follow-up to help rule out pneumonia

Emergent Treatment

- Ensure adequate oxygenation
- Provide analgesia

- Apply ice
- Binding with elastic wrap may help

Tests

- Chest x-ray and specific rib-view x-rays
- X-rays may not show all fractures

Definitive Treatment/Follow-up/
Return to Play

- Analgesia to allow normal respiration
- If fracture apparent clinically and initial film negative, treat as fracture and repeat films in follow-up
- Pulmonary toilet if needed to clear secretions
- Follow to ensure clinical healing of fractures
- May return to play when there is normal painless range of motion of trunk, extremities, and spine and minimal tenderness to palpation over sites of fractured ribs
- Continue to watch for late development of complications

Complications

- Pneumothorax, tension pneumothorax, hemothorax, pulmonary contusion, respiratory failure, pneumonia, atelectasis, flail chest, pleural effusion

ICD-9 Codes

- 807.0 Rib fracture, unspecified
- 807.1 One rib
- 807.2–807.7 Two to seven ribs
- 807.8 Eight or more ribs
- 807.9 Multiple ribs, unspecified

FLAIL CHEST

Mechanism of Injury/Pathology

- Definition: three or more ribs fractured at two or more places
- Freely moving segment of chest
- Results in paradoxical chest wall movement with respiration, limiting inspiration and expiration
- Occurs with extreme chest compression (trauma)

Diagnostic Keys

- Pain over flail segment
- Pulmonary contusion can occur with flail chest
- Both flail chest, with a mechanical disruption to breathing, and pulmonary contusion contribute to respiratory insufficiency
- Pulmonary contusion contributes more to respiratory insufficiency than flail chest in most cases
- Diagnosis can be delayed by patient's own splinting of the flail segment due to pain
- 31 percent not recognized within the first 6 h
- Paradoxical motion becomes evident later

Examination

- Visible evidence of flail segment
- Bleeding from open fractures
- Paradoxical motion may be evident or may be hidden by intentional splinting due to pain

Emergent Treatment

- Airway, breathing, circulation (ABCs)
- Binding with wide elastic wraps can provide support to assist with respiration
- Analgesi

Tests

- Chest x-ray
- Pulse oximetry
- Arterial blood gases
- May need CT if pulmonary contusion suspected.

Definitive Treatment/Follow-up/ Return to Play

- Hospital management
- Intubation may be needed
- Analgesia
- Steroids and prophylactic antibiotics have shown no proven benefit
- No benefit from rib belts or rib stabilization
- Intercostal nerve blocks
- Continuous positive airway pressure (CPAP) by mask may help avoid intubation

- Athlete may return to play following clinical and radiologic healing of fracture, possibly in 6–8 weeks

Complications

- 20 percent mortality in flail chest, depending on severity of associated injuries

ICD-9 Code

- 807.4 Flail chest

PENETRATING PROJECTILE

Mechanism of Injury/Pathology

- Penetration into the chest of a projectile
- Has occurred in the javelin throw
- Any major or minor structure or organ may be injured

Diagnostic Keys

- History/observed injury
- Physical assessment will guide immediate action

Examination

- ABCs
- Assess for bleeding
- Auscultate for signs of pneumothorax or hemothorax

Emergent Treatment

- Medical emergency, activate emergency action plan
- Follow advanced cardiac life support (ACLS) protocols
- EMS
- Place intravenous line, administer oxygen
- Transport may require cutting the penetrating object. **DO NOT** remove impaled object.
- Excessive movement of the projectile may cause further injury

Tests

- X-rays and other necessary imaging to be done in the ER setting
- Follow blood count
- Follow oxygenation

Definitive Treatment/Follow-up/ Return to Play

- Medical stabilization, analgesia, and removal of projectile
- Surgery may be required
- Return to competition plans depend on specific injuries

Complications

- Devastating complications may result from blood loss or direct injury to tissue or vital organs
- Hypoxia, exsanguination, dysrhythmias all possible

CARDIAC (MYOCARDIAL) CONTUSION/CHEST WALL CONTUSION/STERNUM FRACTURE

Mechanism of Injury/Pathology

- Blunt chest trauma
- Projectile trauma
- Fall onto a football or other object
- Direct injury to the myocardium
- Compression between sternum and vertebrae
- Displacement of abdominal viscera against heart during blunt abdominal trauma
- True cardiac contusion causes injury to myocardial tissue

Diagnostic Keys

- High suspicion for more serious injuries following chest trauma
- Less severe chest wall contusions are commonplace
- True cardiac contusion occurs in less than 3 percent of cases of blunt chest trauma
- Cardiac contusion rarely causes angina
- ECG

Examination

- Pallor
- Hypotension
- Diaphoresis
- Thready or faint pulse
- Tender chest wall
- Bony tenderness over sternum associated with fracture; most sternal fractures not displaced but quite painful

Emergent Treatment

- Transfer if cardiac injury suspected
- Activate emergency action plan
- EMS with intravenous line and oxygen during transfer
- ACLS protocols
- Blunt chest wall trauma with abnormal ECG requires admission with cardiac monitor

Tests

- Diagnostic methods are controversial for cardiac contusion
- Normal initial ECG does not rule out cardiac contusion
- Some experts state that early echocardiography is not helpful, since wall motion abnormalities are often clinically insignificant and often resolve
- Others recommend that an ECG pattern of myocardial infarction requires inpatient echocardiography
- Use of cardiac enzymes (troponins and CPK-MB) varies by center
- Sternal fracture may require good lateral sternal x-ray view

Definitive Treatment/Follow-up/ Return to Play

- Admission to monitored floor if cardiac contusion suspected
- Chest wall contusion (uncomplicated) may require only local and anti-inflammatory measures
- Sternal fractures (nondisplaced) are treated conservatively
- Analgesia to allow clearing of respiratory secretions/avoidance of pneumonia
- Return following clinical and radiologic healing of fractures
- Return following cardiac contusion depends on specific case

Complications

- Wall motion abnormalities
- Dysrhythmias and complications of cardiac contusion similar to those of myocardial infarction
- Myocardial infarction can result directly from traumatic occlusion of coronary arteries with or without coronary atherosclerosis
- Chambers may rupture, resulting in tamponade or bleeding with hemothorax

ICD-9 Codes

- 807.2 Sternal fracture
- 861.01 Myocardial contusion
- 922.1 Chest wall contusion

COMMOTIO CORDIS (SUDDEN TRAUMATIC CARDIAC DEATH)

Mechanism of Injury/Pathology

- Blunt nonpenetrating chest trauma
- 81 percent from blunt projectile, most often a baseball
- Typically low-energy/low-velocity projectile contact
- No obvious gross or microscopic pathology
  - This differentiates commotio cordis from cardiac contusion
- Dysrhythmias are the problem
- 107 fatalities of 128 total cases recorded in the U.S. Commotio Cordis Registry as of September 1, 2001
- Ventricular fibrillation occurred in 33 of 82 cases
- Ventricular tachycardia occurred in 3 of 82 cases
- Bradycardia occurred in 3 of 82 cases
- Complete heart block occurred in 1of 82 cases

Diagnostic Keys

- Dysrhythmia is the most common key problem

Examination

- Athlete is semiconscious or unconscious
- Athlete changes in appearance immediately following projectile trauma
- Irregular, rapid, or slow pulse
- Point of contact of projectile may be visible on skin
- Pallor

Emergent Treatment

- Automatic external defibrillator (AED)
- Activate emergency action plan
- EMS transfer

Tests

- AED
- Rhythm strip
- Monitor

Definitive Treatment/Follow-up/ Return to Play

- ABCs
- AED
- EMS transfer to ER
- Newer designs for chest protection may protect better
- Return is rare

Complications

- Limited window of time to provide appropriate treatment
- Anoxic injury
- Survivors may sustain permanent neurologic or cardiac pathology

ICD-9 Codes

- 426.0   Complete heart block
- 427.1   Ventricular tachycardia
- 427.41 Ventricular fibrillation
- 427.89 Bradycardia

PNEUMOTHORAX/HEMOTHORAX/ TENSION PNEUMOTHORAX

Mechanism of Injury/Pathology

- Air leak into pleural space causes a pneumothorax
- May occur spontaneously or with trauma
- Bleeding into the pleural space from any vessels causes hemothorax

- Both together = hemopneumothorax
- Tension pneumothorax caused by tissue functioning as a one-way valve
  - Pressure increases on side of pneumothorax
  - Causes mediastinal shift, compromising function of other lung
- Fractured rib may puncture the pleura, resulting in pneumothorax, or may lacerate intercostal vessels, leading to hemothorax, pneumothorax, or both
- Spontaneous rupture of blebs or bullae (familial) is considered the common atraumatic etiology
- Pneumomediastinum rarely occurs in sports

Diagnostic Keys

- Patient may have a combination of chest discomfort, dyspnea, decreased breath sounds, and dullness to percussion

Examination

- Decreased breath sounds over pneumothorax or hemothorax
- Tachycardia, tachypnea, pallor
- Dullness to percussion in hemothorax, hyperresonance in larger pneumothoraces
- Trachea and midline structures may shift in tension pneumothorax

Emergent Treatment

- Tension pneumothorax requires emergent decompression
  - 16-gauge angiocatheter inserted into second intercostal space at midclavicular line allows venting
  - Catheter to remain taped in place during transfer
- Activate emergency action plan
  - Transfer for chest x-ray, possible chest tube placement

Tests

- Chest x-ray
- Pulse oximetry
- Arterial blood gas (ABGs)
- Cardiac monitor
  - Hypotension and cyanosis can occur quickly in tension pneumothorax; these are ominous signs

Definitive Treatment/Follow-up/ Return to Play

- Small pneumothorax without tension can simply be observed, follow with serial chest x-rays
- Chest tube to reexpand lung if >15–20 percent loss of lung volume
- Hemothorax with pneumothorax requires chest tube drainage
- Return to sports in 2–3 weeks after athlete is asymptomatic
- Return to scuba diving is not recommended
- Discomfort, especially associated with fracture, may last 6 weeks
- Follow-up chest x-ray in 6 weeks

Complications

- Spontaneous pneumothorax associated with blebs is often recurrent
- These conditions can cause respiratory failure
- Blood can collect between parietal and visceral pleura (in pleural space) if pneumothorax is not reexpanded; may require additional procedures to clear

ICD-9 Codes

- 511.8 Traumatic hemothorax
- 512.0 Tension pneumothorax
- 512.8 Spontaneous pneumothorax
- 860.0 Traumatic pneumothorax
- 860.4 Traumatic pneumothorax with hemothorax

CARDIAC RUPTURE/TRAUMATIC AORTIC INJURY/RUPTURE OF GREAT VESSELS

Mechanism of Injury/Pathology

- Blunt chest wall trauma

Diagnostic Keys

- High suspicion is the key

Examination

- Rupture of vessels or heart can cause rapid circulatory collapse
- Traumatic aortic injury (TAI) may present subtly

Emergent Treatment

- Activate emergency action plan

Tests

- Chest x-ray, CT of the chest
- Chest x-ray findings suggesting TAI may include:
    - Wide mediastinum, obliteration of aortic knob, deviation of trachea to right, deviation of NG tube to right, left hemothorax, obliteration of space between pulmonary artery and aorta, sternal fractures, upper rib fractures, thoracic spine fractures

Definitive Treatment/Follow-up/ Return to Play

- Stabilization and transport to trauma center with cardiovascular capabilities
- Evaluation and treatment by thoracic surgeon
- Return to play dependent largely on extent of injury and evaluation by thoracic surgeon

Complications

- Exsanguination and death
- Cardiac tamponade
- Aneurysm

ICD-9 Codes

- 417.8 Pulmonary artery rupture
- 441.5 Traumatic aortic injury

STERNOCLAVICULAR (SC) JOINT DISLOCATION

Mechanism of Injury/Pathology

- 47 percent in motor vehicle accidents, 31 percent in sports
- Anterior or anterosuperior displacement of medial clavicle most common
    - Indirect force with the shoulder rolled backward
- Posterior displacement (into mediastinum and major vessels) is *uncommon*

- ○ Direct force pushing on medial clavicle
- Less severe injury may result in subluxation or SC joint sprain

Diagnostic Keys

- Pain over the SC joint
- Physical examination

Examination

- Tenderness, asymmetry, deformity at SC joint
- Severe SC pain with arm motion when supine
- Shoulder appears short and rolled forward

Emergent Treatment

- Anterior dislocation can be reduced in the supine patient with direct pressure and a pad between shoulders
- Posterior dislocation may require reduction by pulling the medial clavicle forward with a towel clip

Tests

- Routine and special x-ray views
- CT is imaging of choice

Definitive Treatment/Follow-up/ Return to Play

- Figure-of-eight strap
- 6–8 weeks for full clinical healing

Complications

- Physeal injuries
- Airway compromise
- Recurrent dislocations
- Pneumothorax
- Compression or laceration of great vessels, esophagus, or trachea

ICD-9 Code

- 839.61 Sternoclavicular (SC) joint dislocation

Bibliography

Bowling WM, Wilson RF, Kelen GD, et al: Thoracic trauma, in Tintinalli JE, Kelen GD, Stapczynski JS (eds): *Emergency Medicine: A Comprehensive Study Guide,* 5th ed. New York: McGraw-Hill, 2000, p 251.

Curtin SM, Tucker AM, Gens DR: Pneumothorax in sports. *Phys Sports Med* 28:8, 2000.

Maron BJ, Gohman TE, Kyle SB, et al: Clinical profile and spectrum of commotio cordis. *JAMA* 287:9, 2002.

Rosen CL, Wolfe RE: Blunt chest trauma, in Ferrera PC, Colucciello SA, Marx JA, et al (eds): *Trauma Management: An Emergency Management Approach.* St. Louis: Mosby, 2001, p 232.

14

Abdominal Trauma

Mark Bouchard

MECHANISM OF INJURY/PATHOLOGY

- 10 percent of all sports-related injuries
- Often unrecognized and poorly treated
- Blunt trauma more common than penetrating
- Occurs more commonly in contact sports and high-speed sports (skiing, cycling)

Abdominal Wall

- Most common and least life-threatening of all abdominal injuries
- Muscle contusions due to blunt trauma, localized tenderness
- More severe trauma may develop large hematomas

Spleen

- 50 percent of all intraabdominal injuries
- Increased risk with splenomegaly (mononucleosis)
- Mechanism: blow to left upper quadrant, deceleration, or overlying rib fracture
- Range of injury: contusion, laceration, rupture of vascular pedicle (most severe)
- Can be life-threatening

Hepatobiliary

- Liver injuries much more common than gallbladder (anatomically protected)
- Increased risk with hepatomegaly
- Mechanism: blow to right upper quadrant, deceleration, or overlying rib fracture
- Range of injury: contusion, hematoma, lacerations of liver; rupture and duct laceration of gallbladder
- Again, lacerations can be life-threatening

Pancreas

- Uncommon but typically severe
- Mechanism: most commonly due to a direct blow in upper midabdomen (football helmet, handlebars, steering wheel)
- Range of injury: contusion, laceration, duct laceration

Hollow Viscus (Intestines, Stomach)

- Mechanism: crush injury against spine or rapid deceleration causing shearing
- Range of injuries: contusion, hematoma, rupture

DIAGNOSTIC KEYS

- Direct blow or deceleration injury
- Acute onset of abdominal pain
- Concurrent abdominal pathology: i.e., hepato- or splenomegaly
- Maintain high index of suspicion for serious injuries

EXAMINATION

Symptoms

- Change in mental status
- Light-headedness
- Presence of pain and location
- Referred pain: shoulder pain due to splenic laceration and resultant diaphragmatic irritation (Kehr's sign)

Signs

- Airway, breathing, circulation (ABCs) (respirations, pulse, BP if able)
- Observation: bruising, redness, lacerations
- Palpation: bone, soft tissue, organs
  - Right upper quadrant (RUQ)—liver, gallbladder
  - Left upper quadrant (LUQ)—spleen
  - Back—kidneys, ribs
- Tenderness—diffuse (intraperitoneal) vs. localized (abdominal wall)
- Rebound tenderness
- Guarding
- Auscultation: hypoactive bowel sounds
- Important: *serial* examinations, monitoring for worsening symptoms

- If unstable (mental status changes, hypotensive, tachycardic), *immediate* hospital transport. One should have a low index of suspicion for intraabdominal injury and should err on the side of transport when warranted.

EMERGENT TREATMENT

- Call for immediate transport
- Make patient comfortable, lying supine
- If orthostatic, elevate legs and start large-bore intravenous line with isotonic fluid if available
- **DO NOT** allow athlete to take anything orally

TESTS

- Performed in hospital
- Labs: Complete blood count (CBC), type and cross, bleeding studies, liver panel, amylase, chem panel, urinalysis
- Imaging
  - Acute abdominal series—free air, rib fractures
  - CT scan of abdomen/pelvis with oral/intravenous contrast—excellent in evaluation of intraabdominal injuries
- Serial labs and CT scans typically performed in managing splenic and hepatic lacerations and hematomas conservatively

DEFINITIVE TREATMENT/ FOLLOW-UP/RETURN TO PLAY

General Guidelines

- Penetrating trauma: object is *not* removed due to risk of hemorrhage upon removal, typically done in OR under controlled conditions
- Blunt trauma: may require CT scan to rule out underlying intraabdominal injury
- Usually, conservative therapy for abdominal wall contusions and hematomas: NSAIDs, relative rest, soft tissue mobilization, stretching
- Return to play once asymptomatic, penetrating trauma guidelines depend on underlying intraabdominal injuries

Spleen

- Conservative treatment with mild injuries (including small lacerations)
- Bed rest, serial CTs and labs, hospitalization for 5–10 days
- Failure of conservative treatment typically occurs within first 3–4 days

- Can have delayed rupture 2–8 weeks after initial injury
- Surgery (repair vs. splenectomy) if unstable or pedicle injured
- Return to play (RTP) in 3–6 months if spleen salvaged (dependent on clinical course); 6–8 weeks if splenectomized

Liver

- Conservative treatment with mild injuries (contusions, subcapsular hematomas)
- Bed rest, serial CTs and labs, hospitalization
- Severe injury (large lacerations, burst/stellate rupture, pedicle injury) or if unstable—requires surgery
- Return to play 1 month after resolution of CT changes in mild injuries. In severe injuries, most recommend no RTP for contact sports *ever*. This is due to risk of recurrent bleeding at site of original injury. (No evidence or studies performed to support this, however.)

Gallbladder

- Injury typically requires cholecystectomy
- RTP in 4–6 weeks

Pancreas

- Typically treated conservatively unless duct/vascular injury. Management as in acute pancreatitis; bowel rest, intravenous fluids, serial amylase/lipase, serial CT scans.
- Occasionally treated surgically, especially if duct is ruptured
- If treated conservatively, RTP once asymptomatic and labs have normalized. If treated surgically, in 2–3 months.

Hollow Viscus

- Most injuries (contusion, hematoma) treated conservatively. Bowel rest until motility returns. RTP once asymptomatic.
- Severe injuries (rupture) require surgical repair and routine postoperative management. RTP 6–8 weeks.

COMPLICATIONS

- Missed injuries not uncommon
- Large hepatic and splenic lacerations and pedicle injuries can lead to hemorrhagic shock and death
- Viscus/gallbladder rupture and severe pancreatic injuries can lead to fulminant peritonitis and sepsis
- Delayed rupture of spleen can develop weeks after injury

ICD-9 CODES

- NEC 868.00 Abdominal organ(s) contusion
- 864.01 Liver contusion
- 864.02 Liver laceration, minor (capsule only)
- 865.01 Splenic contusion
- 865.02 Splenic laceration, capsule
- 922.2 Abdominal wall contusion

Bibliography

Amaral JF: Thoracoabdominal injuries in the athlete. *Clin Sports Med* 16(4):739–753, 1997.

Diamond DL: Sports-related abdominal trauma. *Clin Sports Med* 8(1):91–99, 1989.

Ryan JM: Abdominal injuries and sport. *Br J Sports Med* 33:155–160, 1999.

15

Genitourinary Injury

William Dexter

KIDNEY INJURY
Mechanism of Injury/Pathology

- Most commonly injured genitourinary organ—usually secondary to direct blow
- Kidney is well protected but mobile—vulnerable to deceleration injury
- Injuries range from contusions (60 percent), lacerations of cortex (30 percent), lacerations of calices (<10 percent), fracture and pedicle injury (<1 percent)

Examination/Evaluation

- Symptoms: pain, severe dull ache, hematoma
- Examination
  - "Gray—Turner's sign" or flank ecchymosis, indicates retroperitoneal bleed
  - Flank tenderness
  - Shock with fracture and pedicle injuries

Emergent Treatment

- Treat shock, establish intravenous line, arrange transport, keep NPO

Tests

- Urinalysis (hematuria)
  - No relationship between degree of hematuria and severity of injury
- Plain x-rays
  - Fracture lower ribs or vertebral transverse processes: think kidney injury
  - Loss of kidney outline ("ground-glass appearance"), loss of psoas shadow

- In children: if lower rib fracture, then high incidence of kidney injury
- CT—test of choice
- IVP
  - May be false-negative with contusion, cortical laceration
  - Intrarenal extravasation of dye with caliceal laceration and fracture
  - Extrarenal extravasation if complete fracture
  - Nonvisualized kidney if pedicle injury (confirm with angiography)

Definitive Treatment/Follow-up/ Return to Play

- Contusions and minor lacerations
  - Bed rest, hydration, analgesics
  - Surgery if: progressive symptoms, falling hematocrit, expanding mass, shock
  - Return to play usually in 3–4 weeks
  - Consider rescan, follow blood pressure and urinalysis
- Fractures and pedicle injury
  - Surgical referral (urgent)
  - No consensus on return to play (contact/collision): 6–12 months (minimum) vs. not at all

Complications

- Delayed bleeding (up to 15 percent with lacerations)
- Rebleed (2–3 weeks postinjury most common)
- Hypertension

ICD-9 Codes

- 866.00 Kidney injury (subcapsular)
- 866.01 Hematoma/contusion without rupture of capsule

BLADDER CONTUSION AND RUPTURE

Mechanism of Injury/Pathology

- Direct blow, rupture requires great force and is rare
- Repetitive/indirect causes contusion:
  - Posterior wall against trigone

Diagnostic Keys

- Symptoms: hematuria, dysuria, void clots, suprapubic pain
- Intraperitoneal rupture: ileus, inability to void

Examination/Evaluation

- Tender suprapubic, guarding
- Intraperitoneal rupture: shock
- Extraperitoneal rupture: suprapubic tenderness, fluctuant mass

Emergent Treatment

- Same as above

Tests

- X-ray: intravesicular gas, ileus, obturator fat pad displaced
- Urethrogram/cystogram: best test

Definitive Treatment/Follow-up/ Return to Play

- Contusions:
  - Minor: watch and wait
  - Severe: Foley catheter for 1–2 weeks
- Extraperitoneal rupture:
  - Minor: Foley catheter for 2 weeks, antibiotics
  - Large: suprapubic catheter 2 weeks
- Intraperitoneal rupture: urgent surgery
- Return to play: not well defined, requires complete healing

Complications

- Early: sepsis
- Late: scarring, UTI, bladder calculi

ICD-9 Codes

- 596.0 Bladder rupture (sphincter)
- 867.0 Bladder injury and urethra

URETHRA

Mechanism of Injury/Pathology

- Straddle injury, bicycle most common
- Strike perineum, crush on pubic ramus/symphysis

- Anterior injury most common
- Posterior injury: usually associated with pelvic fracture, inability to void
- Buck's fascia is key
  - If intact, urine extravasates locally
  - If ruptured, urine extravasates to scrotum and abdominal wall

Diagnostic Keys

- Symptoms: painful; good urine stream usually maintained

Examination/Evaluation

- Blood at meatus, ecchymosis, boggy "floating" prostate with posterior injuries

Emergent Treatment

- Transport for definitive care

Test

- Retrograde urethrogram

Definitive Treatment/Follow-up/ Return to Play

- Anterior injury: 20 percent resolve spontaneously; suprapubic catheter, 14 days
- Posterior injury: suprapubic catheter; usually requires surgery
- Return to play requires resolution, probably minimum 1 month

Complications

- Short term: edema, necrosis, sepsis
- Long term: strictures (common), incontinence, impotence

ICD-9 Code

- 867.0 Urethral injury

MALE GENITALIA

Penile Injuries

Mechanism of Injury/Pathology

- Direct trauma
- Danger of injury: corpus cavernosum rupture, laceration, amputation (rare)

Diagnostic Keys

- Clinical
- Symptoms: swollen, bruised, pain, difficulty voiding
- May develop traumatic priapism (requires urgent treatment)

Examination/Evaluation

- Ecchymosis, penile shaft bent to injured side

Test

- Doppler ultrasound

Definitive Treatment/Follow-up/ Return to Play

- Contusion: conservative, return to play with cup
- Corpus rupture: urgent surgical decompression or arterial embolization

Complications

- Dupuytren's, Peyronie's, thrombosis

Testicular Injury

Mechanism of Injury/Pathology

- Direct trauma most common cause
- Range of injuries: contusion, laceration, fracture, dislocation, torsion
  - Torsion may occur with vigorous activity
  - Fracture/rupture of tunica albuginea
  - Dislocation: scrotum forced against abdominal wall

Diagnostic Keys

- Symptoms: swelling, ecchymosis, pain, light-headedness, nausea/vomiting, possibly urinary retention

Examination/Evaluation

- Torsion: scrotal edema, high-riding testicle, tender
  - Pain relieved by elevating scrotum (patient supine)
  - Pain intensified if testes lifted and supported with patient standing (unlike epididymitis)
- Fracture: epididymis cannot be separated from testicle
- Laceration
  - significant swelling, hematoma/hematocele
- Dislocation: testes under abdominal wall

Emergent Treatment

- Support, control bleeding, transport

Tests

- Transillumination
  - Evaluate for hydrocele
- Ultrasound
  - Useful test, may be false-negative
- Radioisotope scanning
  - Checks viability of testes—90 to 100 percent accurate

Definitive Treatment/Follow-up/ Return to Play

- Contusion: ice 24–48 h, return to play as able, protect with cup
- Fracture: repair if partial, orchiectomy usually required
- Dislocation: surgical fixation
  - Identification key: 72-h window for fixation
  - Can be confused with cremaster reflex
- Torsion: timing is key
  - 4- to 6-h window to treat with manual detorsion, usually requires surgical fixation

Complications

- Possible testicular loss
- Increased estradiol levels may be seen after blunt trauma (controversial)

ICD-9 Codes

- 878.0 Penile open wound
- 878.1 Complicated
- 922.4 Penile contusion
- 959.1 Penile injury

PERINEAL /VULVAR/VAGINAL INJURIES

Mechanism of Injury/Pathology

- Blunt trauma, straddle injury (bike, gymnastics, sledding)
- Can occur with high speed water sports

Diagnostic Keys

- Symptoms: pain, bruising, lacerations (uncommon), dysuria

Examination/Evaluation

- Hematoma, laceration, vaginal evisceration (rare)
- Requires careful pelvic examination

Definitive Treatment/Follow-up/ Return to Play

- Usually conservative
- Ice, pain control
- Repair of lacerations; surgery if there is evisceration

Complications

- Early: salpingitis; miscarriages have been reported
- Late: perineal numbness (up to one-third), urethral strictures (2 percent), fistulas

ICD-9 Codes

- 922.4 Vaginal/vulval contusion
- 959.1 Vaginal/vulval injury

HEMATURIA AND PROTEINURIA

Mechanism of Injury/Pathology

- Common problem (over 70 percent incidence), usually benign
- May be caused by any trauma to GU system
- Foot-strike hemolysis
- Intrinsic genitourinary system disease
- Dehydration
- NSAIDs

Diagnostic Keys

- Timing of (gross) hematuria may help locate injury
  - Initial stream—ureter
  - Terminal stream—bladder
  - Continuous hematuria—upper tract disease
- Thorough history and physical examination

Tests

- Urinalysis
  - Do not do routinely as part of preparticipation physical
- Urine culture
- BUN and creatinine
- Consider 24-h urine for creatinine and protein
- CT and/or IVP
- Cystoscopy

Definitive Treatment/Follow-up/ Return to Play

- Usually benign and self-limited
  - Will resolve in 2 or 3 days
- Return to play, no follow up needed
- Underlying pathology must be identified and treated

ICD-9 Codes

- 599.7 Hematuria
- 791.0 Proteinuria

Bibliography

Lynch JM: Renal and genitourinary problems, in Mellion MB, Walsh WM, Shelton GL (eds): *The Team Physician's Handbook,* 2d ed. Philadelphia: Hanley & Belfus, 1997.

Rich BSE: Genitourinary injuries, in Safran MR, McKeag DB, Van Camp SP (eds): *Manual of Sports Medicine.* Philadelphia: Lippincott-Raven, 1998.

16

Lacerations, Suturing, and Sunburn

Ken Honsik

NORMAL WOUND HEALING

Three Overlapping Phases

- Inflammation
  - Immediate
  - Release of mediators that attract/activate macrophages, neutrophils, and fibroblasts
- Tissue formation
  - Begins within hours
  - Reepithelization, granulation, and neovascularization
- Tissue remodeling
  - Occurs during second week of healing
  - Wound contraction and strengthening

LACERATIONS

Mechanism of Injury/Pathology

- Sharp trauma laceration
  - Penetration of epidermis with a foreign object
- Blunt trauma laceration
  - Crush injury of skin against bony edge
    - Commonly cheekbones and eyebrows
- Clean wound
  - Primary closure should be performed within 6 h
  - May consider primary repair for clean wounds within 12–24 h
- Contaminated wound
  - Primary closure must be within 6 h after thorough cleansing
  - Healing by secondary intention after 6 h

Evaluation

- Control bleeding first. Then proceed with evaluation
  - Stop the bleeding with direct pressure over the wound

History

- Mechanism
- Time since injury
- Medications (i.e., anticoagulants)
- Anesthetic, antibiotic, latex allergies
- Tetanus status

Examination

- Local anesthetic useful at this point
  - Use 1% lidocaine, 0.25% or 0.50% bupivacaine
  - Epinephrine may help with hemostasis in well-vascularized regions
  - Do not use epinephrine in fingers, toes, nose, penis, earlobes
  - Consider regional nerve blocks for larger wounds

Exploration

- Depth of wound
- Assess if damage to tendons, muscle, nerves, or bone
  - Operative repair should be considered if any of these structures are involved
- Cosmetic landmarks
- Tension on wound edges
- Wound preparation for repair
- Cleanse wound
- Remove gross contamination
  - Scrub gently with a wound-cleansing solution
- 18-g needle with 60-mL syringe (provides high pressure)
  - Use normal saline
  - 60 mL of saline should be used per centimeter of wound length
  - Do not irrigate with iodine products or hydrogen peroxide; these may impede healing
- Debride
  - Remove all foreign particles and hair from wound
  - Cut away all devascularized tissue
- Revise
  - If wound edges are ragged and irregular, consider trimming wound with a scalpel to provide clean wound edges that will approximate well

REPAIR TECHNIQUES

Suture

- When to use:
  - Wounds under tension
  - Perpendicular to natural stress lines
  - Joints
  - Complicated/complex lacerations
  - Cosmetically challenging wounds
  - Vermilion border of lips
  - Eyebrow
  - Eyelids
- Properties
  - High tensile strength
  - May cause reaction with tissue
  - Time-consuming
  - Nonabsorbable sutures require removal
- Suture materials
  - Nonabsorbable (nylon, polypropylene, silk)
    - Epidermal/dermal closures
  - Absorbable
    - Subcuticular closures
  - Sizes:
    - 3-0 or 4-0—trunk
    - 4-0 or 5-0—extremities
    - 5-0 or 6-0—face, scalp

Techniques

Basic

- Approximate wound edges but do not strangulate the tissue
- Align cosmetic reference points first
- Achieve hemostasis to avoid hematoma

Simple Interrupted (See Fig. 16.1)

- Effective for most wounds
- Fast/easy

Deep Suture (See Fig. 16.1)

- Helps to approximate edges of deep wounds, prevents dead space, decreases surface tension on superficial sutures

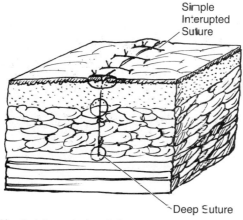

Figure 16.1 Simple interrupted and deep sutures.

Vertical Mattress (See Fig. 16.2)

- Provides increased strength
- Improves eversion of edges

Horizontal Mattress (See Fig. 16.3)

- Provides increased strength
- More effective for thinner skin

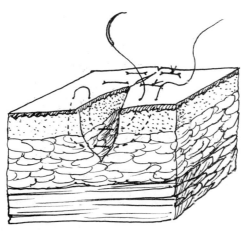

Figure 16.2 Vertical mattress suture.

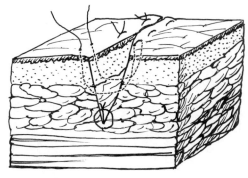

Figure 16.3 Horizontal mattress suture.

Half-Buried Horizontal Mattress (See Fig. 16.4)

• Approximates free flap corners
• Avoids pressure ischemia of flap

Subcuticular Suture (See Fig. 16.5)

• Cosmetic closure of low tension wound

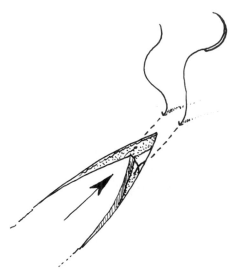

Figure 16.4 Half-buried horizontal mattress suture.

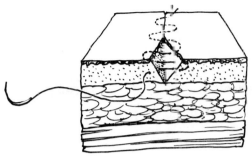

Figure 16.5 Subcuticular suture.

Special Situations

- Lips
  - Approximate vermilion border first
  - Regional anesthesia (nerve blocks) minimize tissue deformity
  - Only *repair* philtrum, *do not* revise
- Eyebrows
  - Do not shave eyebrow
  - Use brow as landmark for repair
- Eyelids
  - Repair if lid margins uninvolved
  - Refer if margins involved
- Ears
  - Be gentle. The cartilage of the pinna is avascular, making it more susceptible to pressure necrosis and requiring that skin be closed over it.
  - Drain auricular hematomas to decrease pressure on cartilage

Wound-Care Instructions

- Observe for infection
- Keep dry 24 h
- Keep clean

Suture Removal

- Face and scalp: 3–5 days
- Scalp, arm, hand: 7–10 days
- Trunk, legs, joints: 10–14 days

Complications

- Dehiscence
- Infection
- Hematoma

Return to Play

- Inform athlete of increased dehiscence risk
- Wound must be covered before participation

Staples

- When to use
  - Scalp wounds
  - Rapid repair required
- Properties
  - Very strong
  - Little tissue reaction
- Techniques
  - Manually approximate and evert skin edge
  - Apply staples in even distribution
- Wound care
  - Same as above

Cyanoacrylate Adhesives

When to Use

- Small, superficial lacerations
- Even edges, easily approximated
- Low-tension wounds parallel to tension lines
- Do not use for mucocutaneous or moist areas
- Do not use for deep wounds without subcutaneous sutures

Properties

- Waterproof once dry
- Max strength at $2\frac{1}{2}$ min
- Nontoxic to tissue, including eye

Technique

- Cleanse wound
- Achieve complete hemostasis
- Manually approximate wound edges and hold
- Crush inner vial and invert
- Brush gently and evenly along laceration
- **DO NOT** apply into the wound. It will seal the edges and prevent healing
- May release wound in 30 s
- Apply two more layers
- Blowing on it does not make it dry faster
- Vinyl gloves get stuck less than latex ones

Troubleshooting

- 10-s grace period to wipe off excess
- If poor approximation occurs:
  - Do not pry apart
  - Apply topical antibiotic or petroleum jelly to loosen and break down adhesive
  - May be possible to peel off after 30 min
- If gets in eye (nontoxic) and lids stuck together:
  - Do not pry lids apart or cut eyelashes
  - Apply ophthalmologic antibiotic ointment for 1–2 days
    - Adhesive should loosen and allow lids to open

Wound Care

- If satisfied with approximation, inform athlete that the adhesive peels off in 5–10 days
- Once dry, **DO NOT** apply topical antibiotic or petroleum jelly, as this could weaken the repair

Return to Play

- Immediate, if wound is not under high tension

Surgical Taping (Butterfly Dressings, Steri-Strips)

- When to use
  - Small, superficial wounds
  - No tension
- Properties
  - Must be kept dry
- Technique
  - Commonly applied with adhesive (benzoin)
- Wound care
  - Keep dry
  - Spontaneously peels off in 7–14 days
  - May be removed manually

Complications

- High rate of dehiscence if tension present

Return to Play

- Immediate, if no tension unless healing by secondary intention is acceptable to athlete if closure fails

SUNBURNS/THERMAL BURNS

Prevention

- Sunscreen SPF 15 or greater
  - Apply 20–30 min before sun exposure
  - Team physicians and trainers should do this as well as athletes!
    - Sunscreen should be part of the medical kit
- Wide-brimmed hat should be worn when possible
- Tight-weave fabric clothing (white T-shirt provides only 5–9 SPF)

Treatment

- Remove from direct sunlight
- Cold compress/bath
- Pure aloe vera
- Cool Silvadene cream for more severe burns
- If no blisters, may consider 1% hydrocortisone lotion
- If severe with blisters, swelling, and exudates: treat as direct contact burn
  - Nonadhesive dressings
  - Consider antibiotics for prevention of cellulitis
  - Provide pain control

EQUIPMENT—SUTURE KIT

Local Anesthetic Supplies

- Lidocaine 1% with and without epinephrine
- Bupivacaine
- 25-, 27-, and 30-g needles
- 5- and 10-mL syringes
- Sodium bicarbonate to buffer lidocaine

Cleansing/Irrigating Supplies

- 60-mL syringe (Luer-Lok type)
- 18-g needles
- Normal saline/sterile water
- Forceps/tweezers
- Cleansing solution
- Surgical scrub brush

Suture Materials

- - Nonabsorbable and absorbable (2-0 through 6-0) sutures
  - Needle driver
  - Suture scissors
  - Tissue forceps
- Cyanoacrylate with plastic tissue approximator
- Steri-Strips/butterfly bandages
  - Tincture of benzoin
- Skin stapler
- Dressings
  - Sterile gauze
  - Paper tape
  - Semipermeable membranes
  - Antibiotic ointment and petroleum jelly
  - Sunscreen SPF 15 or higher, waterproof/sweatproof
  - Headlamp (camping/hiking type)
  - Small tackle-box tray with lid is ideal for organizing these supplies in your medical kit
  - Preprepared suture kits and trays are available
  - *Always check the expiration dates on the medicines and supplies in your kit*

Bibliography

Forsch RT: Soft-tissue injury and laceration repair: Office management of trauma. *Clin Fam Pract* 2(3):551–564, 2000.

Ramsey ML, Wappes JR: Soothing your summer skin problems: From sun abuse to bug bites to plant plagues. *Phys Sports Med* 26(7):75, 1998.

Rubin A: Suture substitutes: Using skin adhesives. *Phys Sports Med* 26(4): 115, 1998.

Yamamoto LG: Preventing adverse events and outcomes encountered using Dermabond. *Am J Emerg Med* 18(4):511–515, 2000.

17

Environmental Injury

R. Tucker Thole

HEAT INJURY
Mechanism of Injury/Pathology

- Heat illness occurs when thermoregulation fails (body heat exceeds heat loss)
- Heat loss and gain regulated by physics of heat exchange:
  - Conduction, radiation, convection, evaporation
  - Related to environmental parameters of ambient air temperature, relative humidity, wind velocity, and radiation
  - Wet-bulb globe temperature (WBGT) is an index of heat stress
    - WBGT = (0.1 × dry-bulb thermometer) + (0.7 × wet-bulb thermometer) + (0.2 × solar radiation globe thermometer)
    - High weighting of wet-bulb thermometer related to importance of relative humidity

Thermoregulation

- Physiologic mechanism of body temperature regulation
- Evaporation is responsible for majority of heat dissipation with maximal exertion
  - Sweating and resulting heat loss through evaporation is slowed at increasing humidity and environmental heat
- Heat illness occurs with failure of thermoregulation to moderate heat dissipation

Risk for Heat Illness

- Risk factors related to impairment of thermoregulation
  - Vigorous physical activity
    - 75 percent of energy conversion at maximal exercise is released as heat
  - High environmental heat and humidity

- Dehydration, diuretic beverages, vapor-impermeable clothing, poor conditioning, poor heat acclimatization, obesity, elderly, children, drugs and medication

EXERTIONAL HEAT SYNDROMES

Heat Cramps

Pathophysiology

- Mechanism under investigation
- Possible total-body salt deficiency

Diagnostic Keys/Examination

- Core temperature normal
- Symptoms—muscle spasms and cramps

Emergency Treatment

- Rest, stretching, massage, ice, mild cooling, oral rehydration

Definitive Treatment/Follow-up/Return to Play

- Athlete may return to play when asymptomatic
- Prevention with prehydration and adding salt to food and drink

Heat Exhaustion

- Pathophysiology
  - Dehydration (water depletion) and/or electrolyte loss (sodium depletion)

Diagnostic Keys/Examination

- Inability to continue exercise
- Core temperature normal to slightly elevated but less than 40°C (104°F)
- Orthostatic vital signs, syncope, dyspnea, weakness, headache, decreased exercise performance
- Profuse sweating, cutaneous flushing, decreased urine output, nausea/vomiting, headache, mild mental status changes (confusion, agitation)

Emergent Treatment

- Stop exercise; rest
- Rapid, moderate cooling
  - Move to cool location, elevate legs, remove excess equipment and clothing, spray with cool water (misters), use fans

- Oral hydration with cool water, 1 L/h
- Intravenous fluids if orthostatic or tachycardic

Tests

- Serum sodium, electrolytes, glucose, urine specific gravity

Definitive Treatment/Follow-Up/Return to Play

- Transport to medical facility if symptoms worsen and/or core temperature rises despite cooling interventions
- Return after rehydration, asymptomatic, and at least 24 h of rest
- For temperature greater than 39°C (102°F), mental status changes, or syncope, no return to play for a minimum of 48 h and then only when asymptomatic, after rehydration, and return with lighter workloads and gradual progression; close monitoring of temperature and symptoms

Heatstroke

Pathophysiology

- Failure of thermoregulation with hyperthermia and neurologic dysfunction

Diagnostic Keys/Examination

- Rectal temperature greater than 40°C/104°F
- Skin temperature hot, possible absence of sweating (late phase)
- Hypotension, sinus tachycardia
- Mental status change and CNS dysfunction (confusion, syncope, coma)

Emergent Treatment

- ABCs
- Start cooling and evacuate to medical facility
- Rapid cooling to core temperature of 39°C (102°F)
  - Provide cool environment; wet with cool mist spray; fan; remove excess clothing; administer ice packs to neck, axillae, groin; give ice-water baths
- Intravenous fluid challenge D_5NS 500 mL/1 L bolus

Tests

- Arterial blood gas (ABG), CBC, electrolytes, glucose, CPK, LFTs, renal function tests, coagulation tests, urinalysis

Definitive Treatment/Follow-up/Return to Play

- Transport to definitive medical care facility immediately
  - ICU and lab test monitoring
- Return to play after resolution of any resultant medical complications, asymptomatic, and with evidence of adequate heat acclimatization and evaluation with a heat tolerance test

Complications

- Chronic central nervous system deficits, coma, cardiopulmonary failure, rhabdomyolysis, disseminated intravascular coagulopathy, acute renal failure, hepatic injury, death

ICD-9 Codes

- 992.0 Heat stroke
- 992.2 Heat cramp
- 992.5 Heat exhaustion

COLD INJURIES

Hypothermia

Mechanism of Injury/Pathology

- Core temperature less than 35°C (95°F)
- Related to decreased heat production, increased heat loss, or impaired thermoregulation
- Generally related to prolonged cold exposure in athletic competitions

Diagnostic Keys

- Cold environmental temperature, lack of appropriate behavioral modifications, wind chill factor, precipitation increase prevalence of hypothermia
- Initial estimate of the degree of hypothermia by level of consciousness and presence of shivering

Examination

- Mild hypothermia: core temperature 32–35°C (90–95°F)
  - Confusion, loss of coordination, apathetic, impaired mentation
  - Shivering, tachycardia
- Moderate hypothermia: core temperature 28–32°C (82–90°F)
  - Severely impaired mentation, muscle rigidity
  - Lack of shivering, hypotension, bradycardia, cardiac arrhythmia, ECG changes with J-point elevation, hypoventilation

- Severe hypothermia: core temperature <28°C (82°F)
  - Comatose, can appear to be dead
  - Pupils fixed and dilated, blood pressure not detectable, slow respirations

Emergent Treatment

- Mild hypothermia
  - Goal—prevent further heat loss
  - Passive rewarming
  - Warm shelter, dry clothes, warm fluids orally, dry blankets
- Moderate/severe hypothermia
  - ABCs, ACLS hypothermia protocol
    - Avoid jostling patient to prevent precipitation of arrhythmia
    - Check for breathing and pulse for 1 min
    - Standard ACLS protocols are often ineffective in hypothermia
    - If in ventricular fibrillation, attempt defibrillation once and if conversion fails, warm core to >30°C before repeating defibrillation
  - Transport to medical facility immediately
  - Rewarming best performed at medical facility
    - Amount of field rewarming is related to availability of evacuation
    - Prevent further cooling
    - Start warm D_5NS IV

Tests

- ECG, cardiac monitoring, ABGs, blood sugar, CBC, electrolytes, BUN, creatinine, coagulation studies, serum calcium, serum magnesium, amylase, lipase

Definitive Treatment/Follow-up/Return to Play

- Emergency/ICU care for moderate to severe hypothermia
  - Active rewarming and close monitoring
    - Heated intravenous fluids [40°C (104°F)], electric blankets, heated humidified oxygen, heated lavage, dialysis, extracorporeal blood rewarming
    - Rewarming endpoint: temperature >35°C (95°F)

Complications

- Atrial and ventricular arrhythmias
- Electrolyte abnormalities
- Sepsis
- Death

Frostbite

Pathophysiology

- Freezing of skin occurs in four phases:
  - Prefreeze
    - Chilling of skin surface prior to ice crystal formation
  - Freeze-thaw
    - Ice crystal formation and tissue temperature below freezing point
  - Vascular stasis
    - Blood vessel damage with plasma leakage
  - Ischemia
  - Thrombosis, ischemia, autonomic dysfunction, gangrene

Diagnostic Keys

- Environmental risk factors:
  - Cold ambient temperature, wind chill, high altitude, prolonged exposure, high humidity, lack of appropriate clothing/environmental avoidance
  - Sensation of cold, then numbness
  - Extreme pain to throbbing pain after rewarming

Examination

- Skin waxy, white-yellow or mottled blue, with frozen appearance
- After thawing, skin hyperemic with return of sensation, vesicle formation, and edema
- Late changes include black eschar and eventual mummification

Emergent Treatment

- Immediate transport to medical facility (optimally within 2 h)
- Avoid thawing until there is no chance of refreezing
- Avoid field reheating with intense, dry heat (campfire and car heaters) and avoid gradual partial rewarming
- Avoid vigorously rubbing or massaging frostbitten tissue
- Remove wet, tight-fitting clothing and use loose, dry material to cover wounds
- Leave vesicles and bullae intact

Definitive Treatment

- Rapid reheating with warm-water immersion [40–42°C (104–108°F)] until skin is pliable and hyperemic (15–30 min)
- Control rewarming pain with adequate analgesia
- Hospital admission
- Debride clear-white vesicles, leave hemorrhagic bullae and vesicles intact, cover both with aloe vera

- Antibiotics, daily hydrotherapy, adequate pain control, tetanus pro-phylaxis, elevation of extremities
- Late treatment can involve surgical debridement and amputation; these should be avoided, if possible, in early treatment course

Tests

- Triple-phase bone scan to assess viable tissue in management deci-sions regarding surgical debridement

Complications

- Cold hypersensitivity, Raynaud's syndrome, hyperhidrosis, skin color change, nail abnormalities, chronic joint pain, premature epi-physeal closure in skeletally immature patients

ICD-9 Codes

- 991.3 Frostbite, unspecified site
- 991.6 Accidental hypothermia

Trenchfoot/Immersion Foot

Mechanism of Injury/Pathology

- Prolonged exposure to cold and wet environment leads to peripheral vasoneuropathy
- Cold above freezing temperature [0–10°C (32–50°F)]

Diagnostic Keys/Examination

- Initially cool to touch, white/yellow color, loss of sensation
- After warming, intense pain, hyperemia, edema, paresthesia

Treatment

- Drying of skin, extremity elevation, and passive rewarming

Complications

- Cold hypersensitivity, paresthesias, pain, hyperhidrosis
- Muscle wasting, nerve damage, permanent disability in severe cases

Raynaud's Syndrome

Mechanism of Injury/Pathology

- Digital vasospasm in response to cold and/or emotion

Diagnostic Keys/Examination

- Ischemic phase associated with cold, numb, pale (white) digits
- Hyperemic phase associated with redness, pain, swelling

Emergent Treatment

- Warming of affected extremity and digits

Definitive Treatment/Tests/Follow-up

- Avoid cold exposure and smoking
- Keep core warm and use warm mittens and footwear
- Complete medical evaluation to rule out primary disease
- Rule out collagen vascular disease, autonomic dysfunction, thoracic outlet syndrome, cold agglutinin disorders, cryoglobulinemia
- Cold-challenge test using high-frequency ultrasound if diagnosis is in question
- Demonstrated by a 45 percent or greater decrease in digital artery diameter after cold exposure
- Some benefits with pharmacologic intervention (vasodilators, calcium channel blockers, ACE inhibitors, and reserpine)
- Refractory cases sometimes require surgical sympathectomy

ALTITUDE ILLNESS

Mechanism of Injury/ Pathology

- High-altitude illness includes the signs and symptoms that occur as a result of ascending to high altitude. This high-altitude environment is characterized by a low barometric pressure, which causes a decreased partial pressure of inspired oxygen. The resulting state of hypobaric hypoxia is the physiologic basis for acute mountain sickness (AMS), high altitude pulmonary edema (HAPE), and high altitude cerebral edema (HACE).

Diagnostic Keys

- AMS
  - Headache, insomnia, nausea, anorexia, lassitude, fatigue or weakness, malaise, dizziness, light-headedness, memory impairment, concentration difficulties
- HAPE
  - 50 percent of HAPE victims experience symptoms of AMS in addition to the following:
    - Severe dyspnea on exertion progressing to dyspnea at rest, nonproductive and persistent cough, chest tightness, fatigue, weakness
- HACE
  - Initially, signs of AMS, which progress in severity

- Headache, lethargy, incoordination, vomiting, disorientation, irrational behavior, visual or auditory hallucinations, semicoma, unconsciousness

Examination

- AMS
  - Nonfocal examination until progression to HACE
- HAPE
  - Cyanosis, tachypnea, tachycardia, crackles on lung examination (classically in right middle lobe)
- HACE
  - Ataxia, inability to perform tandem gait walking (heel to toe), altered mental status, confusion

Emergent Treatment

- Descent to lower altitude is primary treatment for severe AMS, HACE, and HAPE
- AMS
  - Mild:
    - No further ascent until symptoms resolved; consider descent of 500 m/1500 ft or more if symptoms persist >24 h
    - Rest and hydrate
    - Symptomatic medications
    - Nonsteroidal anti-inflammatory drugs or acetaminophen for headache
    - Antiemetics (prochlorperazine) for nausea, vomiting
    - Acetazolamide 125 mg–250 mg every 8–12 h to aid acclimatization and symptomatic relief (usually within 24–48 h)
  - Moderate to severe AMS or continued mild AMS symptoms:
    - In addition to treatment of mild AMS, descend at least 500 m/1500 ft or until symptoms improve
    - Consider low-flow oxygen at 2–4 L/min
    - Consider dexamethasone at 4 mg PO, IM, or IV every 6 h until symptoms resolve
    - After stopping dexamethasone, ensure that the patient remains symptom-free for 24–48 h before reascending, as rebound symptoms of AMS can occur after discontinuing steroid use
    - Consider use of hyperbaric therapy if oxygen not available or descent is impossible and symptoms severe
    - A hyperbaric bag is a portable, inflatable hyperbaric chamber
    - Symptom relief is generally experienced after 2–4 h in bag and is comparable to supplemental oxygen use
  - If above treatment not effective and symptoms persist or worsen, evaluate patient closely for the presence of HAPE and HACE and descend immediately

- HAPE
  - Descent
    - Assisted descent of at least 900–1200 m/3000–4000 ft should occur as soon as the diagnosis of HAPE is suggested
    - Early recognition of HAPE symptoms is essential to initiate immediate descent and/or evacuation
  - Oxygen
    - Use of high-flow oxygen at 4–6 L/min is essential with goal to keep oxygen saturation >90%
  - Nifedipine
    - If descent impossible and/or symptoms are severe or worsening, consider nifedipine 10 mg sublingual every 4 h until symptoms improve or 10 mg sublingual once and then 30 mg extended release every 12–24 h
  - Hyperbaric therapy
    - Hyperbaric therapy for 4–6 h can be used if immediate descent is impossible and oxygen unavailable
  - Symptomatic medications as in AMS can be used
  - Check for HACE or severe AMS
- HACE
  - Descent and/or immediate evacuation mandatory
  - Supportive measures before descent
    - High-flow oxygen at 4–10 L/min
    - Hyperbaric therapy
  - Acetazolamide 250 mg qid
  - Dexamethasone 4 mg qid or slow IV drip
  - Periodically record vital signs (pulse, blood pressure, respiration rate, urine output)
  - Check for concomitant HAPE

Tests

- HAPE
  - Homogenous or patchy confluent infiltrate in right middle lobe with no cardiomegaly
- HACE
  - MRI can demonstrate white matter edema and cortical atrophy

Definitive Treatment/Follow-up

- Evacuation to medical facility for HACE and HAPE
  - Hospital admission for oxygen, monitoring, and imaging studies
- Preventive measures for future ascents to high altitude:
  - Acclimatization and gradual ascent is paramount
  - Avoid heavy exertion for 2–3 days upon arrival to high altitude
  - Maintain adequate hydration
  - Frequent small high-carbohydrate meals
  - Avoid alcohol, sedative/hypnotics, smoking

- Consider pharmacologic prophylaxis with history of AMS, HACE, or HAPE
  - HACE and AMS prevention: acetazolamide 125–250 mg PO bid starting 24 h prior to arrival at high altitude, dexamethasone 2 mg PO q4h or gingko biloba 120 mg PO bid
  - HAPE prevention: nifedipine 30 mg extended release PO q12h
- Prevention, proper planning, and reasonable goals can prevent most incidents of altitude illness

ICD-9 Code

- NEC 993.2 High altitude illness

Bibliography

Auerbach PS: *Wilderness Medicine,* 4th ed. St Louis: Mosby, 2001.

Giesbrecht GG: Prehospital treatment of hypothermia. *Wilderness Environ Med* 12:24–31, 2001.

Hackett PH, Roach RC: High altitude illness. *N Engl J Med* 345(2):107–114, 2001.

McCauley RL, Heggers JP, Robson MC: Frostbite: Methods to minimize tissue loss. *Postgrad Med* 88:67, 1990.

Part 2

Orthopedic Concerns

18

Fractures

Mark R. Hutchinson
Joseph Tansey

OVERVIEW
Definition—Structural Failure of Bone

Classification

Complete vs. Incomplete

- Complete—radiographically evident with structural discontinuity, displacement, and/or alignment change
- Incomplete—may or may not be radiographically evident, no discontinuity is present, single cortex can be involved. nondisplaced fractures, stress reaction, and stress fractures. Bone scans positive within 3 days.

Open vs. Closed (Formerly Compound vs. Simple)

- Closed—no bleeding or break in skin
- Open—any fracture with an associated break in skin. Open fractures are orthopedic emergencies and require irrigation and subsequent antibiotic prophylaxis.
  - Grade 1—puncture or small wound <1 cm
  - Grade 2—mild to moderate soft tissue injury with lacerations <10 cm
  - Grade 3—severe soft tissue injury, all lacerations greater than 10 cm, all severely contaminated wounds, any fracture on a farm or related to a tornado, and all fractures with arterial injuries

Skeletally Mature vs. Immature

- Mature—fractures in adults when physis is closed
- Immature—in skeletally immature athletes, where the physis is the weak link (Fig. 18.1)

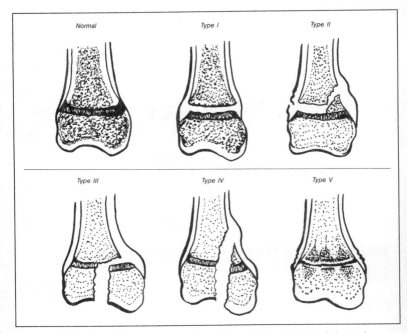

Figure 18.1 The Salter-Harris classification system used in epiphyseal injuries. (From Simon RR, Koenigsknecht SJ: *Emergency Orthopedics: The Extremities*, 4th ed. New York: McGraw-Hill, 2001. Used by permission.)

- Salter-Harris type I: a fracture purely through the physis
- Salter-Harris type II: a fracture predominantly through the physis with an associated metaphyseal component
- Salter-Harris type III: a fracture predominantly through the physis with an associated epiphyseal component. These are intraarticular fractures; they must be anatomically reduced to reduce the risk of arthritis.
- Salter-Harris type IV: a rare fracture in which the fracture line crosses perpendicular to the physis and includes both metaphyseal and diaphyseal components. These must be anatomically reduced to reduce the risk of arthritis and growth arrest.
- Salter-Harris type V: a compression injury to the physes in which the growth cells are crushed
- Other fracture patterns in the skeletally immature include:
  - Greenstick fractures—nonphyseal incomplete fractures of skeletally immature long bones in which the tension side cracks or splits like a living tree branch when bent; however, the opposite side has a permanent plastic deformation. These

fractures may have to be completed to correct the plastic deformity.

- Torus fractures or buckle fractures—nonphyseal incomplete fractures of skeletally immature long bones in which the compression side is crushed (like an aluminum can) and the tension side remains intact

Descriptive Terminology

- *Comminution*—how many pieces. Simple fractures have two pieces, comminuted fractures indicate a higher-energy injury.
- *Angulation*—how crooked. Some authors describe angulation as a flexed or extended, varus or valgus deformity. It is much easier to describe angulation in reference to which way the apex (the point of the fracture) is pointing. For example a tibial fracture with the distal fragment flexed 30 degrees relative to the proximal fragment would be described as 30-degree angulation, apex anterior. Angulation is always described in degrees (best measured with a goniometer).
- *Translation*—the amount a fracture is offset side to side. There may be no angulation or crookedness, yet the fracture is still unstable because only one cortex of each fragment is touching (almost 100 percent translated).
- *Shortening*—when a fracture is 100 percent translated, muscle tension tends to shorten the fracture. The amount of shortening should be documented.
- *Avulsion*—the ripping or tearing away of a part. Both ligaments and tendons originate or insert onto bone via Sharpey's fibers. The ligaments and tendons can fail in midsubstance, through Sharpey's fibers at their insertion or by pulling off a piece of bony insertion (avulsion injury). In children, this is usually an apophyseal injury.
- *Pathologic fracture*—a fracture due largely to an underlying weakness in the bone, leading to an increased risk of fracture. Pathologic fractures are relatively rare in athletes. Causes include tumors, metabolic bone disease, and osteoporosis. (An eating disorder is also a possible cause.)

Mechanism of Injury—
Macrotrauma vs. Microtrauma

- Macrotrauma—often the cause of fractures occurring in contact and collision sports. Such a fractures can occur directly, as by being hit by a stick, ball, or opponent; or indirectly, as when a football player is thrown down, hitting the lateral border of his acromion against the ground and fracturing his clavicle. In the general population, macrotraumatic fractures are commonly associated with falls or motor vehicle accidents.
- Microtrauma—often seen in athletes, especially those in noncontact sports, these fractures are related to repetitive overuse. Runners face an increased risk of stress fractures in their feet and legs if their

shoes become old, if they increase their mileage or the intensity of training too quickly, or if they begin to run on a harder surface than before. Poor nutrition and energy balance as well as eating disorders have also been related to an increased risk of microtraumatic fractures.

Physical Examination

- Inspection may reveal gross deformity
- *Examination should ALWAYS include an assessment of neurologic and circulatory function distal to the suspected fracture*
- Functional motor testing may exacerbate pain if avulsion or a complete fracture has occurred
- Loading or stressing the bone will exacerbate pain
- Pain to palpation is usually localized at the fracture site and not diffusely over the bone
- *Exam should ALWAYS include the joint above and below the suspected fracture*
- The vibrations of a tuning fork or the use of ultrasound directly over a suspected stress fracture will frequently exacerbate pain
- Gross instability or the sensation of "potato chips crunching" is an obvious sign of fracture

Radiographic Examination

- *Two clear views of the suspected fracture should ALWAYS be obtained.* In long bones, this is commonly an anterposterior (AP) view and a lateral view. For some bones, additional views are necessary to visualize the fracture clearly; e.g., for patellar fractures a patellar sunrise or Merchant's projection is necessary to get an unobstructed second view. For scapular or clavicular fractures, internal and external rotation views of the proximal humerus are inadequate, as they provide only a single view of the suspected fracture.
- *The joint above and below the suspected fracture should ALWAYS be included.* The fracture pattern may extend into the joint and be missed unless these views are routinely obtained.
- *Comparison views of the opposite side should ALWAYS be obtained in the skeletally immature*
- Additional special views may be beneficial for certain anatomic sites.
- Bone scans may be helpful in confirming the presence of subtle fractures and stress fractures even when radiographs are negative. However, they may not be positive for 3–4 days postinjury. Bone scans (by single photon emission tomography, or SPECT) are particularly sensitive for stress fractures of the lumbar spine in some athletes.
- MRI is rarely indicated to diagnosis fractures or stress fractures but may reveal bone edema before bone scans are positive. They also help to clarify the extent of soft tissue injury.
- CT scans and tomography may be used by the orthopedic surgeon to assist in preoperative planning of the most complex fracture patterns

General Recommendations: Acute Fractures:

- *Always begin by assessing the airway, breathing, circulation (ABCs) and the cervical spine* (see Chaps. 3, 4, and 5)
- When in doubt, immobilize
- Ice and cryotherapy can reduce swelling and relieve pain
- Elevation of a limb above the level of the heart will reduce throbbing and pain; however, in the case of a possible compartment syndrome, the extremity should remain at heart level
- Immobilization should include the joint above and below the fracture
- Splinting is usually safer (if less rigid) than circumferential casting, reducing the risk of compartment syndrome and allowing for swelling
- All open fractures require surgical irrigation and a course of antibiotics
- Intraarticular fractures require anatomic reduction to minimize the risk of arthritis
- The amount of acceptable angulation, displacement, and shortening depends on the patient's age, potential for remodeling, the specific bone involved, and the direction of angulation
- Early motion when possible will reduce muscular atrophy, may encourage bone healing, and may speed return to sport
- Some fractures that might well heal with conservative treatment may benefit from surgical intervention in certain populations of athletes to avert the risk of delayed healing or recurrence—e.g., stress fractures of the scaphoid, Jones's fractures of the fifth metatarsal
- *Avoid use of nonsteroidal anti-inflammatory drugs in fractures as they have been shown to delay bone healing*
- Use of bone-stimulation devices in acute fractures has been said to return high-level athletes to their sports more quickly, but no prospective blinded study has been able to prove its effectiveness in large populations
- Return-to-play decisions are made based on the stability of the fracture, the specific sport's demands of the athlete, functional testing prior to participation, and a gradual and progressive return to sport

Potential Complications of Fractures

- Infection
- Major nerve or vessel injury
- Malalignment and deformity
- Posttraumatic arthritis
- Delayed union or nonunion
- Respiratory distress syndrome and fat emboli syndrome
- Reflex sympathetic dystrophy

FRACTURES OF THE SPINE

Cervical Spine (See Chap. 20)

Mechanism of Injury

- More common in contact and collision sports (football, rugby, ice hockey, motor racing)
  - Axial loading occurs with spear tackling in football (when a defender tackles with the crown of his helmet). Rule changes in 1976 outlawing spear tackling resulted in a significant reduction in catastrophic injuries.
  - Checking from behind in ice hockey (now illegal) can cause a player to run head-first into the boards, causing a cervical spine injury
  - Catastrophic cervical spine injuries in motor racing have been related to severe neck flexion during a crash impact. This risk may be reduced with the introduction of head and neck safety (HANS) apparatus systems (see Chap. 41).
- Fractures of the cervical spine are also common secondary to falls from heights or the use of apparatus (gymnastics, cheerleading, pole vaulting, diving)
  - Risk reduction in diving has targeted head-first diving restrictions in shallow water
  - Risk reduction in gymnastics and cheerleading has focused on a gradual progression of skills on apparatus and the elimination of some stunts in cheerleading, such as the double back flip with basket tosses, and restrictions on pyramid heights to $2\frac{1}{2}$ people

Diagnosis and Treatment

- *ALL athletes with midline neck pain and a traumatic injury should be considered to have a cervical spine fracture until proven otherwise*
- *ALL athletes with bilateral burners, stingers, or neurologic findings should be considered to have a cord lesion and an unstable spine until proven otherwise*
- *Any unconscious athlete or any athlete with head injury and impaired sensorium should be considered to have a cervical spine injury until proven otherwise*
- Field-side treatment includes:
  - Immobilization
  - Gentle in-line traction/stabilization
  - Palpation of the midline and assessment of peripheral nerve function; if abnormal, complete emergent spine treatment is required
  - Team log-rolling onto spine board
  - Rigid collar placement
  - Taping to spine board

- *For adult helmeted sports, the helmet and shoulder pads are left in place until a spot lateral c-spine view is obtained. If airway access is necessary, the face mask should be removed.*
- *For pediatric helmeted sports, blankets should be placed beneath the child's torso on the spine board—or a specially designed spine board with a head cutout should be used. Children's heads are relatively larger and the spine board forces them into flexion rather than a neutral position.*
- Imaging studies include:
  - A screening lateral prior to helmet removal
  - AP, lateral, oblique, and odontoid views after helmet removal if the screening lateral is normal
  - Active (patient-controlled) flexion and extension views if all studies are normal

Treatment

- All cervical spine fractures should be referred and treated by an expert in the field

ICD-9 Codes

- Closed fracture vertebra
  - 805.01 C1
  - 805.02 C2
  - 805.03 C3
  - 805.04 C4
  - 805.05 C5
  - 805.06 C6
  - 805.07 C7

Lumbar Spine

- Macrotraumatic fractures of the thoracic and lumbar spine are rare in athletes
- Examination reveals pain along the midline focally over the fracture
- Imaging studies should include AP, lateral, and oblique views
- Microtraumatic fractures of the lumbar spine are much more common in athletes
  - Spondylolysis—a stress fracture of the pars interarticularis
    - More common in sports and positions demanding repetitive hyperextension
      - Gymnastics and rhythmic gymnastics
      - Wrestling
      - Football (linemen)
      - Weight-lifting
      - Cheerleading
    - May be associated with rotation-demanding sports such as golf

- Radiographs are frequently negative; tomographic bone scanning (SPECT) is the imaging study of choice
- Examination reveals
  - Midline spine tenderness
  - Pain with back extension and rotation
  - Pain with single leg extension (stork test)

Treatment

- Acute (onset less than 6–8 weeks):
  - Goal is cure and fracture healing
  - Custom thoracolumbosacral orthosis for 8–12 weeks followed by lumbosacral corset and core stabilization exercises
  - Some authors follow via serial bone scans
  - Return when strong and asymptomatic
- Chronic (onset greater than 2–3 months):
  - Likely fibrous nonunion
  - Treat symptomatically with lumbosacral corset and core stabilization exercises
  - Return to sport as tolerated

ICD-9 Codes

- 805.4 Closed fracture of lumbar vertebra
- 806.4 With spinal cord injury

UPPER EXTREMITY

Clavicular Complex

- Medial clavicle and sternoclavicular (SC) separations
  - Pain on medial clavicle
  - Mechanism is usually blow on lateral blow of shoulder such as being slammed into the boards in hockey or thrown to the ground in martial arts
  - Medial clavicular physis is last to close at age 23; therefore injury prior to that is likely physeal and not an SC separation
  - Posterior displacement places great vessels and trachea at risk. If no symptoms, treat conservatively. If symptoms, reduction with vascular surgeon on standby. It may be necessary to convert to anterior displacement.
  - Anterior displacement: may attempt reduction but frequently unstable. Athletes usually do fine if left alone.
  - General consensus for chronic medial snapping is conservative treatment. Surgery has many risks.

Clavicular Fractures

- May be secondary to direct (hit by a stick) or indirect trauma (as above)
- The most common cause of clavicular nonunion is surgery; therefore primary surgery should be avoided in most clavicular fractures except those that are open
- Sling treatment is usually adequate, although some authors still prefer figure-of-eight strapping
- Fracture healing may take 8–12 weeks, followed by protection from contact for an additional 1–2 months to prevent recurrence

ICD-9 Codes

- Clavicular fracture
  - 810.01 Sternal end
  - 810.02 Mid third
  - 810.03 Acromial end

Shoulder

Body of Scapula

- Usually secondary to high-energy impact
- Rare in sports unless due to direct contact from a helmet
- Look for associated neurovascular injury
- Routine radiographs should include an AP view in the plane of the scapula and a Y scapular view
- Extraarticular injuries are usually treated conservatively

Glenoid

- Usually associated with dislocation in contact or collision sports
- Routine shoulder views should include an axillary view, which will reveal the lesion
- Treatment is usually conservative if large fragment is anatomically reduced
- If intraarticular displacement is present, surgical reduction is necessary
- Small fragments are likely bony Bankart lesions, which portend a high risk of recurrent shoulder instability in young overhead athletes. They should be fixed surgically.

ICD-9 Codes

- Closed fracture of scapula
  - 811.00
- Glenoid fracture
  - 811.03

Proximal Humerus

- Usually classified into four parts: head, shaft, and greater and lesser tuberosities
- Imaging studies should include internal and external rotation views of the proximal humerus
- In the skeletally immature, comparison views of the opposite arm are essential to diagnose "Little Leaguer's shoulder," an overuse physeal injury of the proximal humeral physis
- Treatment of Little Leaguer's shoulder is conservative, with rest for 6–8 weeks followed by a gradual progressive return to throwing after 12 weeks
- Tuberosity displacement of greater than 1 cm requires fixation secondary to an increased risk of impingement
- Significantly displaced three- and four-part fractures pose an increased risk of avascular necrosis of the head. Nonetheless, fixation should still be attempted in the young athlete if possible.
- In recreational athletes or exercise-active individuals over age 60 with displaced four-part fractures, hemiarthroplasty is the procedure of choice

ICD-9 Codes

- Closed fracture of upper humerus
  - 812.03 Greater tuberosity
  - 812.09 Head
  - 812.09 Lesser tuberosity

Humerus

- Imaging studies should include AP and lateral views of the entire humerus, including the shoulder and elbow. Midshaft humeral fractures can occur secondary to direct trauma in contact and collision sports.
- If a midshaft humeral fracture occurs in a throwing or noncontact sport, suspicion should be raised for the potential of underlying bony pathology
- Closed fractures with intact neurovascular examination are usually treated conservatively with cast bracing (a coaptation splint) or a light hanging arm cast

ICD-9 Codes

- 812.21 Closed fracture of shaft of humerus

Elbow

- Fractures about the elbow may be secondary to macrotrauma (collision and contact sports) or microtrauma (throwing sports)

- Imaging studies should include AP and lateral views of the arm
- Comparison views of the opposite elbow should ALWAYS be obtained in children, as the maturing physes can be confused as fractures
- Examination should include an assessment of distal neurovascular function and a good examination of the wrist
- Intraarticular, displaced, and angulated fractures must be anatomically reduced and fixed
- Throwing athletes create a repetitive valgus-extension overload force across the elbow. This, in turn, can lead to stress or avulsion injuries of the medial epicondyle, stress or avulsion injuries of the olecranon process, and compression stress injuries of the radial head and capitellum.
- Displacement of the medial epicondyle or olecranon process in throwing athletes is an indication for surgical fixation

ICD-9 Codes

- Closed fracture of elbow
  - 812.41 Supracondylar
  - 812.42 Lateral epicondyle
  - 812.43 Medial epicondyle
  - 813.01 Olecranon
  - 813.05 Radial lead

Forearm

- Imaging studies for suspected forearm fractures should include AP and lateral views of the entire forearm, including the wrist and elbow
- Bone scans can reveal stress fractures in athletes with a particularly high forearm demand, such as gymnasts
- Isolated fractures of the midshaft of the ulna (a nightstick fracture) can occur if an athlete attempts to block a blow from an opponent's stick. Minimally displaced fractures can be treated conservatively with a protective splint.
- Displaced radial fractures and both bone fractures in adults require surgical fixation for optimum functional return of the upper extremity. Pediatric patient can be treated conservatively depending on the level of fracture, age of patient and potential for remodeling and the amount of deformity.
- Fractures of the midshaft ulna with dislocation or injury about the radial head are called Monteggia fractures and require surgical fixation (Fig. 18.2)
- Fractures of the midshaft radius with dislocation of injury about the distal ulna are called Galleazi fractures and require surgical fixation (Fig. 18.3)

ICD-9 Code

- 813.23 Closed fracture of shaft of radius and ulna

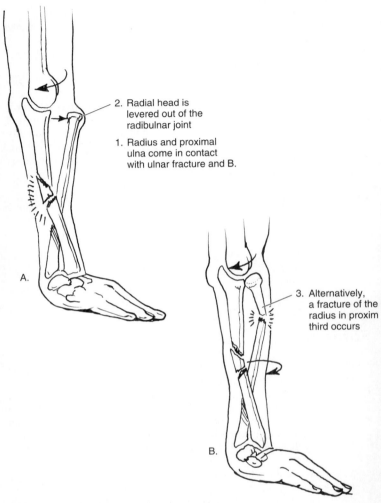

2. Radial head is levered out of the radibulnar joint

1. Radius and proximal ulna come in contact with ulnar fracture and B.

3. Alternatively, a fracture of the radius in proxim third occurs

A.

B.

Figure 18.2 *A.* Monteggia fracture. *B.* Alternative Monteggia fracture.

Wrist and Hand

- Injuries to the wrist and hand are most common in sports that demand weightbearing on the upper extremities (gymnastics), ball sports, and grabbing/tackling sports (football, wrestling, rugby)
- Mechanism can be overuse, a fall on an outstretched arm, or misgrabbing or catching an apparatus or opponent
- Standard imaging studies include AP, lateral, and oblique views of the affected area

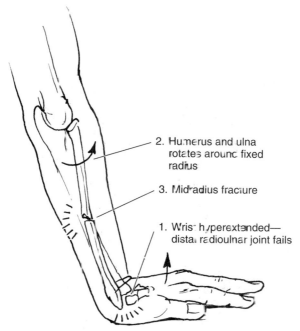

2. Humerus and ulna
   rotates around fixed
   radius

3. Mid-radius fracture

1. Wrist hyperextended—
   distal radioulnar joint fails

Figure 18.3 Galleazi fracture.

- The most common fracture of the wrist is a scaphoid fracture (Fig. 18.4)
  - Athletes present with pain with dorsiflexion and radial deviation of their wrist
  - Pain is present dorsally over the scaphoid and in the "anatomic snuffbox" at the base of the first metacarpal on the radial aspect of the wrist
  - Imaging studies can include a scaphoid view, which is a magnified coned-in view of the scaphoid
  - Initially, imaging studies may be negative; nonetheless, in the face of clinical suspicion, the athlete should be immobilized in a thumb spica cast until repeat films 2 weeks later or a bone scan 3–4 days postinjury is negative
  - Aggressive immobilization is required secondary to an elevated risk of avascular necrosis and nonunion with this fracture
  - A short arm thumb spica cast may be used for 12 weeks although an initial treatment of 4–6 weeks of a long arm thumb spica cast may improve and speed healing potential
  - Some authors propose initial treatment, for even nondisplaced scaphoid fractures in athletes, with cannulated screw fixation. This allows almost immediate range of motion and an earlier return to sport.

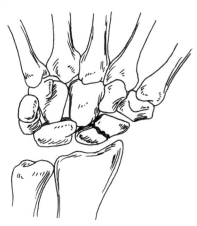

Figure 18.4 Scaphoid fracture. (From Simon RR, Koenigsknecht SJ: *Emergency Orthopedics: The Extremities*, 4th ed. New York: McGraw-Hill, 2001. Used by permission.)

Hook of the Hamate

- Related to bat and stick sports. Athlete presents with pain on the ulnar aspect of the palm at the wrist.
- Along with the traditional studies, imaging studies should include a carpal tunnel view. Others suggest CT or MRI.
- Treatment can be conservative, although this fracture tends to heal with a fibrous union, leading to additional pain. Surgical excision has proven to be effective.

Physeal Injuries of the Distal Radius (Gymnast's Wrist)

- Seen in skeletally immature athletes in upper extremity weight-bearing sports
- Present with pain with wrist extension and weight bearing on wrist
- Imaging should include comparison views of the opposite wrist and usually reveal physeal widening and irregularities
- Treatment includes restriction from all weight-bearing activities for 4–6 weeks
- Cast immobilization is not necessary but can relieve pain in the acute setting
- Return to sport should not occur until after 12–16 weeks and then only with a gradual progressive return to weight bearing
- Dorsal extension block splints and braces can reduce the risk of recurrence

ICD-9 Codes

- Closed fracture distal radius
  - 813.42
- Closed fracture of carpal bones
  - 813.44 Distal radius
  - 814.01 Scaphoid
  - 814.08 Hamate
  - 815.00 Metacarpal
  - 816.00 Phalanges

LOWER EXTREMITY FRACTURES

Pelvis and Hip

Pelvic and Acetabular Fractures

- Require significant energy
- Rare in sports
- Acetabular fractures are intraarticular and associated with hip dislocations
- Intraarticular displacement must be reduced anatomically

Avulsion Fracture (Fig. 18.5)

- Most common pelvic injury in athletes
- Sartorius can avulse from anterosuperior iliac spine
- Ischial tuberosity can be avulsed by hamstrings
- Adductors can avulse small fragments from inferior pubic ramus
- Treatment is conservative for most avulsion fractures, even displaced ones. Some authors have recommended open reduction and internal fixation of large displaced ischial avulsion in sprinters and jumpers.

ICD-9 Codes

- Closed fracture of pelvis
  - 808.00 Acetabulum
  - 808.2 Pubis
  - 808.42 Ischium
  - 808.43 Pelvis (multiple)

Hip Fracture

- Macrotraumatic fractures are rare in athletes
- Microtraumatic stress fractures of the femoral neck are more common in runners and in females
- A high index of suspicion is necessary
- Plain radiographs are usually negative

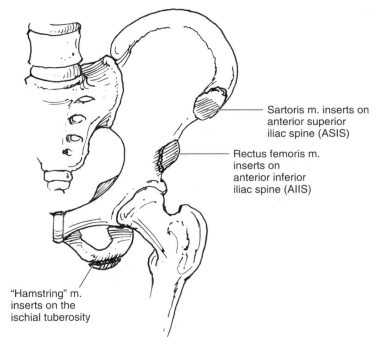

Sartoris m. inserts on anterior superior iliac spine (ASIS)

Rectus femoris m. inserts on anterior inferior iliac spine (AIIS)

"Hamstring" m. inserts on the ischial tuberosity

Figure 18.5 Pelvic avulsion fractures.

- Bone scans (SPECT) are diagnostic
- Tension side fractures are at increased risk of progression to complete fracture and may require pinning
- All athletes should be evaluated regarding their training program, changes in shoe wear, training surface, and training intensity
- All athletes should be evaluated regarding their energy balance and nutrition
- Females should be screened for menstrual irregularities and the female athlete triad
- Return to sport is dictated by an absence of complaints and a gradual progressive return to full training

ICD-9 Codes

- Closed fracture of neck of femur
  - 820.11 Transepiphyseal
  - 820.13 Base of neck
  - 820.21 Intertrochanteric
  - 820.22 Subtrochanteric

Femur

- Femoral fracture is relatively rare in sports but can be seen in collision and contact sports
- Imaging studies should include AP and lateral views of the entire femur, including the hip and knee
- Classic treatment for complete, displaced, angulated, and/or pathologic fractures in adults and most teenagers is intramedullary rodding
- Injuries of the distal femoral physis are commonly missed, being mistaken for ligamentous injuries in the skeletally immature. Stress views should reveal widening with varus or valgus stressing. Treatment is cast immobilization or occasionally pinning.

ICD-9 Code

- 821.01 Closed fracture of femur

Knee

- Intraarticular
  - Displaced intraarticular injuries including fractures of the distal femoral chondral and tibial plateau must be anatomically reduced (Fig. 18.6)
  - CT scans and tomograms are frequently helpful in identifying the extent of displacement and assisting in preoperative planning
  - Careful examination should include an evaluation for associated ligamentous injuries

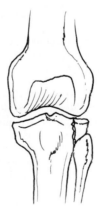

Figure 18.6 Tibial plateau fracture.

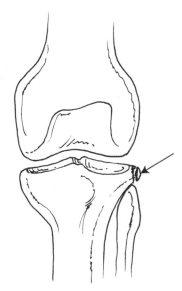

Figure 18.7 Segond fracture.

Avulsion Injuries

- Segond's sign—the appearance of a small fragment off the lateral tibial plateau is called Segond's sign. Historically, this has been correlated with ACL injuries. In actuality, it is an avulsion of the middle-third capsular ligament, which is a part of the posterolateral complex and related to posterolateral rotatory instability (Fig. 18.7).
- Avulsion fragments off of the medial epicondyle represent avulsion of the medial collateral ligament. This is usually treated conservatively if isolated and easy to fix if surgery is required for other ligaments.
- Avulsions of the medial tibial eminence in the intracondylar notch indicate an injury to the insertion of the ACL. Intrasubstance injury to the ligament has also occurred; nonetheless, treatment is open reduction and internal fixation (possibly with recession) of the displaced fragment (Fig. 18.8).
- Avulsions of the tibial tubercle are uncommon in adults but may be seen in mature adolescents. Near anatomic reduction is necessary to ensure that the extensor mechanism is of an appropriate functional length (Fig. 18.9).

ICD-9 Codes

- Closed fracture of distal femur
  - 821.21 Chondyle
  - 821.22 Epiphyses

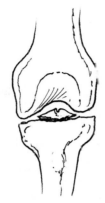

Figure 18.8 Tibial spine fracture.

- 821.23 Supracondylar
- 823.00 Tibial plateau
- 824.80 Tibial physis

Tibia and Fibula

Complete Fractures (Macrotraumatic)

- More common in collision and contact sports
- Imaging studies should include the joint above and below the fracture

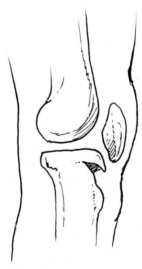

Figure 18.9 Tibial tubercle fracture.

- Stable fractures can be treated with casting
- Unstable fractures are treated with intramedullary nailing or other alternative techniques (plating, external fixation)

ICD-9 Codes

- 823.20 Closed fracture of shaft of tibia
- 823.22 With fibula

Stress Fractures (Microtraumatic)

- More common in runners, gymnasts, endurance athletes
- Pain is worse with impact
- May be associated with energy balance and nutrition
- Most common cause is a change of intensity in training
- Females should be screened for the female athlete triad
- Focal pain on examination exacerbated with ultrasound or the vibration of a tuning fork
- Imaging studies may be positive if carefully reviewed. Bone scans are definitive in confirming diagnosis.
- Treatment
  - Reduction of stresses
  - Cryotherapy
  - Avoid the use of NSAIDs, as they may slow healing
  - Pneumatic braces can be used for midshaft stress injuries and lower. If athlete has pain relief, he or she can safely complete the season using braces.
  - There are anecdotal reports of accelerated healing with bone stimulation, although no prospective, blinded study is available to confirm this

ICD-9 Codes

- 733.93 Stress fracture of tibia

Foot and Ankle

Ankle

Bi- and Trimalleolar Fractures

- Macrotraumatic fractures can occur in all sports with running, jumping, tackling, collision, and contact
- Imaging studies include AP, lateral, and mortice views
- Need for obtaining radiographs can be determined on sidelines with some confidence. If athlete has pain over bone, especially posterior border of fibula, radiographs are necessary. If the ath-

lete has pain only distal to the tip of the fibula, over ligaments, no radiographs are necessary.
- Must be anatomically reduced with no wideningof the mortice
- 1–2 mm offset increases loads, significantly increasing the risk of arthritis

Triplane and Physeal Fractures

- When adolescents are approaching skeletal maturity, they are at risk for complex variations of physeal fractures
- Imaging studies should include comparison views of the opposite side
- Any intraarticular component must be anatomically reduced

Talar Dome Fractures (Fig. 18.10)

- Ankle sprains can lead to shearing forces over the corners of the talus, leading to nondisplaced fractures or osteochondral loose fragments
- Loose bodies should be removed arthroscopically. Large fragments may be fixed

ICD-9 Codes

- Closed fracture of ankle
  - 824.00 Medial malleolus
  - 824.20 Lateral malleolus
  - 824.50 Bimalleolar
  - 824.60 Trimalleolar

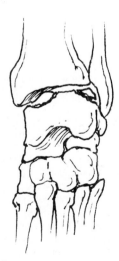

Figure 18.10 Talar dome fracture.

Foot

Hindfoot and Midfoot Fractures

- Calcaneal, talar, and other hindfoot fractures can be associated with impact or traumatic injuries
- Imaging studies should include AP, lateral, and oblique views of the foot. Special calcaneal views and subtalar joint views (Brodin's views) can also assist in picking up subtle fractures. CT scan is an excellent way to better elucidate the complexity of hindfoot fractures.
- Talar neck fractures must be treated especially aggressively, because displacement introduces a great risk of avascular necrosis and nonunion
- The Lisfranc fracture is a traumatic disruption of the tarsometatarsal joint with a fracture through the base of the second metacarpal. This is a significantly disabling injury that must be reduced and pinned anatomically to give the athlete the best chance of returning to function.

Navicular Stress Fracture

- Most common hindfoot bone injury in athletes
- Plain imaging studies can be equivocal
- MRI scan will clearly elucidate bone changes
- Bone scan is also diagnostic
- Treatment is rest, immobilization, and a period of non weight bearing. These fractures can take 2–3 months to heal.
- Occasionally, screw placement is necessary to stabilize the bone for healing

Forefoot Fractures

- Metatarsal stress fractures (March fractures)
  - Historically related to military recruits who sustained stress fractures in their feet secondary to the increased stresses and intensity of basic training
  - Most common in track, runners, and dance athletes
  - Most commonly occur in second metatarsal (the longest metatarsal)
  - Athlete should be screened for change of shoe wear, intensity of training, training surface, and nutritional habits (for females, in addition, a menstrual history should be obtained)
  - Treatment is a reduction in impact stresses. A hard-soled shoe or postsurgical wooden shoe may help to reduce pain.
  - Orthotics have been tried with poor success in returning an athlete to sport. Occasionally, some athletes with rigid, conforming shoe wear (figure skaters, ice hockey players, and skiers) have competed successfully.

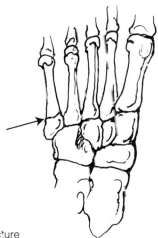

Figure 18.11 Jones fracture

- Jones fracture (fracture of the base of the fifth metatarsal) (Fig. 18.11)
  - A unique metatarsal injury that occurs between 0.5 and 1.5 cm distal to the proximal tip of the fifth metatarsal
  - This relatively avascular zone of bone is at increased risk for nonunion and delayed union
  - Mechanism is impact loading, but fracture may occur with a pivot in the opposite direction as the planted foot
  - Classic treatment is non-weight-bearing short leg cast for 6–8 weeks followed by progressive weight bearing in a cast or boot for 6 weeks. Rehabilitation may take an additional 2 months before return to play.
  - Surgical fixation with an intramedullary screw has been advocated for high-demand athletes, especially basketball players who want an earlier recovery and to reduce the risk of recurrence

Phalangeal Fractures

- The great toe is most commonly injured
- Mechanism is usually direct trauma or axial load, such as stubbing the toe or impacting the toe within the toebox of the shoe
- For minor toes, simple buddy taping is usually effective for treatment, with return to play when symptoms disappear
- Intraarticular fractures may require reduction
- Athletes with fractures involving the phalanges of the great toe tend to take longer to return to play secondary to the high demands placed on the great toe during push-off of walking, running, or jumping

ICD-9 Codes

- Talar dome fracture
  - 825.21
- Foot fracture
  - 825.00 Calcaneus
  - 825.22 Tarsal navicular
  - 825.25 Metatarsals
  - 826.00 Phalanges

Bibliography

DeLee JC, Drez D: *Orthopaedic Sports Medicine: Principles and Practice.* Philadelphia: Saunders, 1994.

Kay RM, Matthys GA: Pediatric ankle fractures: evaluation and treatment. *J Am Acad Orthop Surg* 9:268–278, 2001.

Matheson GO, Clement DB, McKenzie DC, et al: Stress fractures in athletes. *Am J Sports Med* 15(1):46–58, 1987.

Morgan WJ, Slowman LS: Acute hand and wrist injuries in athletes: Evaluation and management. *J Am Acad Orthop Surg* 9(6):389–400, 2001.

Orava S, Hulkko A: Stress fractures in athletes. *Int J Sports Med* 8:221–226, 1987.

Rockwood CA, Green DP (eds):. *Fractures in Adults and Children.* New York: Lippincott, 2001.

19

Emergency Splinting and Bracing

Ken Honsik

FUNDAMENTALS OF SPLINTING

- Joint injury—splint or brace should include bones above and below the joint
- Bone injury—splint or brace should incorporate joints above and below the bone
    - Always check the neurovascular status of an injured limb before applying a splint or brace and after application
    - Splints are meant as temporary immobilizers in the acute setting that allow for swelling and stabilize the injury until the extent of the injury is confirmed and a definitive plan of care is made

MATERIALS

Ready-Made Splints

- Ready-made splints are currently available from many different companies
    - They are portable and fit easily into a team physician's sideline kit
    - Consist of fiberglass or plaster layers, precut and contained in a padded sleeve
    - Can be applied rapidly with little mess and cleanup
    - Author's preferred material for sideline splinting
- Splints can also be custom-made with raw plaster or fiberglass materials cut to length and layered
    - More layers needed for bigger/heavier bones and joints
    - Apply over a layer of cast padding to protect skin
    - Use extra padding over bony areas
- Either splint type can be held in place by an elastic bandage (not too tight!)

Temporary Splints

- Temporary splinting can be done with any rigid object, such as tongue blades, cardboard, rolled-up magazine or newspaper
- Splinting can also be performed with ready-made materials; e.g., SAM splint, Aircast, knee immobilizer, air splints, and vacuum splints
- Refer to Table 19.1 for specific splints

Table 19.1 Splints and Braces

Region	Splint/Brace Type	Indications	Application Tips	Picture/Diagram
Fingers	Buddy tape	IP/MCP and interosseus sprains (2d–5th digits)	Tape the injured finger to the supporting digit above and below the injured joint	See Fig. 19.1.
	Aluminum splints	IP/MCP sprains and dislocations (2d–5th digits)	Dorsal application more functional than volar	See Fig. 19.2.
	Stack splints	DIP injuries, tuft fracture, mallet finger	Finger should be kept in extension on flat surface if and when splint is removed or changed	See Fig. 19.3.
	Radial gutter splint	Suspected phalangeal or metacarpal (Boxer's) fractures (2d and 3d digits)	Goal of splinting these injuries is anatomic "holding a can" position	See Fig. 19.4.
	Ulnar gutter splint	Suspected phalangeal or metacarpal (Boxer's) fractures (4th and 5th digits)	Goal of splinting these injuries is anatomic "holding a can" position	See Fig. 19.5.
Wrist/finger	Thumb spica splint	Suspected thumb fracture, 1st MCP collateral ligament injury (gamekeeper's thumb), possible scaphoid and/or lunate fracture	Extra padding at snuff box/De Quervain's region avoids irritation and injury by splint	See Fig. 19.6.
Wrist/hand	Volar wrist splint	Wrist sprains, suspected metacarpal fractures	Dorsal splint may also be applied for increased strength and improved stability	See Fig. 19.7.
Wrist/forearm	Sugar-tong splint	Distal radius/ulnar fractures, midshaft forearm fractures	Extend to distal metacarpal necks, limits pronation/supination	See Fig. 19.8.
Wrist/forearm/ elbow	Double sugar tong splint	Distal radius/ulnar fractures, mid-/ proximal forearm fractures, elbow fractures/dislocations	Best immobilizer; limits pronation/supination and elbow flexion/extension	See Fig. 19.9.

(continued)

Table 19.1 Continued

Region	Splint/Brace Type	Indications	Application Tips	Picture/Diagram
Elbow/Arm	Long arm posterior splint	Proximal forearm, elbow, or distal humerus fractures	Best if used with sling; double sugar-tong provides better stability	See Fig. 19.10
Shoulder	Sling	Dislocation/subluxation, sprain, AC joint separation, suspected fracture of proximal humerus, scapular injury	Easily fashioned with triangular bandage in medical kit or with pinning sleeve to shirt with safety pins	
Neck	Cervical collar Spine board SAM splint	See Chap. 20		
Back	Spine board			
Hips	Spine board/crutches	Hip dislocation	If possible, early reduction may decrease risk of avascular necrosis	
Femur	Traction splint	Suspected femur femoral fracture	Early traction decreases the potential space for bleeding and hematoma formation	
Knee	Posterior knee splint (long leg post splint)	Knee dislocation, completely unstable knee	Rarely kept in kit (too big); speak with trainer about having available at events	
	Knee immobilizer brace	Knee sprain, suspected patellar fracture, patellar dislocation/subluxation	Side bars may be bent to comfort before brace applied	
	ROM brace (hinged brace)	ACL/PCL/LCL/MCL injuries	Many models are adjustable and can block knee within specific ROM Best choice if early ROM will quicken recovery time	

Ankle/Leg	Posterior ankle splint	Fracture of distal tibia/fibula, ankle dislocation or bad sprain tarsal or metatarsal fracture, Achilles tendon injury/rupture	Splint in equinus position for Achilles injuries	See Fig. 19.11.
Ankle	Stirrup ankle splint	Ankle sprains, fractures of distal tibia/fibula	Best splint for acute ankle sprains	See Fig. 19.12.
	Air stirrup brace, lace-up brace	Ankle sprains	Allow for participation while providing support	
Misc.	Vacuum splints, air splints	May be used to immobilize just about any medium/large joint and/or bone	Too large to keep in medical bag. Discuss with trainer about having it at events with risk of high-energy trauma.	
	Orthoplast (moldable hard plastic)	Injuries that will allow athlete to play if they are protected/supported: contusions, sprains, nondisplaced stable fractures	These hard splints must be adequately padded to allow for safe play	
	Wilderness splints ("SAM" splint)—anything available: backpack frames, ski poles, sticks/branches, blankets, triangular bandage	These splints can be fashioned or improvised for just about any injury where immediate medical care and supplies are not available.	Just follow the fundamentals of splinting	

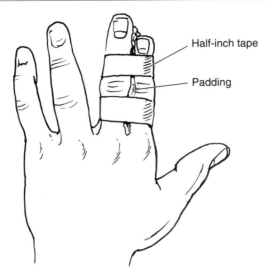

Figure 19.1 Buddy tape.

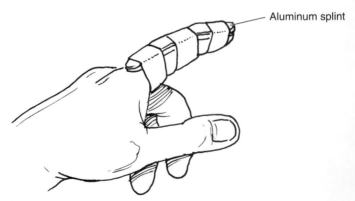

Figure 19.2 Aluminum splint.

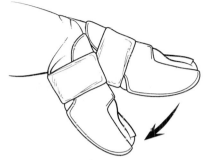

Splint DIP – allow PIP motion

Figure 19.3 Stack splint. (From Lewis CG: *Orthopaedic Pocket Procedures: General Orthopaedics*. New York: McGraw-Hill, 2003. Used by permission.)

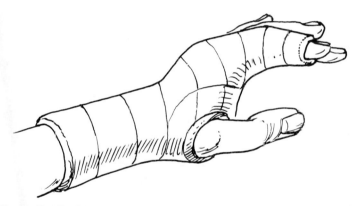

Figure 19.4 Radial gutter splint.

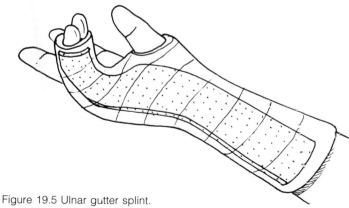

Figure 19.5 Ulnar gutter splint.

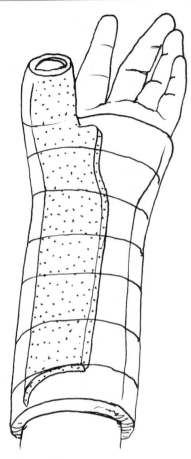

Figure 19.6 Thumb spica splint.

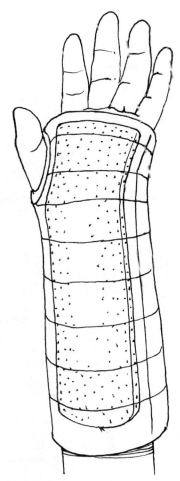

Figure 19.7 Volar wrist splint.

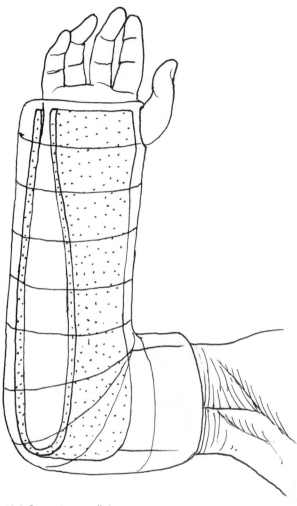

Figure 19.8 Sugar tong splint.

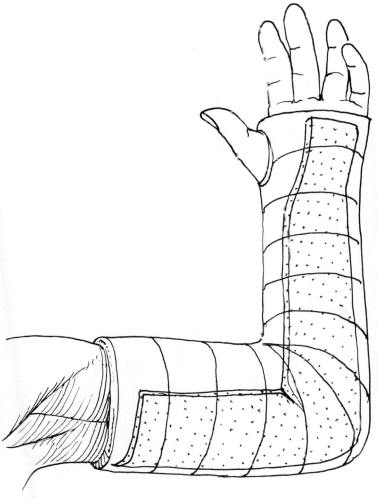

Figure 19.9 Double sugar-tong splint.

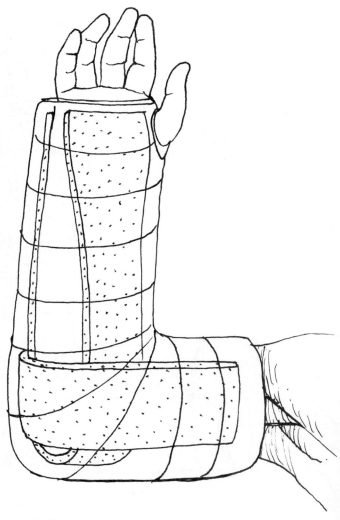

Figure 19.10 Long arm posterior splint.

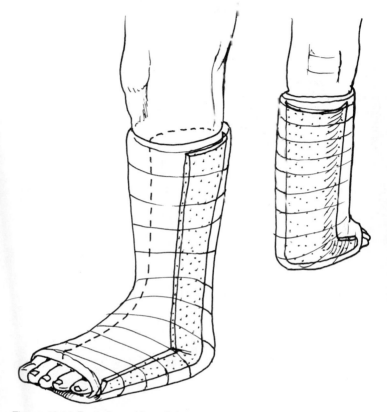

Figure 19.11 Posterior ankle splint.

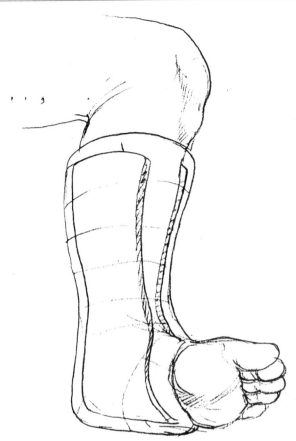

Figure 19.12 Stirrup ankle splint.

20

Cervical Spine Injury

Quincy Wang

INTRODUCTION

- Assessing and managing cervical spine injury is among the most frightening scenarios the sports medicine team can encounter
- Fortunately, catastrophic cervical spine injury is uncommon. The sports medicine team should rehearse the proper techniques of cervical spine management prior to each season and review them periodically to reduce the chances of permanent injury to the athlete.

ON-THE-FIELD MANAGEMENT OF CERVICAL SPINE INJURY

General Principles

- Every downed athlete should be approached as having a cervical spine injury until proven otherwise. Head and neck stabilization techniques must be implemented if an athlete is unconscious or suspected to have a cervical spine injury.
- It is important that the first examiner from the sports medicine team not move the athlete until it is determined that the athlete does not have a cervical spine injury
- Equally, it is important that players be instructed not to move, lift, or assist a fallen teammate on the playing field. Such movement can create a permanent injury if an unstable cervical spine injury is present.

Unconscious Athlete

- The unconscious athlete must be presumed to have a life-threatening injury. Head and neck stabilization techniques must always be used with the unconscious athlete.
- Do not move the athlete

Primary Survey

- Check airway, breathing, circulation (ABCs) (see Chaps. 3, 4, and 5)
- Remove the mouthpiece if present. If treating a football athlete, DO NOT remove the helmet and chin strap.
- Begin CPR and activate EMS if respiration and/or pulse is absent
- A senior member of the medical team should take control of the athlete's head
- Remove face mask for airway access with the football-helmeted athlete. Hockey, lacrosse, and motor vehicle athletes may require helmet removal if access to the airway is required.
- If shoulder pads are present, cut through the front of the jersey and laces or straps connecting the fronts of the shoulder pads. Separate the fronts of the shoulder pads and begin chest compressions.
- If defibrillation is needed, cut the axillary straps of the shoulder pads and separate them further for defibrillation
- While maintaining proper head and neck stabilization, logroll the athlete, using proper technique, onto a spine board. Secure the head and neck as well as the torso and extremities and transport the athlete to the designated trauma facility.

Conscious Athlete

- Assume that athlete has a cervical spine injury

Primary Survey

- Check ABCs: determine whether the athlete is awake and breathing
- Stabilize the head and neck
- DO NOT move the athlete, DO NOT remove helmet or chin strap (if present)

Secondary Survey

- Obtain a brief history of the injury from the athlete
- Ask if there is any neck pain
- Ask athlete if there is any numbness, burning, or tingling down the arms and/or legs
- Palpate the neck gently, feeling for point tenderness of the spinous processes and paraspinal musculature of the cervical spine
- Ask the athlete to sense for touch in order to assess the associated nerve root dermatomes (see Table 20.1)

Table 20.1 Sensory Dermatomes

C2	Back of scalp	T4	Nipple line
C3	Anterior neck	T10	Umbilicus
C4	Anterior chest	L1	Upper thigh
C5	Deltoid	L2	Midthigh
C6	Radial forearm and thumb	L3	Lower thigh
C7	Middle finger	L4	Medial shin
C8	Ulnar aspect of hand and forearm	L5	Anterior shin
T1	Medial side of upper arm	S1	Lateral shin

Table 20.2 Motor Function of Nerve Roots

C5	Deltoid and biceps	L2	Hip flexion
C6	Wrist extension	L3	Knee extension
C7	Wrist flexion and triceps	L4	Ankle dorsiflexion
C8	Flexing fingers to make a fist	L5	Great toe extension
T1	Interossei (abduct fingers)	S1	Ankle plantarflexion

- Perform motor examination
    - If the athlete is breathing with diaphragmatic motion, neurologic function is present at least down to neurologic level C4
    - Ask the athlete to move his or her extremities to assess the associated nerve roots (see Table 20.2)

Tertiary Survey

- Perform a brief examination to check for any other associated musculoskeletal or internal injury
- If neck pain is present along with sensory and/or motor nerve loss, maintain cervical spine stabilization and activate EMS
- Using proper logrolling technique, move athlete to a spine board and secure his or her head, neck, torso and extremities
- Remove the face mask (if present) before loading the athlete into an ambulance in case airway access is needed during transport

HEAD AND NECK STABILIZATION TECHNIQUES

- The team physician or certified athletic trainer should be the medical provider responsible for head and neck stability

Lateral Head Hold (See Fig. 20.1)

- With the provider in the kneeling position, straddling the athlete's head, the provider's hands are placed on the lateral sides of the head or helmet, holding firmly
- The provider should rest his or her elbows on his or her thighs for additional stability
- The provider's index finger can be inserted into the ear hole of the helmet to ensure a good grip

Forearm Cradle Hold

- In this technique, the provider kneels and straddles the athlete's head, as in the previous technique. The provider's hands are placed at the base of the athlete's neck with the fingers supporting the trapezius region and the thumbs wrapped anteriorly along the lateral aspects of the neck base.

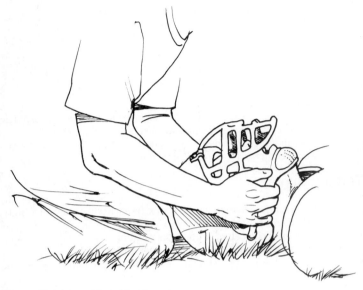

Figure 20.1 Lateral head hold.

- The provider's elbows are rested on his or her thighs for additional support
- Either technique is effective in maintaining cervical spine stabilization until the athlete can be moved onto a spine board and strapped securely

LOGROLLING TECHNIQUE

- All commands for movement must come from the team physician or certified athletic trainer stationed at the athlete's head
- Execution of the logroll technique requires at least four medical providers
- Ideally, the athlete should be moved only once when being transferred to a spine board. However, if the athlete is prone or without a pulse, he or she will have to be logrolled to the supine position to start resuscitation efforts. If the athlete is breathing with a pulse and either conscious or unconscious, he or she should remain in place until they can be safely logrolled to a spine board.

Supine Logroll

- The providers who will logroll the athlete are placed along one side of the athlete—at the chest, pelvis, and legs—in the kneeling position

- The spine board is placed on the other side of the athlete
- Under the direction of the provider in charge, the athlete's head, shoulders, chest, pelvis, and legs are logrolled simultaneously until the athlete is perpendicular to the board
- Additional helpers can slide the spine board under the athlete and the athlete can then be lowered onto the spine board. The middle provider at the pelvis can reach for the spine board if no additional help is available.
- The head or helmet should be secured to the spine board with tape and straps as well as foam or sandbag rests at the sides

Prone Logroll

- The providers on the sports medicine team should assume the same positions as the supine logroll except that the spine board should be placed on the same side as the providers as they kneel on it to begin
- The provider at the athlete's head must stabilize the head with the crossed-arm technique. This allows the provider's hands to "unwind" his or her arms as the athlete is logrolled.
- Upon the direction of the lead provider, the head, shoulders, chest, pelvis and legs are logrolled simultaneously until the athlete is perpendicular to the ground
- After the spine board is placed in position, the logroll onto the spine board can be completed
- The athlete's head and body can be secured to the spine board

FACE MASK REMOVAL

- The modern football face mask can be removed easily and quickly with minimal head motion by using the proper tools
- The modern football helmet uses four or more plastic loop straps to anchor the face mask. No longer are face masks bolted to the helmet. Any helmet in which the face mask is bolted to the helmet and cannot be removed SHOULD NOT be used.
- The anvil-pruning shear is the recommended tool for removing the football face mask. The "Trainer's Angel" (Riverside, CA) (see Fig. 20.2) and FM Extractor are other tools used for removing the football face mask. Screwdrivers, utility knives, scissors, or bolt cutters are not recommended as their use causes too much head motion and potential injury to the rescuers and athlete.
- The face mask must be fully removed. It must not be hinged, as the face mask would then become a powerful lever arm if it were accidentally struck, greatly increasing the chance of secondary spinal injury.
- Cutting the loop straps
    - Forehead loop straps

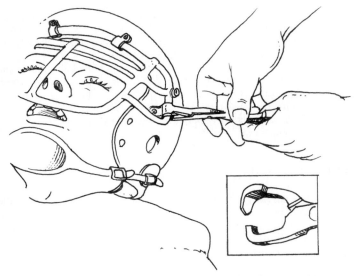

Figure 20.2 Cutting face mask loop straps with "Trainer's Angel."

- The forehead loop straps can be cut at their midportion between the anchoring screw and loop holding the face mask. Only one cut is required at this location.
- Another method is to cut the loop portion of the strap. Here, two cuts are required to remove the front of the loop.
- Lateral loop straps
  - These are often the most difficult to cut, as their positioning is usually between the bars of the face mask, making access to the midportion of the loop straps difficult
  - The loop portion of the strap must be cut in two places. The cuts must be wide enough to offer no resistance when the face mask is lifted and removed from the helmet. Make sure that the first cut is anterior enough so there is no anterior lip that blocks the mask from being lifted from the helmet.

HELMET AND SHOULDER PAD REMOVAL

- Football helmets and shoulder pads should not be removed in the field unless indicated. They should be removed in a controlled environment after the athlete reaches the hospital. Both the football helmet and shoulder pads work as a unit, keeping neutral spinal alignment by maintaining equal head and shoulder elevation when the athlete is supine. Both must be removed together.
- Motor vehicle helmets should be removed in the field, as airway access can be limited and—because as the helmet elevates the head

above the level of the shoulders—neu ral spinal alignment is difficult to obtain, thus causing neck flexion

- Hockey, lacrosse, rollerblading, skateboarding, and similar helmets
also should be removed, as these are typically loose-fitting helmets
that do not immobilize the head when strapped to a spine board

General Guidelines for on-the-Field Removal

Helmet Removal

- This should be done
  - If the airway is inaccessible
  - If the helmet is loose-fitting and does not immob lize the head when
    the helmet is secured
  - If the helmet prevents immobilization
  - If neutral spine alignment is prevented

Shoulder Pad Removal

- This should be done
  - If the helmet is removed
  - If neutral spine alignment is prevented
  - If securing the athlete to the spine board is difficult
  - If full access to chest and shoulder area is required

Helmet and Shoulder Pad Removal Technique

- All movement must be coordinated under the instruction of the
  sports medicine team leader. Ideally, four or more medical
  providers should assist with helmet and shoulder pad removal.
- Cut the jersey from the neck to the waist along the front midline
  and from the neck to the end of each sleeve
- Cut the laces or straps over the sternum of the shoulder pads and
  under each axilla
- While maintaining head and neck stabilization, cut the chin strap
  and deflate the air bladder inside the helmet (if it has one) with
  an air pump needle or by opening the valve
- Remove the cheek pads by prying them off their snap attach-
  ments, using a tongue blade or any flat-blaced object between
  the pad and the helmet
- As the lead provider is maintaining head and neck stabilization
  at the top of the athlete's head, a second provider facing cephalad will give additional support by holding each side of the neck
  and occiput while resting his or her forearms on the athlete's
  chest and clavicles

- The lead provider can then slide the helmet off the athlete with slight forward rotation of the helmet. The helmet should not be spread apart by the ear holes as it may then tighten around the athlete's forehead and occiput.
- With the helmet off, providers on each side of the athlete slide their hands between the chest and the posterior portion of the shoulder pads
- With the direction of the lead provider, the athlete is lifted slightly, just enough for the lead provider to slide the shoulder pads over the athlete's head. The provider facing cephalad ensures head and neck stabilization. He or she must lift the athlete's head and neck simultaneously with the chest and shoulder to maintain neutral spinal alignment.
- The athlete is lowered. Ideally, this maneuver is done while the athlete is on a spine board. However, in emergent situations where the helmet and shoulder pads are removed for immediate airway access, the athlete will have to be placed on the spine board with a second maneuver.

ICD-9 Codes

- 805. Fracture of vertebral column
- 952. Spinal cord injury without evidence of spinal injury

Bibliography

Dietz JW Jr, Lillegard WA: Cervical spine injuries, in Lillegard WA, Butcher J, Rucker KS (eds): *Handbook of Sports Medicine: A Symptom Oriented Approach.* Woburn, MA: Butterworth-Heinemann, Burlington, MA 1999, pp 63–79.

Prehospital Care of the Spine-Injured Athlete, Inter-Association Task force for the Appropriate Care of the Spine-Injured Athlete. Dallas, TX www.nata.org National Athletic Trainers' Association, 1998.

Roberts WO: Helmet removal in head and neck trauma. *Phys Sports Med* 26(7):77, 1998.

Warren WL, Bailes J: On the field evaluation of athletic neck injury. *Clin Sports Med* 17(1):99–111, 1998.

21

Thoracic and Lumbar Spine Injury

Frank Winton

THORACIC SPINE INJURY
Mechanism of Injury/Pathology

- Thoracic spine injuries are rare in athletics. They are usually seen in high-velocity or high-impact sports (auto racing, football, downhill skiing, diving).
- Pathology includes soft tissue injury, fractures, dislocations, thoracic disk disease, Scheuermann's disease, ring apophyseal injury, and cord injury

Diagnostic Keys

- Most injuries of the thoracic spine involve soft tissues; they are musculoligamentous strains or sprains or contusions related to a direct blow. A large, diffuse area of tenderness is more suggestive of muscle strain.
- History of a direct blow with a discrete area of tenderness likely represents a contusion or possible underlying fracture
- Any neurologic change or muscular weakness after injury must be treated as a possible cord injury, with the patient appropriately immobilized
- Athletes should generally be immobilized in their helmets or other equipment for transportation to hospital
- Athletes in significant pain after injury should be transported immobilized on a spine board. Those with too much muscle spasm pain should be immobilized for diagnostic evaluation.
- On-field examination should not be rushed and should include as much evaluation as needed to convince the examiner that there is no evidence of serious injury. Any concern for serious injury to the spine should prompt proper immobilization and transportation to the appropriate facility for further testing and treatment.

Examination/Evaluation

- After adequate history, examination includes inspection, palpation, range-of-motion testing, and neurologic evaluation
- If feasible, have the patient standing and adequately disrobed and look for curvature deviation in all planes
- Palpate along the spinous processes, paraspinous muscles, and rib bases. The suspected area of maximum tenderness should be palpated last. Attempt to identify the primary structure involved, deep or superficial.
- Range-of-motion testing is done with flexion, extension, lateral flexion and rotation, noting limitations, pain, changes in normal curvature, spasm, and radiation
- Neurologic examination of thoracic nerves is limited due to sensory overlap and multiple levels of innervation. Sensation is best tested with light touch examination.
- Pediatric and adolescent patients can have significant spinal injury with normal radiographs. MRI may be helpful in these cases.

Emergent Treatment

Potential Cord Injury

- Airway, breathing, circulation (ABCs) of life support must be maintained while ascertaining if significant spinal injury has occurred
- Full spinal immobilization with backboard and neutral positioning. As with cervical spine injury, prevention of further injury is the key.
- Proper oxygenation and blood pressure must be ensured
- Consider giving methylprednisolone 30 mg/kg shortly after injury—may improve neurologic outcome

Thoracic Musculoligamentous Strains, Sprains, and Contusions

- Initial cold therapy, rest, medications for pain and spasm, back brace if needed

Thoracic Spine Fractures

- With any neurologic changes, suspicion of instability, or unclear diagnosis, immobilize on spine board and transfer for diagnostic studies and treatment

Thoracic Disk Herniation

- Rare. Acute onset with neurologic findings require immobilization pending evaluation. Usually vague history of onset allows guided exam and evaluation without spine precautions.

Tests

- X-rays: anteroposterior and lateral projections for initial evaluation of potential fractures or dislocations and after any neurologic alterations after injury
- CT scanning: used to confirm findings from history and physical. Useful in evaluation of bony abnormalities or significant trauma involving fractures to determine spinal canal involvement.
- MRI: excellent for visualizing disk disease, nerve root compression, ligamentous injury with hemorrhage, primary spinal cord and nerve root changes, intramedullary tumors, and syringomyelia. Useful in adolescent trauma when radiographs are normal due to greater flexibility and cartilaginous content of young spine.

Definitive Treatment/Follow-up/ Return to Play

Thoracic Sprains/Strains and Contusions

- Aggressive rehabilitation with strengthening and stretching
- Return to play is permitted when adequate range of motion is attained and the athlete is comfortable enough to participate safely. Protective equipment may be needed in some sports. Contact sports require full return of range of motion for the player's personal protection.

Thoracic Disk Herniation

- If no neurologic deficits: trial of rest, pain control, bracing in thoracic orthosis, and possibly epidural injections. Surgical treatment is reserved for failed conservative care and patients with neurologic deficits.
- Return to play is determined by the surgery done and the sport played. If no fusion has been performed, the athlete can return to all sports after adequate rehabilitation. If fusion after disk excision has been performed, many surgeons will not allow contact sports. Once the patient is healed and pain-free, all other sports are allowed.

Thoracic Fractures

Transverse Process Fracture (Rib Base)

- Stable injury requiring no special bracing or immobilization. Protect from further trauma. Athlete may return to play when full range of motion is restored and activities of sport cause no pain.

Compression Fracture

- Most common thoracic fracture

- Requires significant trauma in young athlete; if no major trauma, suspect underlying pathology
- Most of these fractures involve less than 25 percent of the anterior vertebral body height. They are treated with analgesia, possible immobilization in a thoracic orthotic device, and sports exclusion until healing is complete, which may take 8–12 weeks in a young athlete.
- 50 percent or greater compression requires CT scanning to evaluate the spinal canal for compromise. May be treated same as above or with early instrumentation and fusion, which may preclude return to participation. Athlete may return to play when he or she is pain-free and full range of motion is restored. Fusion may preclude contact sports.

Fracture/Dislocation

- High-energy injury rare in athletics except for sky-diving, automobile racing and highdiving
- Spinal cord injury in 85–100 percent. Rare case of fracture/dislocation without neurologic deficit treated with posterior open reduction with internal fixation and limited fusion to stabilize the spine. Controversy in cases with incomplete and complete neurologic deficit. Treatment may include open reduction and internal fixation with fusion or conservative treatment with thoracolumbar spinal orthoses (TLSO). These athletes will require coordinated treatment, therapy, and specialized spinal rehabilitation to maximize function.

LUMBAR SPINE STRAIN/ SOFT TISSUE INJURY

Mechanism of Injury/Pathology

- More common than thoracic injury but generally involves minor strains from extension, flexion, or rotation and soft tissue injury due to direct blow
- Lumbar pathology includes soft-tissue injury, fracture, dislocation, disk disease, spondylolysis, spondylolisthesis, cord injury

Diagnostic Keys

- Same as for thoracic spine injury

Examination

- Same as for thoracic spine with inclusion of sacroiliac joints, sciatic notches, and deep posterior thighs

- Neurologic testing of the lower extremities to include motor strength testing, light touch sensation, reflex testing, sciatic and femoral nerve tension signs, and assessment of sacral motor and sensory function
- Muscle and reflex testing of the lower extremities:
  - L1 and L2—hip flexion, no reflex
  - L3—knee extension, no reflex
  - L4—foot dorsiflexion, knee extension, knee jerk reflex
  - L5—great toe extension, foot eversion posterior tibial reflex
  - S1—foot plantarflexors, knee flexion, ankle jerk reflex
- Sciatic nerve irritation tested with straight-leg-raising test. Positive test if pain occurs between 30 and 70 degrees of elevation with pain along anatomic course of nerve (lower leg, ankle, foot). Back pain does not indicate positive test. Femoral nerve tension tested with patient prone, knee flexed to 90 degrees, hip extended while pelvis fixed to table. Radicular pain in the anterior thigh is a positive test.
- If history or situation warrants, testing of sacral motor and sensation may be necessary. Testing includes perianal sensation, sphincter tone and contractility, and superficial anal reflex mediated by S2–4 nerve roots.

Emergent Treatment

- Lumbar musculoligamentous injury:
  - Rest, cold therapy, pain and antispasmodic medications as needed; lightweight lumbosacral corset may help control spasm

Tests

- Usually not needed

Definitive Treatment/Follow-up/ Return to Play

- Light stretching and strengthening of abdominal and paraspinous muscles. Avoid exercises that exacerbate pain. Moist heat and massage may be helpful.
- Return to play:
  - Noncontact sports when pain allows
  - Contact sports allowed with some pain remaining but tolerable with modalities. Range of motion needs to be adequate for athlete to protect himself or herself. Lumbosacral corset brace may be allowed in competition.

LUMBAR FRACTURE

Mechanism of Injury/Pathology

- Direct trauma or high-energy impact
- Hyperextension forces leading to stress fracture of pars interarticularis—spondylolysis (see next section)

Diagnostic Keys

- Same as thoracic spine injury (above)

Examination

- As above

Emergent Treatment

- Lumbar spine fractures: often spine board immobilization required due to great pain on examination. Athlete will not allow changes in position, range-of-motion testing, or percussion over injury. Consider evaluation for renal, spleen, and other intraabdominal injury as well.

Tests

- X-ray: AP and lateral
- CT scanning: may visualize fractures not seen on plain films, delineate extent of fractures and bone fragment displacement
- MRI: (see above, under "Thoracic Spine Injury")

Definitive Treatment/Follow-up/ Return to Play

Lumbar Spine Fracture

- Classify by "three-column spine stabilization classification" of Denis
  - Anterior column—anterior longitudinal ligament and anterior vertebral body
  - Middle column—remainder of vertebral body and posterior longitudinal ligament
  - Posterior column—pedicles and including remaining bony and soft tissue structures

Posterior Column Fracture

- Always stable, treat with local measures to decrease pain and aid in fracture healing
  - Return to play:
    - Noncontact sports: when normal range of motion returns and pain is diminished
    - Contact sports: when there is no pain on palpation or with range of motion

Anterior Column Fracture

- Compression fracture less than 50 percent (of vertebral body height)
  - Brace in TLSO and no sports until healed
- Compression greater than 50 percent
  - Often treated with posterior distraction instrumentation and fusion

Anterior and Middle Column Fracture

- Burst fracture represents failure of anterior and middle column in compression and is often responsible for bony retropulsion into spinal canal. Considered unstable but may be treated conservatively.
  - Less than 50 percent compression, less than 50 percent canal impingement, and less than an acute 20-degree kyphosis may be treated with rest and TLSO for 12 weeks
  - Compression greater than 50 percent, more than 50 percent canal impingement, or more than 20 degrees of kyphosis requires surgery. Type varies, but after surgery patient is immobilized in TLSO for 3 months, then rehabilitated as tolerated.

Anterior and Posterior Column Fracture

- "Seat-belt injury" or Chance fracture. Uncommon in sports
  - Failure of anterior column in compression and posterior column in distraction
  - If more than 50 percent compression on anterior column or greater than 20 degrees of acute kyphosis, surgery is considered

Fracture/Dislocation:

- Rarest of all injuries. Usually high-energy injury
  - Always requires surgical care, usually posterior open reduction and instrumentation with fusion. Consideration of the patient's neurologic status is paramount.

OTHER THORACOLUMBAR INJURIES

Mechanism of Injury/Pathology

- Disk disease: disk degeneration and disk herniation
- Spondylolysis/spondylolisthesis
- Scheuermann's disease
- Ring apophyseal injury

Diagnostic Keys

- Disk herniation: radiation of pain or numbness along path of nerve root involved
- Bilateral signs, bowel or bladder incontinence may be cauda equina syndrome
- Ring apophyseal injury seen in adolescents, causing transient nondescript pain. Also called atypical or lumbar Scheuermann's disease.

Examination

- As above. Spasm may cause flattening of lumbar contour. Disk degeneration has normal lower extremity examination.
- Disk herniation: patient more comfortable lying than standing, stands with list to opposite side from pain
- Spondylolysis pain worse with extension to side of defect (single leg extension test or "stork" test), often tight hamstrings

Emergent Treatment

- Lumbar disk disease:
  - Disk degeneration: usually not acute or emergent in nature; pain control and active motion initially
  - Disk herniation: early management involves program of bed rest in position of greatest comfort, pain control, anti-inflammatory and anti-spasmodic medication
    - Evaluate for cauda equina syndrome by looking for bilateral leg numbness, weakness, and bowel or bladder symptoms such as incontinence or retention
    - If cauda equina syndrome or progressive neurologic deficit is found, rapid consultation is indicated
- Spondylolysis/spondylolisthesis: usually not emergent problem, suspicion for early diagnosis needed with proper history and physical findings

Tests

- Disk degeneration
  - X-rays show loss of disk height. Advanced disease may show facet joint arthrosis. MRI not indicated.
- Disk herniation
  - MRI—increasingly the test of choice. Myelogram and CT less commonly.
- Spondylolysis
  - X-ray: AP, lateral, and oblique, looking for pars defect ("Scottie dog collar" if chronic)
  - Radionuclide scanning (bone scan): useful in conjunction with plain films to evaluate if acute, subacute, or chronic defect
  - Spinal CT helpful for acute condition
- Scheuermann's disease
  - Plain lateral X-rays show anterior wedging of vertebral body, Schmorl's nodes common. Diagnostic if three or more consecutive vertebrae wedged more than 5 degrees.
- Apophyseal injury
  - Radiographs suggest chronic vertebral end-plate wedging, irregularities of the end plates, and changes in the disk space

Definitive Treatment/Follow-up/ Return to Play

Disk Degeneration

- Active exercise program emphasizing range of motion and muscle strengthening of abdominal and paraspinous muscles. Moist heat, tissue massage, and ultrasound may help reduce spasm and pain. Return to play based on pain control and return of range of motion, especially for contact sports.

Disk Herniation

- When pain allows, patient is mobilized and physical therapy program emphasizing extension and reconditioning begun. Epidural injection may be considered if inadequate pain relief with rest. Various treatments available for failed conservative care include percutaneous diskectomy, microsurgical diskectomy, and standard laminotomy and diskectomy. Rehabilitation is sport-dependent. Athlete may return to play when pain allows and range of motion returns. This may take longer with surgical patients, usually at least 6 weeks for noncontact sports.

Scheuermann's Disease

- Generally anterior thoracic spine, presents with backache and thoracic kyphosis. Pain worse with flexion. Patient develops "roundback" deformity. If involving three or more vertebrae and kyphosis exceeding 30 degrees, Milwaukee bracing likely indicated and refer to orthopedics. Extension strengthening and stretching indicated. Sports are allowed as long as aggravating activity is avoided. Patient is followed until vertebral growth is complete.

Apophyseal Injury (Atypical Scheuermann's Disease)

- Generally midthoracic to midlumbar. Thought to be direct result of microtrauma with resultant multiple growth-plate fractures or possible anterior disk herniation through the anterior ring apophysis and secondary bony deformation of the vertebrae. Seen in adolescent athletes involved with vigorous training with flexion-extension activity. "Flat back" deformity with no appreciable kyphosis at involved areas. When vertebral wedging is noted or pain is persistent, a bracing program may be indicated for symptomatic treatment. Also use of rest, NSAIDs, and strengthening/flexibility program. Return to play when pain and motion allow.

Spondylolysis/Spondylolisthesis

- Treated with rest and avoidance of hyperextension, sometimes with use of lumbosacral orthosis. Takes 6 weeks to 6 months to heal. Treatment guided by pain alone. Spondylolisthesis treated similarly except if progressive, age less than 16 years, greater than 50 percent slippage, or intractable radicular pain with nerve root entrapment. These are treated surgically. Rehabilitation is started when patient is pain-free and out of any brace; includes flexion of spine, strengthening of abdomen, and stretching of hamstrings. Slow, graduated return to sports, delayed return to impact loading of spine, followed by addition of hyperextension activity and then by full participation.

Complications

- Pain, cord injury, weakness, chronic/recurrent pain, abdominal injuries

ICD-9 Codes

- Sprain/strain
  - 847.1 Thoracic spine
  - 847.2 Lumbar spine
  - 922.3 Contusion
- Fracture without neurologic injury
  - 805.2 Thoracic
  - 805.3 Lumbar
- Fracture with neurologic injury
  - 806.2 Thoracic
  - 806.4 Lumbar

- Dislocation
  - 756.11 Spondylosis
  - 756.12 Spondylolisthesis
  - 839.21 Thoracic
  - 839.2 Lumbar
- Back pain
  - 722.2 Intervertebral disk herniation
  - 722.6 Intervertebral disk degeneration
  - 724.1 Thoracic
  - 724.2 Lumbar
  - 732.0 Scheuermann's disease

Bibliography

Chance GQ: Note on a flexion fracture of the spine. *Br J Radiol* 21:452–453, 1948.

Clark P, Letts M: Trauma to the thoracic and lumbar spine in the adolescent. *Can J Surg* 55(5):337–345, 2001.

Eismont FJ, Kitchel SH: Thoracolumbar spine, in DeLee JC, Drez D (eds): *Orthopaedic Sports Medicine: Principles and Practice.* Philadelphia: Saunders, 1994, pp 1018–1062.

Garrick JG, Webb DR: *Sports Injuries: Diagnosis and Management,* 2d ed. Philadelphia: Saunders, 1999.

Savitsky E, Votey S: Emergency department approach to acute thoracolumbar spine injury. *J Emerg Med* 15(1):49–60, 1997.

Wilberger JE: Athletic spinal cord and spine injury: Guidelines for initial management. *Clin Sports Med* 17(1):111–120, 1998.

Yancy RA, Micheli LJ: Thoracolumbar spine injuries in pediatric sports, in Stanitski CL, DeLee JC, Drez D (eds): *Pediatric and Adolescent Sports Medicine.* Philadelphia: Saunders, 1994, pp 162–174.

22

Finger, Hand, and Wrist Injuries

Quincy Wang

Introduction

- Injuries of the fingers, hand, and wrist are very common. Some injuries allow for continued participation provided that adequate protective measures are taken. Recognition and proper management of such injuries can prevent permanent disability.

Subungual Hematomas

- Definition: A subungual hematoma is a very painful injury that arises when a hematoma develops underneath the nail
- Mechanism: Typically the mechanism is a crush injury that creates a fracture of the nailbed (e.g., the finger is hit with a ball or crushed between colliding helmets)
- Evaluation: The athlete will complain of severe, throbbing finger pain; the fingertip tender and swollen. The nail will be discolored due to the hematoma
- Treatment:
  - Decompression of the hematoma (Fig. 22.1)
    - Create two to three burr holes in the nail using an electric cautery unit, heated paper clip, or heated large-bore injection needle
- Return to Play: Once tenderness subsides, allowing participation without discomfort
- Complications:
  - Nailbed laceration—If the hematoma is large and separates 50 percent of the nailbed from the nail, there is likely to be a significant nailbed laceration requiring nail removal and laceration repair
  - Distal tuft fractures—Unstable fingertips or those with continued pain despite hematoma decompression may have a concomitant distal tuft fracture. Radiographs aid in diagnosis.

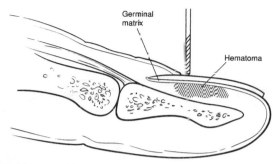

Figure 22.1 Subungual hematoma. (From Lewis C: *General Orthopedics.* New York: McGraw-Hill, 2002. Used by permission.)

Distal Phalanx/Tuft Fractures

- The distal phalanx is the most commonly fractured bone of the hand
- Mechanism: Typically a crush injury
- Evaluation: The fingertip will be swollen and painful with possible extensive soft tissue damage to the finger pulp and nailbed
  - Three-view radiographs should be obtained to determine fracture pattern
- Treatment:
  - Closed fractures usually have minimal displacement and are stable Often treating the soft tissue injury and splinting for 3–4 weeks is adequate. Participation is possible provided that the finger is adequately protected from further injury
  - Open fractures will require wound debridement, irrigation, soft tissue repair, and possible bone fixation. Splinting for 4–6 weeks may be required for healing.
- Complications: Intraarticular fractures involving one-third or more of the articular surface warrant orthopedic evaluation, as operative fixation will be required

ICD-9 Code

- 927.3 Crushing injury of finger

Mallet Finger

- Definition: Mallet finger is a flexion deformity of the distal interphalangeal joint (DIPJ) due to a disruption of the extensor mechanism. Also known as a "drop finger" or "baseball finger."
- Mechanism: Injury occurs when the DIPJ is forcibly flexed during active extension. There are two forms of mallet finger: a tendinous mal-

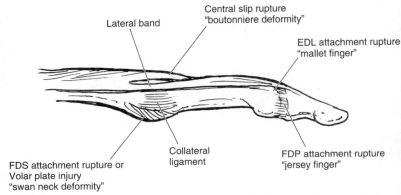

Figure 22.2 Common sports finger injuries: mallet, jersey, swan neck, and boutonniere injuries.

let involving only the extensor tendon and bony mallet involving an avulsion fracture of the distal phalanx.

- Evaluation: The athlete will present with a painful and swollen distal finger and will be unable to actively extend the DIPJ. Three-view radiographs are recommended, as a bony mallet is difficult to diagnose by physical examination only. (Fig. 22.2)
- Treatment: Nonoperative, continuous splinting for 6 to 8 weeks is the treatment of choice in most mallet finger injuries. Splinting should hold the DIPJ in neutral; it *must never* be allowed to drop in flexion at any time during treatment.
- Complications: Large, bony avulsions that are unstable despite closed reduction or involve one-third or more of the articular surface of the distal phalanx require orthopedic referral, as operative treatment may be required

"Jersey Finger"

- Definition: Jersey finger is a rupture or avulsion of the flexor digitorum profundus (FDP), causing an inability to flex the DIPJ
- Mechanism: Injury occurs when the actively flexed DIPJ is forced into extension. This often occurs in football when a player grabs a fleeing opponent's jersey. Most commonly seen in the ring finger.
- Evaluation: Athlete will present with pain in the distal finger and possibly the palm. With the finger in extension to isolate the FDP, active DIPJ flexion is absent. Three-view radiographs are recommended, as bony avulsion from the volar aspect of the distal phalanx can occur (Fig. 22.2).
- Complications: Proper diagnosis is important, as jersey finger requires operative repair. Delayed treatment may jeopardize the final outcome.

Bony avulsions require operative repair as well, and pure tendinous injury may retract down to the level of the palm, requiring surgical exploration and repair.

ICD-9 Code

- 842.1 Sprain or strain of hand

Middle and Proximal Phalanx Fractures

- Mechanism: Phalangeal fractures are usually caused by direct trauma, such as a direct blow or crush, twist, or axial load
- Evaluation: Presentation can range from minimal pain with swelling to gross deformity with angulation. Check for rotational deformity by observing if the fingernails all lie in the same plane. Check for laxity with gentle AP and lateral stress, feeling for gross movement and crepitus. Three-view radiographs are recommended to determine the fracture pattern.
- Treatment: Buddy taping is appropriate for phalangeal fractures that are stable, nondisplaced, and nonangulated. Buddy taping should continue for about 4–6 weeks. Return to play should be allowed when radiographs show adequate healing and the athlete can perform all skills competently at full speed and strength without pain. Angulated and displaced fractures can be closed reduced and immobilized for 4–6 weeks. Irreducible, unstable, and open fractures warrant orthopedic referral and operative fixation.

ICD-9 Code

- 816 Fracture of phalanges of hand

Acute Boutonniere Injury

- Definition: Boutonniere injuries are due to rupture of the central slip tendon of the extensor mechanism at the proximal interphalangeal joint (PIPJ). If left untreated, the finger will develop the characteristic boutonniere deformity of PIPJ flexion and DIPJ extension. Acute central slip tendon injuries do not present with boutonniere deformity (Fig. 22.2).
- Mechanism: Central slip tendon ruptures are due to forced flexion of the PIPJ during active extension. The athlete will present with a painful and swollen PIPJ. Weak or absent PIPJ extension suggests a central slip injury. Extension of the PIPJ does not rule out central slip injury, as the lateral bands of the extensor mechanism are often intact. If left untreated, the lateral bands migrate volarly, creating the classic boutonniere deformity. Three-view radiographs are recommended to evaluate for avulsion fracture or fracture/dislocation.

- Treatment: Dorsal splinting of the PIPJ for 5–6 weeks to allow healing of the ruptured central slip. DIPJ and MCPJ should be allowed to move freely.
- Complications: Operative treatment required for unstable fracture/dislocation, irreducible avulsion fracture, or late-presenting injury (after about 8 weeks)

Swan-Neck Deformity

- Mechanism: Rupture or entrapment of the flexor digitorum superficialis (FDS) or volar plate injury results in dorsal subluxation of the collateral ligaments. This causes PIPJ hyperextension and DIPJ flexion (Fig. 22.2).
- Treatment: Individualized
- Complications: Permanent deformity

Proximal Interphalangeal Joint— Sprains and Dislocations

- Mechanism: The most common dislocation of the hand is at the PIPJ. Dorsal dislocation is most common but can be lateral or volar. Dorsal dislocations are due to hyperextension forces across the PIPJ and lateral dislocations are due to abduction or adduction forces across the PIPJ. Volar dislocations are rare.
- Evaluation: The athlete presents with acute pain and gross deformity of the PIPJ. Palpate the finger, noting any bony crepitus or instability that may signify the presence of a fracture. If there appears to be no fracture but only pure dislocation, reduce the dislocation closed. For a dorsal dislocation, exaggerate the hyperextended position of the middle phalanx with longitudinal traction, then flex the middle phalanx, causing the PIPJ to reduce. Reassess by palpating for tenderness and check for laxity by stressing the PIPJ in the AP direction and laterally. Check active and passive range of motion. Three-view radiographs are recommended to assess for fracture and evaluate adequacy of reduction.
- Treatment: It is possible to return to play with simple buddy taping of the injured finger if the PIPJ has full range of motion, no laxity, and minimal pain on performance. If the PIPJ is unstable or fracture is suspected, the athlete should be removed from competition. After dislocation, splinting for 3–4 weeks—followed with buddy taping for 4 weeks and active range-of-motion exercises—is recommended.
- Complications: For complete collateral ligament or volar plate rupture, splinting is appropriate if the PIPJ is stable and congruous on radiographs. Open fixation may be necessary if the joint is unstable or nonreducible, as soft tissue can entrap in the joint.

Ulnar Collateral Ligament Injury of the Thumb (Gamekeeper's/Skier's Thumb)

- Definition: Gamekeeper's/skier's thumb is a partial or complete tear of the ulnar collateral ligament (UCL) of the metacarpophalangeal joint (MPJ) of the thumb
- Mechanism: A valgus hyperextension stress to the thumb, from a fall with an outstretched thumb
- Evaluation: The athlete will complain of a very swollen and painful thumb after trauma. There is tenderness directly over the UCL. To test the UCL's integrity, valgus stress the MPJ while in 30 degrees of flexion. If the MPJ can be opened 30 degrees more on the one side than on the other, the UCL is likely to be completely ruptured.
- Treatment: UCL sprains can be taped and the athlete can return to competition if the MPJ is stable, has minimal pain with full range of motion, and can perform all the necessary skills. Partial tears may require thumb spica casting for 3–6 weeks.
- Complications: Complete UCL rupturing requires operative fixation because the abductor aponeurosis can engage between the UCL and its point of insertion, creating what is called a Stener's lesion. Intraarticular fractures or avulsion fractures greater than 1mm may warrant operative fixation.

Metacarpal Fractures

- Mechanism: Metacarpal fractures generally occur from an axial load (e.g., punch with a closed fist) or a direct blow/crush injury
- Evaluation: The athlete will complain of acute hand pain, finding it painful to make a fist and having poor grip strength. Gross deformity may be evident. There is tenderness over fracture site. Universal precautions are mandatory with open fractures.
- Treatment: Splint the hand in a position of comfort using cardboard, an inflatable air splint, malleable splint, or plaster if available. Send to medical facility for evaluation and radiographs.

Types of Metacarpal Fractures

- Metacarpal head—intraarticular fractures requiring anatomic reduction and fixation, often with operative intervention
- Metacarpal neck—termed "boxer's fracture" and usually occurring at the fourth or fifth metacarpal. Fractures at the second and third metacarpal necks require anatomic reduction, while some angulation is allowable with the fourth and fifth metacarpal.
- Metacarpal shaft—transverse, oblique, or spiral type. Anatomic reduction with operative intervention is often required.
- Metacarpal base—these fractures are generally stable, but malrotation may require surgical intervention

ICD-9 Code

- 815.0 Fracture of metacarpal, closed

Scaphoid Fracture

- Also known as navicular fracture
- Mechanism: Forced hyperextension with wrist in ulnar deviation
- Evaluation: Acute tenderness to the radial aspect of the wrist—specifically, tenderness to the anatomic snuffbox. Poor grip strength. Routine radiographs of the wrist with addition of scaphoid views recommended. Initial radiographic assessment can be misleading, as no fracture line may be visible (see Fig. 18.4).
- Treatment: Thumb spica splinting advisable for suspicion of fracture with negative radiographs. Repeat radiographs in 1–2 weeks should reveal fracture if suspicion is correct. Nondisplaced stable fractures can be treated with thumb spica casting for 8–12 weeks. Displaced scaphoid fractures >1 mm may require operative intervention if closed reduction cannot be maintained. If timing of return to play is a problem, consultation with orthopedics for operative options is advisable.

ICD-9 Codes

- 814.0 Fracture of carpal bone
- 814.01 Fracture of navicular of wrist

De Quervain's Tenosynovitis

- Definition: Tenosynovitis at the first dorsal compartment of the wrist housing the abductor pollicis longus (APL) and extensor pollicis brevis (EPB)
- Mechanism: Repetitive activity of the wrist requiring radial deviation of the wrist with abduction and extension of the thumb
- Evaluation: Pain to the radial aspect of the wrist and pain with radial deviation. Positive Finkelstein test.
- Treatment: Rest, bracing, NSAIDs, and stretching are the staples of treatment. Steroid injection may be of benefit in prolonged cases. Surgical intervention with release of the first dorsal compartment may be required if conservative measures fail.

Scapholunate Instability

- Definition: Midcarpal instability due to disruption of the scapholunate ligament
- Mechanism: Generally from chronic repetitive activities; patient may not have a history of acute trauma

- Evaluation: Complaints of aching pain to the wrist that worsens with activity. Tenderness over the scapholunate region. Positive Watson's maneuver. AP clinched-fist radiographs may show scapholunate widening (the "Terry Thomas" sign).
- Treatment: Operative repair indicated

Distal Radius Fracture

- Mechanism: Fall on outstretched hand
- Evaluation: Acute pain, swelling, tenderness, with possible deformity. Three-view radiographs recommended.
- Treatment: Generally closed reduction and casting; however, operative intervention is needed if reduction is difficult to achieve and maintain

ICD-9 Code

- 813.4 Fracture of lower radius

Tears of the Triangular Fibrocartilage Complex (TFCC)

- Definition: The TFCC is the complex of connective tissue supporting the distal ulna and the ulnar-sided carpal bones.
- Mechanism: Forced hyperextension of the wrist with forearm in full pronation.
- Evaluation: Pain to the ulnar aspect of the wrist on palpation. Instability of the ulnar head, as it can be manually subluxed and relocated with a painful "clunk." CT and MRI are useful if results are positive.
- Treatment: Long arm casting for 4–6 weeks is advocated by some; however, operative intervention is warranted for failed conservative treatment.

Bibliography

Lairmore JR, Engber WD: Serious, often subtle, finger injuries: Avoiding diagnosis and treatment pitfalls. *Phys Sports Med* 26(6):57, 1998.

McCue FC, Schuett AM: The wrist and hand—soft tissues, in Safran MR (ed): *Manual of Sports Medicine*. Philadelphia: Lippincott-Raven, 1998, pp 388–392.

McDevitt ER: On-site treatment of PIPJ dislocations. *Phys Sports Med* 26(8):851, 1998.

Rettig AC, Patel DV: The wrist and hand—bone and ligament injuries, in Safran MR (ed): *Manual of Sports Medicine*. Philadelphia: Lippincott-Raven, 1998, pp 381–387.

Wang QC, Johnson BA: Fingertip injuries. *Am Fam Physician* 63(10): 1961–1966, 2001.

23

Acute Elbow Injuries

Marc R. Safran

ELBOW DISLOCATION
Mechanism of Injury/Pathology

- Posterior elbow dislocation—most common (80–90 percent are posterior or posterolateral)
  - Fall on outstretched hand with elbow/wrist pronated
  - Ulnar collateral ligament tear (always)
  - Anterior capsular injury (sometimes)
  - Lateral ulnar collateral ligament tear (often)
- Anterior elbow dislocation
  - Anterior blow to olecranon with flexed elbow
- Associated injuries
  - Fractures (coronoid, radial head, lateral condyle)
  - Avulsion fractures (medial epicondyle)
  - Median nerve
  - Ulnar nerve
  - Brachial artery
  - Brachialis rupture

Diagnostic Keys

- Mechanism of injury
- Hold elbow in flexion
- Severe elbow pain increased with attempted elbow motion
- Deformity
  - Extremity foreshortened
  - Antecubital fossa "full"
  - Prominent olecranon and radial head posteriorly
  - Indentation above the tip of the olecranon
- Previous elbow dislocation
- Check median and ulnar nerve function and pulses at wrist before and after reduction

Emergent Treatment

- Reduce the dislocation.
  - May be done on the sideline without sedation if subject is relaxed and before spasms set in
  - Do in controlled setting with sedation
    - Technique for reduction of posterior dislocations
      - Correct any medial or lateral displacement
      - Can be done prone or supine
      - Stabilize the distal humerus with one hand
      - Apply longitudinal traction with the other hand to the proximal forearm
      - Gentle anterior force until a pronounced clunk into flexion is achieved
      - Pronation is helpful
      - The thumb of the hand stabilizing the distal humerus may be used to push the olecranon to assist reduction
      - Flexion of the elbow should be avoided until reduction is achieved to avoid damage to the brachial artery
- Sling
- Ice for 20 min four times a day

Tests

- Radiographs—AP, lateral, oblique
  - Rule out fracture of coronoid, radial head, or distal humerus
  - Confirm reduction

Definitive Treatment/Follow-up/ Return to Play

- Valgus stress to assess stability
  - May splint for 5–10 days
  - If unstable, hinged brace for 4–6 weeks
    - Extension lock at 45 degrees for 1–2 weeks
    - Then extension lock at 30 degrees for 1 week
    - Then full extension in brace for 2–3 weeks
  - Strengthen at 3–6 weeks
- Return to play
  - Full return of strength
  - Pain-free range of motion
  - May hasten by use of brace

Complications

- Stiffness (loss of extension)—most common

- Missed fracture of coronoid, radial head, medial epicondyle, or lateral condyle
- Nonreduced dislocation
- Median nerve, ulnar nerve, or brachial artery injury
- Recurrent instability
  - Rare
  - Associated with coronoid fractures
- Persistent pain
- Heterotopic ossification

ICD-9 Codes

- Closed elbow dislocation
  - 832.01 Anterior
  - 832.02 Posterior
  - 832.03 Medial
  - 832.04 Lateral
- Open elbow dislocation
  - 832.11 Anterior
  - 832.12 Posterior
  - 832.13 Medial
  - 832.14 Lateral

ACUTE ULNAR COLLATERAL LIGAMENT RUPTURE

Mechanism of Injury/Pathology

- Valgus stress to elbow
  - Throwing
  - Dislocation of elbow
- Most often acute rupture of chronically attenuated ligament

Diagnostic Keys

- Mechanism of injury
- Pop with valgus stress
- Pain at medial elbow
- Pain with throwing or unable to throw 100 percent
  - Particularly in the late cocking or early acceleration phase
- Loss of ball control with throwing
- Medial epicondylitis
- Ulnar nerve symptoms
- Ecchymosis at medial elbow
- Previous ulnar collateral ligament symptoms
  - Medial elbow pain with throwing
  - Medial epicondylitis

- Ulnar nerve symptoms
- Intermittent locking of the elbow
- Posterior elbow pain

Examination

- Ecchymosis
- Pain with valgus stress
- Tenderness to palpation 2 cm distal to medial epicondyle
- May have laxity to valgus stress
- May have pain with resisted wrist flexion
- May have numbness in ulnar nerve distribution

Emergent Treatment

- Sling
- Ice for 20 min four times a day
  - Care not to apply ice directly to medial elbow—risk of injury to ulnar nerve

Tests

- Consider radiographs—AP, lateral, oblique
  - Rule out fracture
  - May see evidence of chronic ulnar collateral ligament injury
    - Osteophytes
    - Loose bodies
- Consider stress radiographs to assess valgus laxity
- Consider arthrogram—positive if done within 48 hours of acute injury
- Consider MRI arthrogram to evaluate ulnar collateral ligament

Definitive Treatment/Follow-up/ Return to Play

- Sling for comfort and to reduce acute inflammation; should be limited to preventing pain
- Early motion to prevent stiffness
- NSAIDs
- Ice
- Rehabilitation program—at least two courses before considering surgery unless elite throwing athlete
- Surgery for ulnar collateral ligament reconstruction
- Return to play
  - Pain-free range of motion
  - Full strength
  - Pass functional sports specific testing/throwing program

Complications

- Ulnar nerve injury
- Loss of motion—especially extension
- Missed avulsion of flexor—pronator muscle group
- Loose bodies
- Arthritis
- Inability to return to play

ICD-9 Code

- 841.1 Acute ulnar collateral ligament injury

MEDIAL AND LATERAL EPICONDYLITIS
Mechanism of Injury/Pathology

- Overuse injury, which may present acutely at an event
- Angiofibroblastic degeneration, not true inflammation
- Microtears
- Lateral epicondylitis (LE)—degenerative process of extensor muscles [EDC (extensor digitorum communis), ECRB (extensor carpi radialis brevis), ECRL (extensor carpi radialis longus)] at insertion at the lateral epicondyle of the distal humerus
- Medial epicondylitis—degenerative process of the flexor-pronator muscles [pronator teres and FCR (flexor carpi radialis)] at insertion at the medial epicondyle of the distal humerus
    - One-fifth as common as lateral epicondylitis

Diagnostic Keys

- Lateral epicondylitis
    - Pain at and distal to the lateral epicondyle
    - Pain with lifting or strong gripping
    - Weakness
    - Pain with twisting motions (tennis, screwdriver, open door or jar)
    - History of recent change (increase) in activities, change in equipment—new tennis racquet
- Medial epicondylitis
    - Pain at and slightly distal to the medial epicondyle
    - Pain with gripping
    - Weakness
    - Pain with twisting motions (screwdriver, golf, bowling)
- Previous medial or lateral epicondylitis

Examination

- Lateral epicondylitis
  - Tender lateral epicondyle
  - Increased pain with resisted wrist dorsiflexion
  - Increased pain with resisted supination
  - Increased pain with passive palmarflexion
- Medial epicondylitis
  - Tender medial epicondyle
  - Increased pain with resisted wrist palmarflexion
  - Increased pain with resisted pronation
  - Increased pain with passive dorsiflexion

Emergent Treatment

- Rest from offending activity
- Ice for 20 min, five times a day
  - Medially, take care not to place ice directly over ulnar nerve
- NSAIDs
- Consider injection of cortisone at epicondyle

Tests

- Radiographs (AP, lateral, oblique)

Definitive Treatment/Follow-up/ Return to Play

- Relative rest
- Injection
- Possibly use wrist splint for lateral epicondylitis
- Stretch wrist/elbow
- Strengthen wrist/elbow
- If 6 months of stretching, strengthening, relative rest, and injections fail, consider surgery
- Return to play
  - Adequate return of strength
  - Pain-free range of motion
  - Pass functional sports specific testing
  - May hasten by use of elbow brace (counterforce brace)
  - Gradual return to sports
  - Warm up (stretch) prior to and after play and practice

Complications

- Missed posterior interosseous nerve injury (lateral epicondylitis)
- Ulnar neuritis (medial epicondylitis)
- Chronic epicondylitis
- Missed injury to ulnar collateral ligament
- Muscle/tendon avulsion (medial or lateral)
- Prolonged healing time if usual activities resumed too soon
- Recurrent problem

ICD-9 Codes

- 726.31 Medial epicondylitis
- 726.32 Lateral epicondylitis

DISTAL BICEPS TENDON RUPTURE

Mechanism of Injury/ Pathology

- Acute rupture of the distal biceps tendon from the radial tuberosity
- Rarely—prodromal symptoms or history of biceps tendinitis
- May be at muscle-tendon junction (much less common)
- Forceful extension of a flexed elbow (eccentric contraction) with sudden overload

Diagnostic Keys

- History of sharp anterior elbow pain associated with sudden overload of flexed elbow
- Dull pain in arm and elbow
- Weakness of elbow, especially with lifting or supinating
- Bulge in distal arm

Examination

- Ecchymosis within 24 h
- Biceps muscle bulge usually palpable
- Weakness of supination and elbow flexion

Emergent Treatment

- Rest from offending activity
- Ice for 20 min, five times a day
- See physician within a few days for consideration of surgical reattachment

Tests

- Radiographs (AP, lateral, oblique)—rule out radial head dislocation
- If any doubt, MRI to rule out distal biceps muscle-tendon junction injury

Definitive Treatment/Follow-up/ Return to Play

- Consider surgical reattachment of distal biceps, especially for athlete
- Return to play
  - Adequate return of strength
  - Pain-free range of motion
  - Usually 3–6 months after surgery

Complications

- Loss of motion
- Weakness of supination (40 percent) and elbow flexion (30 percent) without surgery
- Retear

ICD-9 Code

- 841.8 Distal biceps tendon rupture

Bibliography

Baker CL, Gottlob, CA: The elbow, in Safran MR, Van Camp SP, McKeag D (eds): *Spiral Manual of Sports Medicine*. Philadelphia: Lippincott-Raven, 1998, pp 368–380.

Caldwell GL Jr., Safran MR: Elbow injuries in the athlete. *Orthop Clin North Am* 26:465–485, 1995.

Safran, MR: Elbow injuries in athletes. *Clin Ortao Rel Res* 310:257–277, 1995.

Safran MR, Bradley J: Elbow injuries, in Fu FH, Stone DA (eds): *Sports Injuries: Mechanisms, Prevention, and Treatment*. 2d ed. Philadelphia: Lippincott Williams & Wilkins, 2001, pp 1049–1084.

24

Acute Shoulder Injuries

Marc R. Safran

SHOULDER INSTABILITY

Mechanism of Injury/Pathology

- Anterior shoulder dislocation—most common (96 percent of all shoulder dislocations)
  - Arm abducted and externally rotated (throwing position)
  - Anterior force to shoulder (from behind) or posterior force at the hand or elbow
    - Bankart lesion—separation of labrum from glenoid or capsule
    - Stretching of capsule/anteroinferior ligaments of the shoulder
- Posterior shoulder dislocation
  - Arm forward flexed (like pushing) and posterior force at the hand
  - Falling, seizures, electrical shock
    - Posterior capsule—ligamentous injury, possible posterior Bankart
- Subluxation
  - Incomplete dislocation, self-reducing
  - May be congenital, atraumatic, "loose jointed.
  - May be due to microtrauma from repeated overhead activity (such as pitching or swimming)
- Multidirectional instability
  - Dislocation or subluxation
  - More than one direction (anterior, posterior, inferior)

Diagnostic Keys

- Mechanism of injury
- Limitation of shoulder motion
- Pain with arm motion
- Previous shoulder dislocation or subluxation
- Subluxation
  - "Dead arm" when throwing
  - Rotator cuff symptoms

Examination

- Deformity
  - Humeral head more prominent (anterior—in axilla or back with posterior dislocation)
  - Acromion more prominent posteriorly with anterior dislocation
  - Coracoid more prominent with posterior dislocation
- Loss of motion
  - Anterior dislocation—loss of rotation, particularly internal
    - Arm held in slight abduction
  - Posterior dislocation—loss of rotation, particularly external, loss of forward elevation
    - Arm locked in internal rotation
- Laxity—helpful for subluxations or after dislocation reduced
  - Load and shift test
    - Grasp humeral head in one hand and the scapula in the other. Gently apply load axially to arm to center the humeral head in the glenoid and then gently shift the humeral head anteriorly and then posteriorly. Compare to opposite side.
  - Apprehension—relocation test (see Fig. 24.1)
    - With patient laying supine, place arm in 90 degrees of abduction and external rotation. Hold that position with one hand and place the other hand under humeral head and apply anterior force. This should cause the subject to note the shoulder feels like it is slipping out (apprehension). Taking the hand from under the underside of the humerus and placing it on top of the humerus, apply a posterior force. This should relieve the symptoms (relocation).
  - Sulcus sign
    - With the subject seated and relaxed, pull down axially on both humerii. Measure the distance of the humeral head from the acromion. Compare both sides.

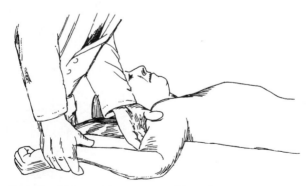

Figure 24.1 Shoulder apprehension test. (From Simon RR, Koenigsknecht SJ: *Emergency Orthopedics: The Extremities*, 4th ed. New York: McGraw-Hill, 2001. Used by permission.)

- Posterior apprehension test
  - With the subject supine, the subject's arm is forward flexed and internally rotated (and elbow bent), and the examiner pushes the arm posteriorly at the bent elbow
- Check axillary nerve function before and after reduction

Emergent Treatment

- Reduce the dislocation
  - May be done on the sideline without sedation if subject is relaxed and before muscle spasms set in
  - Do in controlled setting with sedation
  - Methods of reduction
    - Rowe technique
      - Lay athlete supine on the ground and have athlete relax
      - Gradually and slowly lift the affected arm overhead, using one hand on the athlete's wrist and one at the elbow/upper arm
      - Pull longitudinal traction up and overhead on the arm at the wrist
      - With your other hand, use your thumb to push the humeral head to assist in unlocking it from the glenoid
      - You may have to rotate the arm internally and externally
    - Double-sheet technique or traction-countertraction technique (see Fig. 24.2):
      - Place one sheet around the athlete's body, going under the affected axilla, and tie it around your assistant's waist with the

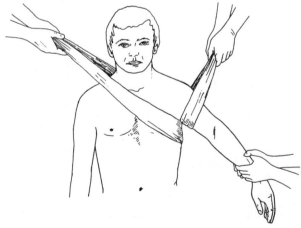

Figure 24.2 Traction-countertraction reduction of shoulder dislocation. (From Simon RR, Koenigsknecht SJ: *Emergency Orthopedics: The Extremities*, 4th ed. New York: McGraw-Hill, 2001. Used by permission)

assistant on the opposite side of the patient from you and the affected arm
- Use another sheet, tie it around your waist, and place it at the anterior part of the athlete's bent elbow on the affected side with the dislocated shoulder abducted
- You should start to lean or move back slowly and gradually to pull longitudinal traction on the arm. Some rotation, internally and externally, will help. Your assistant should provide countertraction to prevent the athlete from sliding.
- Sling
- Ice for 20 min, four times a day

Tests

- Radiographs—AP, transscapular Y, axillary (West Point or Velpeau)
  - Rule out fracture of humeral head or glenoid
  - Confirm reduction
- If above age 40, consider MRI to rule out rotator cuff tear

Definitive Treatment/Follow-up/ Return to Play

- Acute, first-time dislocations treat with sling immobilization
  - If below age 20, high recurrence rate: immobilize 4–6 weeks
  - If 20–40 years old, immobilize 2–3 weeks
  - If above age 40, low risk of recurrence: immobilize 1 week
- Subluxation or recurrent dislocation—immobilization for comfort
- If recurrence, may consider surgery
- Follow-up should ensure the full motion and normal muscle and nerve function
- Return to play
  - Full return of strength
  - Pain-free range of motion
  - Must pass functional sport-specific testing
  - May hasten by use of brace

Complications

- Missed fracture
  - Glenoid rim
  - Greater tuberosity
- Missed dislocation or nonreduced dislocation
- Axillary nerve injury
- Recurrent instability
- Missed rotator cuff tear

ICD-9 Codes

- Closed shoulder dislocation
    - 831.01 Anterior
    - 831.02 Posterior
    - 831.03 Inferior

ROTATOR CUFF INFLAMMATION
Mechanism of Injury/Pathology

- Impingement/overuse tendinitis
    - Primary
    - Due to instability
- Contusion
    - Fall to outstretched hand
    - Fall on shoulder
- Rotator cuff tear
    - Overuse
    - Attritional (older subjects)
    - Traumatic
        - Land on shoulder
        - With dislocation

Diagnostic Keys

- Mechanism of injury
- Unable to lift arm, especially without pain
- Pain with abduction or overhead activity
- Previous rotator cuff symptoms

Examination

- Ecchymosis
- Pain with abduction, at 70–120 degrees
- Weakness—external rotation, forward elevation, abduction
- Impingement sign
    - Pain with full forward elevation
- Jobe's sign
    - Pain and/or weakness with resisted abduction in the scapular plane
- Hawkins's sign
    - Pain with forward elevation at 90 degrees and forceful internal rotation
- Impingement test
    - Relief of pain with subacromial injection of lidocaine
    - If pain relieved and still weak = rotator cuff tear or nerve injury

- Check distal neurosensory
  - Scapular function
  - Axillary nerve
  - Suprascapular nerve
- Shoulder instability

Emergent Treatment

- Sling
- Ice for 20 min, four times a day

Tests

- Consider radiographs—AP, outlet, axillary
- Consider MRI to rule out rotator cuff tear

Definitive Treatment/Follow-up/ Return to Play

- Sling for comfort, to reduce acute inflammation; should be limited to preventing pain
- Early motion to prevent stiffness
- NSAIDs
- Rehabilitation
- Surgery for rotator cuff tear
- Return to play
  - Pain-free range of motion
  - Full strength
  - Pass functional sport-specific testing

Complications

- Missed nerve injury
  - Axillary nerve—direct contusion, causes weakness
  - Suprascapular nerve—weakness of rotator cuff
  - Long thoracic nerve—rotator cuff inflammation due to serratus weakness
- Missed rotator cuff tear
- Missed fracture
  - Greater tuberosity
  - Acromion
  - Coracoid
- Missed shoulder dislocation or subluxation
- Missed deltoid detachment

ICD-9 Codes

- 726.10 Rotator cuff impingement and contusion
- 727.61 Rotator cuff tear, traumatic

ACROMIOCLAVICULAR (AC) SEPARATION

Mechanism of Injury/Pathology

- Sprain of the coracoclavicular ligaments due to fall and landing on shoulder
- May occur from landing on outstretched hand
- Grade I—mild sprain, normal relationship between clavicle andacromion
- Grade II—moderate sprain, acromion lower than normal but not below clavicle
- Grade III—severe sprain, acromion lower than clavicle
- Grade IV—severe sprain, clavicle behind acromion, often into trapezius
- Grade V—severe sprain with deltotrapezial and periosteal injury resulting in acromion significantly below clavicle (>300 percent of clavicular diameter), often tenting the skin
- Grade VI—clavicle below the acromion, often below the coracoid

Diagnostic Keys

- Mechanism of injury
- Physical examination
- Previous shoulder injuries

Examination

- Swelling or bump on top of shoulder (at AC joint)
- Ecchymosis—at AC joint, occasionally to chest (by 48 h)
- Point tenderness at AC joint
- Loss of strength and/or pain with overhead activity or reaching across body
- Check distal neurosensory condition

Emergent Treatment

- Sling for comfort
- Ice for 20 min, five times a day
- Pain medications

Tests

- Radiographs (AP, Y scapular, axillary, AP of both clavicles with and without weights)

Definitive Treatment/Follow-up/ Return to Play

- For type I and II injuries, the treatment is nonoperative
- For type IV, V, and VI injuries, the treatment is surgical repair or reconstruction of the ligaments
- Treatment of type III is controversial—surgery for heavy laborers and throwing athletes and those who have failed nonoperative treatment
- Contact or collision athletes (football, hockey, motocross, etc.) with plans to return to play, nonoperative treatment is usually recommended
- For nonoperative treatment, immobilization should be limited to preventing pain
- Rehabilitation with or without surgery
- Return to play
  - Adequate return of strength
  - Pain-free range of motion
  - Pass functional sport-specific testing
  - May hasten by use of padding to offload pressure to the AC joint

Complications

- Missed clavicular fracture
- Weakness and fatigue of the arm
- Prolonged healing time if usual activities resumed too soon
- Recurrent injury

ICD-9 Codes

- 831.04 Closed dislocation of AC joint
- 831.14 Open dislocation of AC joint
- 840.0 AC joint sprain

Bibliography

Allen AA, Warner JJP: Shoulder instability in the athlete. *Orthop Clin North Am* 26:487, 1995.

Blevins FT, Hayes WM, Warren RF: Rotator cuff in contact athletes. *Am J Sports Med* 24:263, 1996.

Warner JJP, Navarro RA: The shoulder—instability and miscellaneous, in Safran MR, McKeag DB, VanCamp SP (eds): *Manual of Sports Medicine*. Philadelphia: Lippincott-Raven, 1998, p 351.

Warren RF: The shoulder—musculotendinous injuries, in Safran MR, McKeag DB, VanCamp SP (eds): *Manual of Sports Medicine*. Philadelphia: Lippincott-Raven, 1998, p 342.

25

Hip Injury

Chris McGilmer

HIP POINTER

Mechanism of Injury/Pathology

- Contusion to the iliac crest caused by direct blow

Diagnostic Keys

- Mechanism of injury
- Acute pain at site of contusion
- Athlete usually unable to continue activity
- Posture often flexed to ipsilateral side of injury

Examination

- Marked tenderness to palpation over anterior or posterior iliac crest
- Pain and weakness with active abdominal muscle and/or hip flexor contraction
- Possible swelling, deformity. and ecchymosis

Emergent Treatment

- Ice, compressive dressing, and pain medication
- Crutches and avoidance of weight bearing as necessary

Tests

- If clinically indicated, plain radiographs with oblique views may be useful to rule out fracture

Definitive Treatment/Follow-up/
Return to Play

- Contact must be avoided in order to encourage healing
- Athlete may return to sports when pain is tolerated and gait is normal
- Padding over affected area advisable upon return to sport

Complications

- Reinjury common without adequate rest and padding
- Compression fracture of iliac crest
- Consider iliac apophysitis in young athlete
  - Typically afflicts those between 9 and 17 years of age
  - Associated with growth spurt and muscle tendon imbalance

ICD-9 Code

- 924.01 Hip pointer

ADDUCTOR MUSCLE STRAIN
Mechanism of Injury/Pathology

- Generally occurs with a violent forced abduction during a fall, also with twisting injury or collision that stretches the adductor muscles past their elastic limit
- Often overlaps with abdominal and hip flexor muscle strains
- Deconditioned and fatigued muscles are more likely to undergo acute strain
- Most common cause of groin pain often seen in sprinting, soccer, and ice hockey

Diagnostic Keys

- Mechanism of injury
- Pain in the region of the adductor muscle group just distal to their origin
- Previous adductor muscle strain

Examination

- Swelling and ecchymosis may be present
- Tenderness to palpation at adductor tubercle or inferior pubic ramus
- Increased pain with passive abduction and resisted hip adduction
- Pain may be increased with situps and resisted hip flexion

Emergent Treatment

- Rest, ice, and pain medication
- Crutches and avoidance of weight bearing may be necessary

Tests

- Radiographs are rarely indicated but may help to rule out avulsion fractures, myositis ossificans, and osteitis pubis

Definitive Treatment/Follow-up/ Return to Play

- Gentle stretching and strengthening of the adductor muscles is very important
- Gradual return to activity is imperative
- Full recovery may take weeks to months

Complications

- Reinjury common if inadequate rehabilitation, stretching, or premature return to competition
- Complete muscle rupture and avulsion fractures of adductor tubercle

ICD-9 Code

- 843.8 Adductor thigh sprain

AVULSION FRACTURES OF THE HIP

Mechanism of Injury/Pathology

- Injuries result from sudden, violent muscle contraction against a fixed resistance
- May also occur with sudden excessive passive lengthening of muscle
- More common in the skeletally immature (<16 years old) and the osteopenic (>35 years old), especially along the iliac crest and ischial tuberosity
- Most commonly seen in sprinters, hurdlers, gymnasts, or others who rely on sudden, forceful acceleration

Diagnostic Keys

- Localized pain, tenderness, and decreased range of motion at avulsion site

- Audible "pop" often reported and athlete is usually unable to continue activity
- Common muscle insertion avulsion sites (See Fig. 18.5)
  - Anterosuperior iliac spine (ASIS)
    - Forceful overpull of sartorius muscle with hip in extension and knee in flexion
  - Anteroinferior iliac spine (AIIS)
    - Forceful pull on rectus femoris muscle with overextension of hip or resisted hip flexion
  - Ischial tuberosity
    - Forceful eccentric contraction of hamstring muscles with knee extended and hip flexed
  - Iliac crest
    - Forceful overpull of abdominal muscles with resisted hip flexion and/or abdominal torque
  - Iliopsoas and piriformis avulsions may occur but are much less common

Examination

- Tender to palpation at suspected avulsion site
- Avulsed fragment may be palpable
- Muscles involved must be assessed for active and passive range of motion
  - ASIS: pain with resisted hip flexion and knee extension
  - AIIS: pain with passive hip hyperextension and active hip flexion
  - Ischial tuberosity: pain with forceful eccentric hamstring contraction with knee in extension and hip in flexion
  - Iliac crest: pain with resisted hip abduction, abdominal muscle contraction, and twisting of torso
  - Iliopsoas: pain with hip flexion, extension, and rotation against resistance
  - Piriformis: pain with resisted abduction of flexed hip in lateral decubitus position

Emergent Treatment

- Rest, ice, and pain medication
- Position involved muscle group to minimize tension at insertion site
- Crutches are usually required acutely

Tests

- Anteroposterior (AP) pelvic radiograph will demonstrate avulsion fracture
- Oblique views are best with suspected iliac crest avulsions
- Ewing's sarcoma and osteomyelitis can resemble a healing avulsion fracture

Definitive Treatment/Follow-up

- Progressive weight bearing with gradual stretching and strengthening program of specific musculotendinous units involved
- Sport-specific training followed by return to sport when pain-free, with normal strength and full range of motion
- Most avulsion fractures heal with conservative treatment
- Surgery with open reduction with internal fixation (ORIF) should be considered when apophyseal fragment is displaced >2 cm
- Ischial tuberosity avulsions most often require ORIF or excision to avoid large reactive fracture callus formation

Complications

- Missed fractures
- Reinjury is common if rehabilitation and stretching are inadequate or return to competition is premature

ICD-9 Code

- 808.49 Pelvic rim, closed fracture

HIP DISLOCATION

Mechanism of Injury/Pathology

- Dislocation of the hip is a rare but significant athletic injury occasionally seen in high-velocity collisions, as in skiing, motor sports, and equestrian events
- Occurs with significant forces acting along the long axis of the femur, driving the femoral head through the labrum
- 90 percent of dislocated hips dislocate posteriorly, usually due to a direct blow to the proximal tibia with the hip and knee flexed
- Anterior dislocation, although extremely rare, is typically caused by a direct blow with the hip abducted

Diagnostic Keys

- Hip dislocations are extremely painful and immediately disabling
- Mechanism usually requires high-energy trauma

Examination

- Posterior dislocations classically present with limb shortening and the thigh held in flexion, adduction, and internal rotation

- Femoral head may be palpated in buttocks region in posterior dislocations
- Anterior dislocations present with thigh held in external rotation, abduction, and either flexion or extension
- Thorough neurovascular examination is indicated, as injury may warrant more urgent reduction
- Complete trauma evaluation is indicated due to the high likelihood of concomitant pelvic rim fractures, ipsilateral knee injury, and associated life-threatening injuries

Emergent Treatment (See Fig. 25-1)

- All hip dislocations should be reduced as soon as possible (<12 h)
- Intravenous anesthesia and muscle relaxant are often required to overcome pain and muscle spasm
- Urgent orthopedic consultation is imperative
- Repeated neurovascular examination is always indicated postreduction

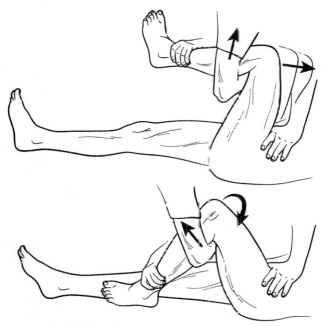

Figure 25.1 Hip reduction. (From Lewis CG, Orthopaedic Pocket Procedures: General Orthopaedics. New York: McGraw-Hill, 2003. Used by permission.)

Tests

- Prereduction x-rays should always be obtained and should include posteroanterior (PA) and true lateral views to determine the exact direction of dislocation
- Postreduction x-ray are needed to confirm reduction
- Additional films may be needed to rule out concomitant injuries
- CT scan should be obtained postreduction to evaluate presence of acetabular fractures and osteochondral fragments

Definitive Treatment/Follow-up

- Postreduction studies and repeat neurovascular examination are essential
- Once hip is reduced, traction is required to prevent recurrent dislocations while capsule heals
- Pain-free range of motion, weight bearing as tolerated, and aggressive physical therapy should be started early
- Important to follow patients with MRI for several years to observe for developing avascular necrosis (AVN)

Complications

- AVN of femoral head (risk directly related to time interval before successful reduction)
- Recurrent dislocations
- Osteoarthritis

ICD-9 Code

- 835.01 Dislocation of hip, closed, posterior

STRESS FRACTURES OF THE FEMUR

Mechanism of Injury/Pathology

- Symptoms may be insidious in onset, but groin or hip pain in a runner should be evaluated aggressively to prevent complications
- Excessive and/or sudden increase in activity surpassing osteoblastic activity and new bone formation
- Uncommon injury in healthy athletes noted mainly in endurance runners, especially in females with athletic triad
- Femoral neck most commonly affected, but subtrochanteric and shaft fractures may occur

Diagnostic Keys

- Athlete presents initially with groin pain, which may progress to involve the hip, thigh, and knee
- Pain worsens with running and is eventually felt with daily activities
- Patient may develop an antalgic gait

Examination

- Limited external and internal range of motion secondary to pain
- Pain with axial loading or standing and hopping on involved leg

Emergent Treatment

- Complete rest is mandatory, with pain control and avoidance of weight bearing
- Orthopedic consultation is strongly recommended
- Displaced fractures are orthopedic emergencies

Tests

- Radiographs usually remain normal for many weeks but may reveal periosteal thickening
- Bone scans are extremely sensitive and can detect lesion 2–8 days after the onset of symptoms
- CT and MRI are also helpful and may demonstrate sclerosis and other subtle signs of displacement

Definitive Treatment/Follow-up

- Conservative therapy includes rest and avoidance of weight bearing, followed by pain-free activity as tolerated, with eventual gradual return to sport activity
- Tension (superior) side stress fractures of the femoral neck usually require ORIF
- Compression (inferior) side stress fractures usually respond to conservative therapy

Complications

- Progression to complete fracture
- Displacement
- AVN of femoral head

ICD-9 Code

- 820.00 Femoral neck fracture

TROCHANTERIC/ILIOPSOAS BURSITIS

Mechanism of Injury/Pathology

- Inflammation and pain in bursal structure caused by excessive friction from repetitive tendon motion passing over a bony prominence; may appear acutely at an event
- Usually caused by insufficient stretching and repetitive activity
- Bursitis of the greater trochanter is usually aggravated by contraction of the tensor fascia (iliotibial band) when moving the hip from full extension to full flexion
- Iliopsoas bursitis is usually aggravated by hip extension, causing the iliopsoas tendon to catch on the pectineal eminence of the pelvic rim or the femoral head

s/p hip replacement

Diagnostic Keys

- Increased risk: running on banked surfaces, adducting beyond midline, and female runners
- Bursitis of the greater trochanter causes lateral hip pain and may cause night pain, difficulty lying on affected side, and pain when first rising in the morning
- Iliopsoas bursitis causes pain in the inguinal region or front of leg with hip flexion and extension, as seen when rising from a seated or recumbent position
- Both may be associated with a "snapping" sensation

Examination

- Greater trochanteric bursitis presents with tenderness just posterior to the greater trochanter and increased pain with adduction of hip in internal rotation
- Iliopsoas bursitis present with tenderness just lateral to femoral neurovascular bundle over the pubic ramus; it is made worse with resisted hip flexion
- Both may demonstrate a reproducible and palpable snapping sensation

Emergent Treatment

- Rest, ice, pain control, and anti-inflammatory medications

Soul - medral pack

Tests

- Radiographs are usually not necessary but may rule out other, more serious pathology

Definitive Treatment/Follow-up

- Once inflammation and pain subside, prevention consists of a stretching and strengthening program of the specific muscle groups involved
- Corticosteroid injection may be tried if conservative therapy fails
- Refractory cases may require bursal excision or lengthening of the involved tendon

Complications

- Without adequate rest and rehabilitation, reinjury is common

ICD-9 Code

- 726.5 Enthesopathy of the hip region

PEDIATRIC CONSIDERATIONS

Mechanism of Injury/Pathology

- Immature athletes are susceptible to all previously mentioned injuries but particularly to AVN and physeal injuries about the femoral head and neck; they therefore require special consideration if presenting with hip or groin pain
- Legg-Calvé-Perthes disease (LCPD) is due to idiopathic AVN of the femoral head; it is most commonly in boys under 10 years of age
- Slipped capital femoral epiphysis (SCFE) is due to slippage of the femoral head relative to the neck about the femoral epiphyseal plate and is most commonly seen in the early teenage years

Diagnostic Keys

- LCPD usually has an insidious onset, presenting with a painless limp, but the child may report groin, anterior thigh, and knee pain that worsens with activity
- SCFE usually presents with hip pain and a limp; there may also be pain referred to the groin, thigh, and knee

- SCFE pain may develop gradually or acutely with dramatic onset and the inability to bear weight; SCFE is often seen in obese or rapidly growing boys

Examination

- LCPD often leads to a decreased range of hip motion, especially with internal rotation and abduction
- A Trendelenburg gait, leg-length discrepancy, and muscle atrophy may be present
- SCFE often presents with an external rotation deformity in slight abduction and limited internal rotation secondary to pain
- Limited abduction, forward flexion, and leg-length discrepancy may also be noted

Emergent Treatment

- Rest, ice, and NSAIDs
- Crutches and avoidance of weight bearing necessary
- Immediate orthopedic referral is indicated, especially with SCFE

Tests

- AP and frog-leg laterals are mandatory in all children with hip pain and/or limp, with careful comparison to the unaffected side
- In LCPD, a smaller femoral head and a widened articular cartilage space is typically seen; however, the picture may be completely normal early on
- Advanced cases may show sclerosis, fracture, fragmentation, and resorption of the femoral head
- In SCFE, a widened physeal plate with posterior and downward displacement of the capital epiphysis relative to the femoral neck is usually demonstrated
- Classification is based on the severity of slippage

Definitive Treatment/Follow-up

- LCPD may be treated nonsurgically with abduction bracing to hold the femoral head in place, but surgery is often required
- It may take up to 18 months for subchondral ossification to be seen radiographically; an extensive rehabilitation program is needed to prevent atrophy and contracture
- SCFE requires surgical stabilization; avoidance of weight bearing postoperatively for 6 weeks is not uncommon

Complications

- Lifelong deformity and disability if not treated early
- Osteoarthritis common in both
- Osteochondrosis dissecans seen in LCPD
- Articular cartilage necrosis and painful fibrous ankylosis of hip joint in SCFE

ICD-9 Codes

- 732.1 Juvenile osteochondrosis of hip and pelvis—LCPD
  - 732.2 Nontraumatic
  - 732.9 Traumatic—SCFE
- 820.01 Fracture-separation—SCFE

Bibliography

Anderson K, Strickland S, Warren R: Hip and groin injuries in athletes. *Am J Sports Med.* 29(4):521–533, 2001.

Bracker M, Rice L, Yassini P: *The 5-Minute Sports Medicine Consult.* Philadelphia: Lippincott Williams & Wilkins, 2001.

Eiff M, Hatch R, Calmbach W: *Fracture Management for Primary Care.* Philadelphia: Saunders, 1998.

Morelli V, Smith V: Groin injuries in athletes. *Am Fam Physician* 64(8):1405–1414, 2001.

Waters P, Millis M: Hip and pelvic injuries in the young athlete. *Clin Sports Med* 1(3):513–525, 1998.

26

Knee Injuries

T. Ted Funahashi
Greg Maletis

LIGAMENT

Mechanism of Injury

- ACL (anterior cruciate ligament)
  - Classically associated with either hyperextension or valgus injuries of the knee
  - May be injured by other mechanisms, including decelerating, pivoting on a planted foot, jumping, twisting, cutting, or landing. Often a noncontact injury.
- MCL (medial collateral ligament)
  - Blow to the lateral aspect of the knee, causing a valgus load
  - With extension injuries, watch for injuries to the PCL and ACL
- LCL (lateral collateral ligament)
  - Blow to the medial aspect of the knee, causing varus load
  - Uncommon as isolated injury, usually seen in combination with ACL, PCL, or posterolateral corner injuries
- PCL (posterior cruciate ligament)
  - Usually a direct blow to front of tibia or by a fall onto a flexed knee
  - Often associated with dashboard injuries
- PLRI (posterolateral rotatory instability)
  - Unusual isolated injury that may be caused by forced external rotation of the tibia
  - Frequently associated with grade II or greater LCL injury
- Dislocation
  - Severe injury may be in any direction; it usually requires injury of three ligaments to occur

Diagnostic Keys

- ACL
  - A "pop" is often heard or felt
  - Swelling occurs usually within 2–3 h of injury

- Athlete is usually unable to continue playing
- Chronic, giving way with pivoting or twisting activity
- MCL
  - Mechanism of injury: knee felt to bend "inward" with a tearing sensation or "pop"
  - Minimal swelling
- LCL
  - Minimal swelling unless associated with ACL or PCL injury
- PCL
  - Mechanism of injury: blow to anterior aspect of the proximal tibia
  - Swelling within first 2–3 h, but less than with ACL
- PLRI
  - Difficult to diagnose; must be kept in mind when evaluating any acute knee injury
- Dislocation
  - Often more than one pop is felt
  - Swelling within first 2–3 h, but effusion may not be present if capsule is disrupted
  - May require manipulation to relocate knee joint

Examination

- ACL
  - Acute knee swelling
  - Lachman's test—anterior force on tibia with knee in 25 degrees of flexion, note laxity and soft endpoint when compared with opposite knee (Fig. 26.1)
  - Pivot shift—extension, valgus, and internal rotation cause subluxation of tibia; moving into slight flexion allows tibia to reduce
  - KT 1000 (knee arthrometer)—manual maximum side-to-side difference of >3 mm is considered abnormal

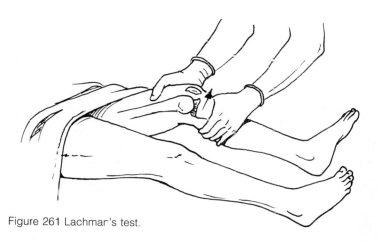

Figure 261 Lachman's test.

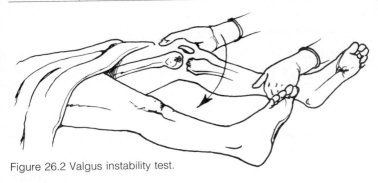

Figure 26.2 Valgus instability test.

- MCL
  - Usually little or no acute swelling; pain along MCL path, valgus instability of knee (Fig. 26.2):
    - Grade I: pain, no laxity
    - Grade II: pain, some laxity but firm endpoint
    - Grade III: gross laxity without endpoint
  - Valgus instability in full extension suggests a more severe injury. Watch for associated ACL, PCL, or posteromedial corner injuries.
- LCL
  - Tender at lateral femoral condyle or fibular head; LCL can be palpated with knee in Fig. 26.4 position
  - Varus laxity in 20–30 degrees of flexion, see above for grading (Fig. 26.3)
  - Grade II and III LCL injuries occur in conjunction with posterolateral corner injuries; they are often also associated with ACL and PCL tears
- PCL
  - Posterior sag (Fig. 26.4)

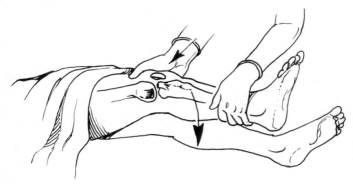

Figure 26.3 Varus instability test.

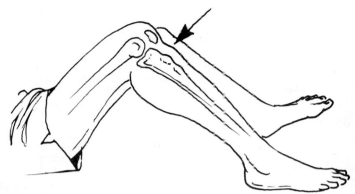

Figure 26.4. Posterior sag.

- Posterior drawer—posteriorly directed force to proximal tibia with knee in >70 degrees of flexion
  - Grade I—anterior tibia still anterior to the femoral condyles
  - Grade II—anterior tibia at the level of the femoral condyles
  - Grade III—anterior tibia posterior to the femoral condyles
- Quadriceps active test: with knee flexed 90 degrees ask patient to slowly slide foot down along table and watch anterior movement of proximal tibia
- PLRI
  - Dial test: with patient prone, externally rotate both tibias with knee flexed at 30 and 90 degrees
    - Increased external rotation at 30 degrees indicates only isolated posterolateral corner injury
    - Increased external rotation at 30 and 90 degrees indicates combined posterolateral corner and PCL injury
- Dislocation
  - Check neurovascular status: there may be intimal tears causing delayed vascular compromise
  - Peroneal nerve often injured; check sensation at ankle and first dorsal web space, dorsiflexion of ankle and toes, and foot eversion

Emergent Treatment

- ACL, MCL, and PCL: Ace wrap and immobilize for comfort; apply ice and start NSAIDs; crutches as needed
- LCL
  - Grade I or less: Ace wrap and immobilize for comfort; apply ice and start NSAIDs
  - Grade II or greater: must rule out associated injury to posterolateral corner; urgent MRI helpful
- Dislocation
  - Check pulse and repeat frequently

- Reduce dislocation with manual traction or in operating room if irreducible
- Emergency room for vascular evaluation, including angiogram if necessary. Vascular repair if indicated.
- Stat MRI to assess extent of soft tissue injury; associated posterolateral corner injuries require operative repair within 10 days

Tests

- ACL, MCL, LCL, PCL
  - Recommend x-rays for all knee injuries to rule out fractures
- Injury-specific tests
  - ACL: may see Segond's fracture ("lateral capsular sign": fleck of bone off of lateral tibial plateau); pathognomic of ACL injury (see Fig. 18.7) in skeletally immature patients, tibial eminence avulsions (see Fig. 18.8)
  - MCL: In skeletally immature patients, rule out Salter II injuries of distal femoral physis; may need stress x-rays
  - LCL: may need stress x-rays; stat MRI if LCL grade II or greater to rule out posterolateral corner injury
  - PLRI: stat MRI to assess area and degree of injury

Dislocation: need vascular surgery consultation; consider angiogram to rule out intimal tears. Intimal tears may cause delayed vascular compromise even in the face of normal initial pulses.

Definitive Treatment/Follow-up/ Return to Play

- ACL
  - Consider bracing in end-of-season or skeletally immature athlete; otherwise plan ACL reconstruction
  - Most athletes with a torn ACL will require ACL reconstruction
  - Return to play (RTP) with an incompetent ACL puts the meniscus and articular cartilage at risk when further episodes of giving way occur
  - Risk of further injury can be assessed based on KT 1000 results and hours of activity at cutting or pivoting sport
  - Rehabilitation after ACL reconstruction is usually 6–8 months; athletes can return after 80–90 percent of the opposite side's strength has been achieved
  - Functional braces are often used for RTP
- MCL: based on degree of injury
  - Grade I
    - NSAID and start PT to recondition knee
    - RTP when pain is tolerable and strength on both sides is equal
    - RTP usually in 3–4 weeks if athlete can do sport-specific activities
    - Consider prophylactic bracing if injury recurs

- Grade II
  - NSAID and start PT to recondition knee
  - Start early full ROM exercises; consider protecting knee in hinged knee brace
  - RTP when is pain diminished, ROM full, and strength equal on both sides, usually 4–6 weeks
  - Consider prophylactic bracing
- Grade III
  - NSAIDs, varus-stressed ROM brace
  - Physical therapy: Start 20–90 degrees and advance as tolerated; aim for full ROM by 3–4 weeks
  - May return to play when knee stable to examination, full ROM is restored, and strength is equal on both sides. Usually minimum of 6–8 weeks.
  - Recommend prophylactic bracing if athlete is returning during same season
- LCL: based on degree of injury
  - Grade I
    - NSAIDs and start PT to recondition knee
    - RTP when pain tolerable and strength equal
  - Grade II
    - Often associated with posterolateral corner injury, needing acute repair within 10–14 days
    - Usual return to sport 9–12 months after repair has healed and knee is fully rehabilitated
  - Grade III
    - Usually associated with posterolateral corner injury, needing acute repair within 10–14 days
    - Usual return to sport 9–12 months after repair has healed and knee is fully rehabilitated
- PCL
  - Grades I and II
    - Nonoperative treatment with early ROM and strengthening
    - Return when nontender, pain-free ROM, adequate strength, able to do sport-specific activities
    - Return to sports at 4–8 weeks
  - Grade III—controversial
    - Displaced avulsion fracture should be fixed acutely
    - When associated with other ligament injuries consider reconstruction
    - Isolated injuries may be treated nonoperatively; if symptomatic instability develops, may require reconstruction
    - If reconstructed, return to sports when 80–90 percent strength is recovered, usually 9–12 months
- PLRI
  - Difficult injuries to treat, especially if not caught early (within 10 days) for repair
  - Most delayed reconstructive efforts are of limited efficacy when compared to early repair
  - RTP dependent upon success of operative repair

- Dislocation
  - Vascular injuries and irreducible dislocations require immediate operative treatment
  - Operative treatment is usually indicated for some or all of the disrupted ligaments; timing of reconstruction is somewhat dependent on which ligaments are involved

Complications

- ACL
  - Missed ACL injuries may lead to subsequent secondary injuries to meniscus and articular cartilage
  - Associated injuries
  - Meniscus tear is commonly associated with ACL tear
  - Missed LCL and posterolateral corner injury may lead to failure of ACL reconstruction
- MCL
  - If tear is proximal, there may be tenderness at the medial femoral epicondyle for 6–8 months
  - Stiffness is often a problem with MCL tears
  - May need stress x-rays to differentiate Salter II fracture from MCL tear in skeletally immature athlete
- LCL
  - Rare injury, often missed
  - Acute repair of LCL and posterolateral corner gives best results
- PCL
  - Sometimes associated with early degeneration of medial and patellofemoral compartment of the knee
  - Rare injury, often missed
- Dislocation
  - Vascular injuries need immediate attention to prevent ischemia and potential amputation
  - Intimal tears can cause delayed vascular compromise
  - Peroneal nerve injuries are common with lateral side injuries

MENISCUS

Mechanism of Injury

- Twisting injury while weight bearing, squatting,
- May be torn with minimal injuries or insidiously

Diagnostic Keys

- Acute onset of knee pain
- Swelling, usually occurs 12–24 hours after injury
- Sharp pain along medial or lateral joint line with certain movements

- Pain with squatting
- Unable to fully extend knee with displaced meniscus
- Knee locks in flexed position

Examination

- May have variable degrees of knee swelling
- Palpate along medial and lateral joint lines looking for tenderness along the meniscus. Mid to posterior joint line tenderness generally more suggestive of meniscal injury.
- Confirm with meniscal stress tests below:
    - McMurray: flex knee, twist knee and gradually extend, look for meniscal click or reproducible pain along suspected meniscus
    - Flick: hyperflex knee and quickly internally and externally "flick" the knee: look for reproducible pain at suspected meniscus

Emergent Treatment

- Rest, ice, and NSAIDs

Tests

- Standard
    - X-rays to rule out other fracture, degenerative joints, osteochondritis dissecans, or other abnormalities
- Special
    - MRI may be helpful in confirming diagnosis or location of meniscus tear
    - Peripheral tears more amendable to operative repairs rather than excision

Definitive Treatment/Follow-up/ Return to Play

- Treatment:
    - May be treated conservatively if asymptomatic
    - Surgical intervention required for symptomatic tears
- If surgically excised:
    - RTP after return of full motion and with minimal swelling, usually in 4–6 weeks
- If surgically repaired:
    - Crutches and brace for 4–6 weeks
    - No deep squatting for 3 months
    - RTP in 6 months

Complications

- Locked knee
- Usually due to displaced bucket-handle meniscus tear
- Should undergo surgical repair semiurgently to prevent further meniscus damage

ICD-9 Codes

- 836.0 Medial meniscus tear
- 836-1 Lateral meniscus tear
- 844.0 Lateral collateral ligament sprain
- 844.1 Medial collateral ligament sprain
- 844.2 Cruciate ligament sprain

PATELLA

Mechanism of Injury

- Dislocation
  - Direct blow to medial aspect of patella or twisting injury to knee
- Extensor mechanism tear
  - Sudden muscular contraction of the quadriceps, such as in jumping or landing, causing rupture of patellar ligament or quadriceps tendon
  - May also be caused by direct blow to anterior knee under quadriceps load

Diagnostic Keys

- Dislocation
  - Patella can be felt to slip out and back in
  - Swelling usually occurs within 2–3 h
  - History of previous dislocations
- Extensor mechanism tear
  - Athlete reports feeling pop,
  - Is unable to ambulate,
  - Is unable to raise straight leg

Examination

- Patellar dislocation
  - Patella palpable on side of knee if unreduced
  - Large effusion
  - Patellar apprehension: Athlete becomes apprehensive when patella is displaced laterally

- There is tenderness at the medial femoral epicondyle and/or along the medial retinaculum
- Extensor mechanism tear
  - Athlete is unable to perform straight leg raise
  - Position of patella is altered
  - Quadriceps tendon tear—patella baja
  - Patellar ligament tear—patella alta
  - Palpable defect at patellar ligament or quadriceps tendon

Emergent Treatment

- Dislocation
  - Attempt relocation by gently extending the knee and by coaxing the patella back into position
  - Wrap, ice, and immobilize for comfort
- Extensor mechanism tear
  - Wrap, ice, and immobilize for comfort
  - Have patient use crutches

Tests

- Dislocation
  - X-rays—AP, lateral, and Merchant view
  - MRI—may help to define location of tear in medial patellofemoral ligament or retinaculum
- Extensor mechanism tear
  - X-rays—lateral view of both knees in approx 45 degrees of flexion
    - With quadriceps tendon rupture, patella will be low compared with normal side
    - With patellar ligament rupture, patella will be high compared with normal side
    - Rule out patellar fracture
- MRI—not usually required but can confirm a tear if examination is questionable

Definitive Treatment/Follow-up/ Return to Play

- Dislocation
  - Immobilization for 2–3 weeks
  - Patellar stabilizing brace when out of immobilizer
  - ROM exercises with PT
  - Quadriceps strengthening
  - RTP when full ROM is reestablished, there is no patellar apprehension, and full strength has been regained
  - RTP usually in 2–3 months

- Extensor mechanism tear
  - Surgical repair of torn tendon
  - RTP usually in 4–6 months, with full ROM and strength regained

Complications

- Dislocation
  - Osteochondral fracture often seen with patellar dislocation
  - Frequently associated with chondral injury to patellar facet or lateral femoral sulcus
- Extensor mechanism tear
  - Avulsion fracture or patellar fracture
  - Delayed repair due to missed rupture leads to poor outcome

ICD-9 Code

- 836.3 Dislocation of patella

FRACTURES

Tibial Plateau

- Usually caused by axial or angular load across tibiofemoral joint
- Angular loads may lead to ligamentous injury, contralateral plateau injury, or both
- Most fractures with intraarticular involvement are treated with open or arthroscopically assisted ORIF

Physeal Injuries of the Distal Femur

- Seen in skeletally immature athletes (with open distal femoral physis)
- Valgus injuries of the knee may result in Salter II injuries of the distal femoral physis
- Undetected or mistreated, these are ominous injuries with serious consequences
- Detection and appropriate treatment, including anatomic reduction and fixation, are essential

Tibial Eminence Avulsions

- Seen in skeletally immature athletes
- Injuries similar to those for ACL in skeletally mature athletes
- Causes acute knee hemarthrosis
- Tibial attachment of ACL causes avulsion of tibial eminence
- May be cause for a locked knee, which cannot be fully extended

- Size and displacement of avulsed fragment determines treatment
  - Smaller and completely avulsed fragment: open or arthroscopic reduction and fixation
  - Larger (McKeever type III) may be treated in extension cast, if acceptable position of fragment is confirmed on postreduction radiographs and the knee can be brought into full extension

Fracture of Patella

- Usually caused by a direct blow to the patella
- In skeletally immature patients, avulsion of the distal pole or proximal pole of the patella may be seen
- Small fragments off of the inferior aspect of the medial patellar facet may be seen with patellar dislocations
- May be treated in a cylinder cast if there is no or minimal displacement
- Any significant displacement or inability to perform a straight-leg raise should undergo operative repair/fixation

ICD-9 Codes

- 822.0 Fracture of patella
- 823.0 Fracture of tibia, upper end, closed

Bibliography

Bergfeld JA, Safran MR: Knee ligaments, in Safran MR, McKeag DB, Van Camp SP (eds): *Manual of Sports Medicine*. Philadelphia: Lippincott-Raven, 1998.

DeLee JC, Drez D (eds): *Orthopaedic Sports Medicine: Principles and Practice*. Philadelphia: Saunders, 1994.

Harner CD, Navarro RA: Knee cartilage, in Safran MR, McKeag DB, Van Camp SP (eds): *Manual of Sports Medicine*. Philadelphia: Lippincott-Raven, 1998.

Rockwood CA, Green DP (eds): *Fractures in Adults and Children*. Philadelphia: Lippincott, 2001.

27

Ankle and Achilles Tendon Injuries

D. Scott Marr

ANKLE LIGAMENT INJURIES

Mechanism of Injury/Pathology

- There are three major ligamentous complexes in the ankle (lateral, medial, and syndesmotic). The lateral ankle ligaments include the anterior talofibular (ATF), calcaneofibular (CF), and posterior talofibular (PTF). Medially the broad-based deltoid ligament attaches to the tibia, talus, and calcaneus. The anterior and posterior tibiofibular ligaments or syndesmotic ligaments join the tibia and fibula.
- The ankle joint is most stable in a neutral dorsiflexed position; therefore most ankle ligament injuries occur when the ankle is in plantarflexion
- Supination usually results in damage to lateral structures; pronation usually results in damage to medial structures
- Rotational injuries often result in injury to the tibiofibular (syndesmotic) ligaments

Diagnostic Keys

- Mechanism of injury is key to understanding likely injured structure (see Table 27.1)
- If concern of an unstable ankle injury exists with normal initial radiographs, weight bearing, external rotation stress and reverse talar tilt stress x-rays should be considered to assess the stability of the ankle joint
- Greater than 4 mm of space between the medial malleolus and talus on the mortise view suggests an unstable injury

Examination:

- Note swelling and ecchymosis. Swelling immediately inferior to the lateral malleolus usually indicates injury to the ATFL. Swelling above the malleolus can be suggestive of a syndesmotic injury or fibular fracture.

Table 27.1 Mechanisms of Ankle Ligament Injury

Mechanism of Injury	Likely Injured Ligament
Plantarflexion with supination	Anterior talofibular, calcaneofibular
External rotation with eversion	Deltoid and syndesmosis
Dorsiflexion with inversion	Calcaneofibular
Dorsiflexion with internal rotation	Posterior tibiofibular ligament and syndesmosis
Dorsiflexion with external rotation	Anterior tibiofibular ligament and syndesmosis

- Immediately after the injury, palpation of specific ligaments may help localize the area of injury. However, the diffuse swelling later in presentation may obscure the specificity of palpation.
- The anterior drawer test is used to evaluate the integrity of the ATFL; however, this test may be difficult to perform in the acute setting secondary to pain. The test is performed by grasping the calcaneus and pulling forward while holding the distal tibia in place. Always compare to unaffected side (Fig. 27.1).

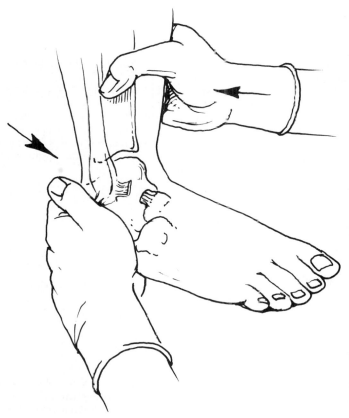

Figure 27.1 Ankle drawer test.

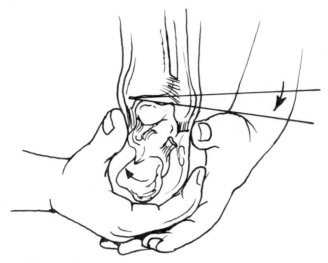

Figure 27.2 Talar tilt test.

- The talar tilt test is used to evaluate the CFL. This test is performed by applying an inversion stress to the hindfoot (Fig. 27.2).
- To evaluate the syndesmosis, the squeeze test (Fig. 27.3) and the external rotation stress test (Fig. 27.4) are commonly used. A positive squeeze test is indicated by pain referring to the ankle with compression of the tibia and fibula at the level of the midcalf. A positive external rotation stress test is indicated by pain referring to the syndesmotic region when the ankle is externally rotated in a neutral position with the knee in 90 degrees of flexion.
- Neurovascular examination

Emergent Treatment

- Rest, ice, compression, and elevation remain the mainstays of early treatment. Aggressive treatment of swelling has been found to improve outcomes.
- Use of a rigid compression splint often allows earlier and less painful ambulation and hence can shorten recovery time
- Encourage early range-of-motion exercises and weight bearing

Tests

- A common question in an acute ankle injury is when to obtain radiographs. The Ottawa ankle rules summarized below can help provide guidance in this setting. See Fig. 27.5 for locating red flag areas of bony tenderness.

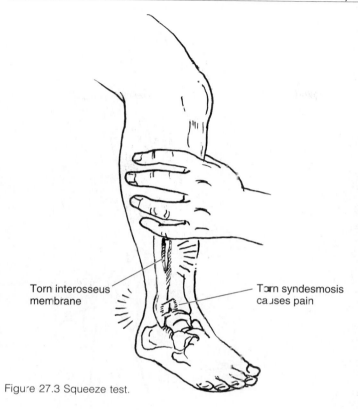

Torn interosseus membrane

Torn syndesmosis causes pain

Figure 27.3 Squeeze test.

- Obtain ankle x-rays if there is:
  - Bone tenderness at the posterior edge of the distal 6 cm of the lateral malleolus
  - Bone tenderness at the posterior edge of the distal 6 cm of the medial malleolus
  - Inability to take four weight-bearing steps immediately after injury
- Obtain foot x-ray if there is:
  - Any pain over midfoot zone
  - Bone tenderness at the base of the fifth metatarsal
  - Bone tenderness over the navicular

Definitive Treatment/Follow-up/ Return to Play

- Ankle rehabilitation program including proprioceptive retraining
- Open reduction with internal fixation (ORIF) usually required for injuries that result in widening of the ankle mortise secondary to tibiofibular diastasis

–227–

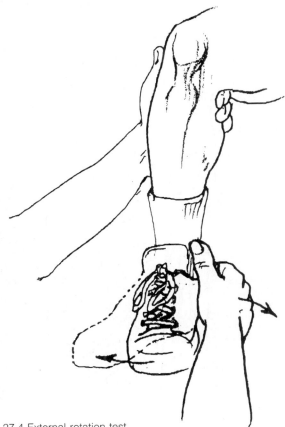

Figure 27.4 External rotation test.

- Return to play (RTP): when there is adequate strength with a full pain-free ROM
- Bracing: Support with tape or brace for 6 months during play
- Orthotics: Consider lateral heel wedge in individual with cavus foot to place the hindfoot in valgus

Complications

- Recurrent ankle sprains secondary to ligamentous instability usually occur because of inadequate rehabilitation
- Posttraumatic synovitis can occur, typically when RTP is too aggressive
- Osteochondral lesions of the talus or tibial plafond are often overlooked at the time of injury. In the case of persistent pain and dysfunction following a properly rehabilitated ankle injury, an MRI or bone scan should be considered.

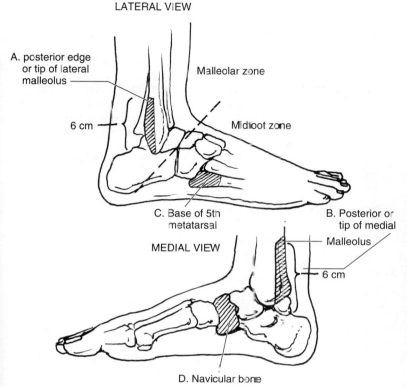

Figure 27 5 Ottawa rules for x-ray of foot and ankle.

- Anterior and anterolateral impingement syndrome can cause "chronic" ankle pain following an ankle injury
  - Anterolateral—meniscoid lesion develops in lateral gutter causing pain and intermittent "catching"
  - Lateral—development of exostoses on anterior lip of tibia or upper surface of talus, often in the setting of joint instability
- Subtalar ligament injury/sinus tarsi syndrome can result in persistent lateral ankle pain, particularly worse in the morning and on uneven surfaces
- Complex regional pain syndrome
- Ankle dislocation can occur but is rare unless a fracture has occurred

ICD-9 Codes

- 845.00 Ankle sprain, unspecified
- 845.01 Deltoid ligament sprain
- 845.03 Tibiofibular (syndesmotic) sprain

ANKLE FRACTURES

Mechanism of Injury/Pathology

- Lauge-Hansen criteria predict probable patterns of ankle injury based on the foot position at the time of injury and the direction of force exerted (Table 27.2). Abduction and adduction injuries occur with falling to the relevant side. External rotation (or eversion) injuries occur when a twisting motion occurs during the injury. Supination results in damage to lateral structures first; pronation results in damage to medial structures first.
- The Danis-Weber system focuses on the fibula injury and classifies injury based on level of the fibular fracture

Diagnostic Keys

- The key to successful management is to distinguish stable from unstable fractures. An unstable fracture results (1) from significant displacement, (2) when both the lateral and medial malleolus are fractured, or (3) when there is a unimalleolar fracture with ligament disruption on the opposite side.
- Oblique or vertical medial malleolar fractures from an inversion injury suggest a lateral ankle ligament injury and thus an unstable fracture. This usually occurs from impaction of the talus against the medial malleolus.
- Oblique fractures of the distal fibula above the level of the syndesmotic ligaments raise concern for disruption of the tibiofibular and deltoid ligaments
- Posterior distal tibial fractures displaced >2 mm or involving >25 percent of the articular surface require ORIF

Table 27.2 Lauge-Hansen Classification of Ankle Injuries

Mechanism of Injury	Progression of Injury
Supination-adduction (Weber A)	1. Injury of lateral collateral ligaments or transverse fibular avulsion fracture below level of syndesmosis 2. Vertical fracture of medial malleolus 3. Impaction or osteochondral fracture of talus
Supination-external rotation (Weber B)	1. Rupture of anterior syndesmosis 2. Spiral fracture at or above level of syndesmosis extending proximally 3. Posterior tibiofibular ligament injury 4. Medial malleolar avulsion or rupture of deltoid ligament
Pronation-external rotation (Weber C)	1. Medial malleolar avulsion or deltoid ligament rupture 2. Anterior tibiofibular ligament 3. Fracture of fibula at or above syndesmosis
Pronation-abduction (Weber C)	1. Medial malleolar avulsion or rupture of deltoid ligament 2. Fracture of fibula at or above syndesmotic ligaments 3. Interosseous membrane rupture up to level of fracture
Vertical loading	1. Tibial plafond 2. Anterior or posterior lip of tibia

Examination

- Tenderness, swelling, and ecchymosis over the bone or joint line can suggest a fracture
- If an unstable injury is suspected, stability of the joint should be assessed with stress radiographs, as this will determine need for operative vs. nonoperative management
- A thorough evaluation of neurovascular structures is always indicated. While injury to these structures is uncommon, damage can occur either by direct trauma or from a compartment syndrome.

Emergent Treatment

- The goal of emergent treatment is to stabilize the fracture and minimize swelling
  - Early application of compressive splint. A Jones dressing is commonly used, as it provides compression and immobilization while allowing for swelling.
  - Elevation and cryotherapy applied for 20 min every 2–4 h are important over the first 48–72 h
  - Avoidance of weight bearing with the use of crutches should be ensured to minimize the likelihood of fracture displacement

Tests

- X-rays: AP, lateral, and mortise views. If the mortise view is normal but an unstable injury is suspected, an external rotation and/or inversion stress view should be obtained to assess the stability of the ankle mortise. This can be done following an injection of anesthetic into the ankle joint.
- If there is a concern for compromised blood flow, compartment pressures and/or sequential Doppler imaging should be used with the clinical examination to determine if further intervention is warranted

Definitive Treatment/Follow-up/ Return to Play

- Stable, nondisplaced unimalleolar fractures are treated in a short leg walking cast or boot for 4–6 weeks. Neutral ankle position is important so as to minimize contracture of the Achilles tendon.
- Unstable fractures usually require ORIF to restore joint stability
- Follow-up radiographs should be obtained every 2 weeks to assess for fracture healing
- Ensure adequate ankle rehabilitation prior to RTP

Complications

- Nonunion
- Posttraumatic arthritis
- Fractures with articular involvement may be complicated by pain and antalgic gait
- Compartment syndrome

ICD-9 Codes

- 824.0 Medial malleolus, closed
- 824.2 Lateral malleolus, closed
- 824.4 Bimalleolar, closed
- 824.6 Trimalleolar, closed

ACHILLES TENDON INJURY

Mechanism of Injury/Pathology

- Injuries to the Achilles tendon include peritendinitis, tendinosis, and partial or complete ruptures. Predisposing conditions include (1) intrinsic factors: varus heel, forefoot supination, poor gastrocnemius-soleus flexibility and (2) extrinsic factors: a sudden increase in training, change of surface, poor footwear.
- Acute rupture is more common following prolonged tendinosis, resulting in a weakened tendon. This usually occurs in an "avascular zone" 2–6 cm proximal to the calcaneal insertion.
- Acute injury usually results from an indirect force such as pushing off while extending the knee or a forceful dorsiflexion of a plantarflexed foot

Diagnostic Keys

- The patient may describe having heard a a loud "pop" at the time of injury or the feeling of being struck in the back of the leg
- Ankle function may be surprisingly maintained secondary to recruitment of other muscle groups. This is particularly the case in partial ruptures.

Examination

- Note the presence of swelling and ecchymosis. Feel for a palpable defect in the tendon (usually 2–6 cm above the calcaneal insertion point).
- The Thompson test is performed with the patient in the prone position, ankles extended off the table. The calf muscle is squeezed, noting the

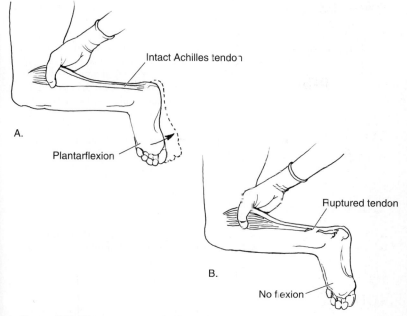

Figure 27.6 Thompson test. *A.* Normal: plantarflexion *B.* Abnormal: no flexion.

presence or absence of plantarflexion. A lack of plantarflexion suggests disruption of the Achilles tendon (Fig. 27.5)
- Strength testing often demonstrates weak or absent ankle plantarflexion

Emergent Treatment

- Rest, ice, posterior compression splint, elevation, crutches
- Analgesia as needed for pain

Tests

- Radiographs to rule out calcaneal avulsion rupture
- MRI or ultrasound should be used if a partial rupture is suspected. This will help guide definitive management.

Definitive Treatment/Follow-up/ Return to Play

- There is some controversy regarding the best treatment for an Achilles tendon rupture. Surgical repair and conservative treatment (casting) both

-233-

have advantages and disadvantages. Both options require an intensive rehabilitation program to restore range of motion and strength.

- Surgical: Surgical repair is generally considered to provide the best functional result (57 percent operative vs. 29 percent nonoperative return to previous functional level) and lowest risk of rerupture (5 percent operative vs. 13 percent nonoperative) in active individuals. There are increased risks, including scar adhesions, overlengthening, persistent equines, DVT, pulmonary embolus, and infection.
- Nonsurgical: Usually reserved for less active or elderly patients and in cases of partial rupture. The literature suggests that conservative management may provide an earlier return to work and fewer complications, but with the trade-off of increased risk of rerupture and a lower likelihood of returning to preinjury level of function.

Complications

- Unrecognized partial tear can result in persistent pain and dysfunction
- Decreased calf strength and power is a common complication following an Achilles rupture, even following treatment

ICD-9 Code

- 845.09 Achilles injury

POSTERIOR TIBIALIS OR PERONEAL TENDON DISLOCATION OR RUPTURE

Mechanism of Injury/Pathology

- Injury to the ankle can result in damage to several tendons, in particular the posterior tibial and peroneal tendons
- Dislocation of the peroneal tendon occurs from forceful passive dorsiflexion, resulting in disruption of the retinaculum
- Dislocation of the posterior tibialis is rare; however, it can occur from a dorsiflexion and inversion ankle injury resulting in forceful contraction of the posterior tibialis, which pulls the tendon from its retinaculum

Diagnostic Keys

- Patients may describe a snapping sensation in the lateral or medial ankle
- Plantarflexion of the ankle usually allows for dislocation of the respective tendon
- Consider dislocation in cases of "typical" ankle sprain that involve persistent pain, swelling, and impairment

Examination

- Posterior tibialis
  - Pain in the area of the navicular tubercle extending posteriorly behind the medial malleolus
  - Inability to raise the heel
  - Flattened medial arch
- Peroneal
  - Tenderness over peroneal tendons
  - Can dislocate tendons, particularly in plantarflexion

Emergent Treatment

- Posterior compression splint, cryotherapy crutches

Test

- MRI

Definitive Treatment/Follow-up/ Return to Play

- Early surgical repair in athletic population
- In those with low activity levels in 60- and 70-year-old age group, immobilization can be tried for 4 weeks in short leg cast that is well molded along the longitudinal arch
- RTP guided by rehabilitation

Complications

- Flattened medial arch
- Decreased strength, with resultant increased risk of recurrent ankle sprains

ICD-9 Code

- 845.00 Ankle sprain/strain, other

Bibliography

Cetti R, Christensen S, Ejsted R, et al: Operative versus nonoperative treatment of Achilles tendon rupture: A prospective randomized study and review of the literature. *Am J Sports Med* 21(6):791–799, 1993.

DeLee JC, Drez D (eds): *Orthopaedic Sports Medicine: Principles and Practice*. Philadelphia: Saunders, 1994.

Hoppenfield S, Murthy VL: *Treatment and Rehabilitation of Fractures*. Philadelphia: Lippincott Williams & Wilkins, 2000.

Kannus P, Renstrom P: Treatment for acute tears of the lateral ligament of the ankle. *J Bone Joint Surg* 73A:305–312, 1991.

Lo IKY, Kirkley A, Nonweiler B, Kumbhare DA: Operative versus non-operative treatment of acute Achilles tendon ruptures: A quantitative review. *Clin J Sports Med* 7(3):207–211, 1997.

Rockwood CA, Green DP, Bucholz RW (eds): *Rockwood and Green's Fractures in Adults*. Philadelphia: Lippincott, 1996.

Stiehll IG, Greenberg GH, McKnight RD, et al: Decision rules for the use of radiography in acute ankle injuries. *JAMA* 269:1127–1132, 1993.

28

Foot and Toe Injuries

Kevin J. Broderick

TURF TOE *1ˢᵗ MTP*

Overview

- Capsuloligamentous injury to the first metatarsophalangeal (MTP) joint
- Severe injuries may involve disruption of the plantar plate and collateral ligaments
  - Grade 1, stretched plantar capsuloligamentous complex
  - Grade 2, partially torn plantar capsuloligamentous complex without articular injury
  - Grade 3, completely torn plantar complex with compression injury to dorsal articular surface

stiff - soled shoes.

Mechanism (Fig. 28.1)

- Forced dorsiflexion of the MTP joint of the toe

Examination/Evaluation

- Erythema and swelling over the MTP joint of the big toe
- Tenderness to palpation at the MTP joint
- Pain with passive movement of the MTP joint

Emergent Treatment

- Rest, ice, compression
- Tape the toe in plantarflexion

Tests

- AP, lateral x-rays of toe to rule out fracture

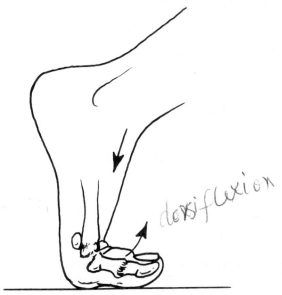

Figure 28.1 Turf toe mechanism.

Definitive Treatment/Follow-up/ Return to Play

- Dependent on the degree of the injury
- Initially, rest, ice, compression, elevation (RICE)
- Early range-of-motion exercises followed by strengthening as symptoms allow
  - Grade 1—return to play as tolerated with stiff-soled shoes to prevent dorsiflexion and taping of the toe
  - Grade 2—refrain from play for 1–2 weeks while wearing stiff-soled shoes, then as in grade 1
  - Grade 3—remove from play for 3–6 weeks while wearing stiff-soled shoes, then as in grade 1
- Consider use of orthotics with rigid forefoot

Complications

- Persistent pain and decreased range of motion

ICD-9 Code

- 845.12 Strain of MTP joint

SESAMOIDITIS AND SESAMOID FRACTURES

Overview

- These lesions involve the sesamoid bones, located in the flexor hallicus brevis tendon under the first metatarsal head

Mechanism

- Sesamoiditis may be secondary to a single traumatic event or due to repeated stress
- Fractures typically follow an acute event resulting in a traumatic force to the sesamoid bones or, less commonly, from forced dorsiflexion of the big toe

Examination/Evaluation

- Tender to palpation under the first metatarsal head over the sesamoid bones
- Pain may be felt with forced dorsiflexion of the toe
- Decrease range of motion of first MTP joint

Emergent Treatment

- Hard-soled postsurgical shoe, rest, ice, and analgesics

Tests

- AP and lateral x-rays of foot with axial views of the sesamoid bones
- Fractures must be distinguished from bipartite or multipartite sesamoid bones

Definitive Treatment/Follow-up/ Return to Play

- Stiff-soled postsurgical or hard-soled shoe
- J-shaped, donut, or metatarsal pad may relieve pressure
- Tape toe in plantarflexion
- Fractures require walking cast for 3–4 weeks, followed by a stiff-soled shoe with unloading via a donut or metatarsal pad
- Surgical excision is a last resort

Complication

- Persistent pain

ICD-9 Code

- 733.99 Sesamoiditis

INTERPHALANGEAL JOINT DISLOCATIONS

Overview

- Often associated with a fracture

interphalangeal joint dislocation

Mechanism

- Direct trauma or axial load

Examination/Evaluation

- Swelling, ecchymosis, and tenderness to palpation at the involved joint
- Decreased range of motion of the involved joint

Emergent Treatment

- Closed reduction using longitudinal traction and gentle downward pressure on the dislocated phalange under a digital block

Tests

- AP, lateral, and oblique x-rays of the foot

Definitive Treatment/Follow-up/ Return to Play

- Buddy tape to next toe for 2–3 weeks
- Refer unstable reductions

Complications

* Recurrent dislocation, instability

ICD-9 Code

* Interphalangeal joint dislocations
  * 838.09 Closed
  * 838.19 Open

PHALANGEAL FRACTURES

Overview

* These fractures most commonly involve the proximal phalange of the big toe
* Interosseous, abductor, adductor, and flexor muscles insert at the bases of the proximal phalanges and may cause displacement of the proximal fragment

Mechanism

* Direct trauma or axial load, such as "stubbing" of the toe

Examination/Evaluation

* Pain, swelling, ecchymosis, and tenderness to palpation in the area of the fracture

Emergent Treatment

* If displaced, closed reduction under a digital block
* Buddy tape to neighboring toe with gauze between the two toes

Tests

* AP, lateral, and oblique x-rays of the foot

Definitive Treatment/Follow-up/ Return to Play

* Refer open fractures or displaced articular fractures

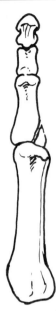

Figure 28.2 Proximal interphalangeal joint fracture.

- Displaced intraarticular fractures of the big toe generally require internal fixation
- Fractures that spontaneously displace after traction is released often require internal fixation and should be referred
- Nondisplaced intraarticular fractures that involve >25 percent of the joint surface should also be referred (Fig. 28.2)

Complications

- Degenerative changes, malunion
- Angulation of the big toe may lead to persistent symptoms, whereas angulation of the lesser toes is generally well tolerated

ICD-9 Codes

- Phalangeal fractures
  - 826.0 Closed
  - 826.1 Open

LISFRANC'S FRACTURE

Overview

- Traumatic disruption of the tarsometatarsal joint
- Often missed

Mechanism (Fig. 28.3)

- Two types—direct and indirect injuries
- Direct injuries are due to a crushing blow to the joint, causing dislocation/subluxation
- Indirect injuries are more commonly seen in sports. These mechanisms include

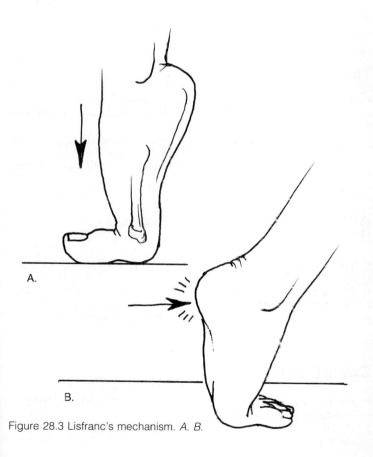

Figure 28.3 Lisfranc's mechanism. *A. B.*

- Forceful abduction of the forefoot while the hindfoot is in a fixed position
- Axial load to a plantarflexed foot ("tip-toe" position)
- A strike from behind by another player on a plantarflexed foot that is fixed on the ground

Examination/Evaluation

- Pain in the dorsum of the midfoot
- Tenderness to palpation and swelling over the tarsometatarsal joint
- Pain with forefoot rotation and abduction while the hindfoot is held fixed

Emergent Treatment

- Non-weight-bearing posterior splint
- Elevation of the involved extremity

Tests

- AP, lateral, and oblique x-rays of the foot must be obtained
- The medial aspect of the second cuneiform should align with the base of the second metatarsal
- The medial edge of the base of the fourth metatarsal should align with the medial edge of the cuboid on the oblique view
- Obtain weight-bearing views of both feet for more subtle injuries if there is clinical suspicion

Definitive Treatment/Follow-up/ Return to Play

- Any diastasis or fracture will require operative reduction and screw fixation
- Orthopedic referral is indicated for any fracture, dislocation, or instability of the tarsometatarsal joint
- Nondisplaced sprains without fracture or diastasis may be treated with non-weight-bearing short leg cast

Complications

- Missed injury results in the loss of normal foot mechanics and function, leading to chronic foot pain
- A high percentage of patients will have chronic pain despite appropriate treatment

ICD-9 Codes

- 825.24 Fracture of cuneiform, closed
- 825.25 Fracture of metatarsal bone, closed

JONES FRACTURE

Overview

- Fracture of the proximal fifth metatarsal diaphysis located >0.5 cm and <1.5 cm from the proximal tip of the fifth metatarsal
- Fracture involves the joint between the base of the fourth and fifth metatarsals
- Three types: I—acute, II—delayed union, III—nonunion (Fig. 28.4)

Mechanism

- May result from a pivot in the opposite direction of the planted foot

Examination/Evaluation

- Pain, swelling, ecchymosis, and tenderness to palpation over the proximal fifth metatarsal

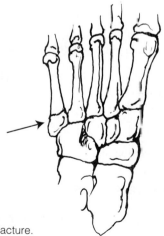

Figure 28.4 Jones fracture.

Emergent Treatment

- RICE (rest, ice, compression, elevation)
- Non-weight-bearing cast for acute fractures

Tests

- AP, lateral, and oblique x-rays of the foot

Definitive Treatment/Follow-up/ Return to Play

- Non-weight-bearing short leg cast for acute fractures
- To allow earlier return to play consider surgical fixation for acute fractures
- Delayed or nonunion fractures may require surgical fixation

Complications

- High rate of nonunion and delayed union

ICD-9 Codes

- 825.25 Metatarsal fracture, closed
- 825.35 Metatarsal fracture, open

AVULSION FRACTURE OF THE FIFTH METATARSAL

Overview

- Located near the insertion of the peroneal brevis at the base of the fifth metatarsal
- Fracture located within 0.5 cm of the proximal tip of the fifth metatarsal
- Often associated with lateral ankle sprains (Fig. 28.5)

Mechanism

- Usually due to an inversion injury

Examination/Evaluation

- Pain, tenderness to palpation, possible swelling at the base of the fifth metatarsal

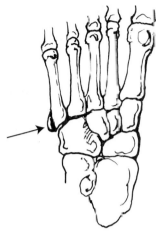

Figure 28.5 Avulsion fracture, fifth metatarsal.

Emergent Treatment

- Cast, cast boot, or stiff-soled shoe
- Crutches until painless weight bearing is possible

Tests

- AP, lateral, and oblique x-rays of the foot

Definitive Treatment/Follow-up/ Return to Play

- Cast, cast boot, or stiff-soled shoe for 3–4 weeks
- Range-of-motion exercises, then strengthening of the peroneal brevis
- Any displaced or comminuted fracture requires referral
- Return to play after 3–4 weeks or when symptoms have resolved

Complication

- Nonunion

ICD-9 Codes

- 825.25 Metatarsal fracture, closed
- 825.35 Metatarsal fracture, open

METATARSAL STRESS FRACTURE

Overview

- These fractures most commonly occur in the second metatarsal
- Most frequent in track, running, and dance
- Patients complain of dull, aching pain in the forefoot that increases with activity

Mechanism

- Repetitive stress injury

Examination/Evaluation

- There may be swelling
- Tenderness to palpation over fracture site
- Pain with mobilization of the affected metatarsal

Emergent Treatment

- Weight bearing as tolerated
- Rest and elevation

Tests

- X-rays may not be positive for 2–3 weeks. AP and lateral x-rays of the foot may show cortical thickening or a radiolucent line.
- Bone scan if there is clinical suspicion and x-rays are negative
- MRI for definitive diagnosis if there is still uncertainty after x-rays and bone scan (generally not indicated)

Definitive Treatment/Follow-up/ Return to Play

- Rest is the definitive treatment
- Postsurgical wooden shoe for 4–6 weeks. No weight bearing if symptoms demand.
- Return to play when pain-free and able to ambulate without a limp

Complications

- Completion or displacement of the fracture, nonunion

ICD-9 Code

- 825.25 Metatarsal fracture, closed

CALCANEAL FRACTURE

Overview

- Relatively uncommon
- 70–75 percent are intraarticular

ecchymosis
ecchymosis

Mechanism

Dx by CT scan.

- Intraarticular fractures typically result from acute trauma, such as a fall from a height
- Extraarticular fractures result from a twisting mechanism or muscular avulsion

Examination/Evaluation

- Tenderness to palpation over the fracture site with associated swelling plus or minus ecchymosis
- Look for associated soft tissue injury, spinal fracture, or additional lower extremity fracture
- Rule out compartment syndrome of the foot, which is suggested by significant swelling in the arch of the foot

Emergent Treatment

- Ice, elevation, analgesics, and compressive splint
- No weight bearing for 48–72 h

Tests

- X-rays: AP, lateral, and axial calcaneal views
- CT if intraarticular fracture is suspected clinically or suggested by x-rays

Definitive Treatment/Follow-up/ Return to Play

- Most nondisplaced extraarticular fractures can be managed conservatively with RICE and compressive dressing, followed by toe-touch ambulation for 4–6 weeks

- Displaced extraarticular fractures that require closed reduction can generally be treated conservatively with a short leg cast for 4–6 weeks, followed by a gradual return to activity
- Exceptions to conservative management include a decrease in the Bohr angle by 10 degrees when compared to the contralateral side or displaced avulsions of the Achilles tendon. These should be referred.
- Intraarticular fractures must be referred.
- All cases of compartment syndrome should be referred emergently

Complications

- Reflex sympathetic dystrophy, nonunion, compartment syndrome, chronic pain, and arthritis

ICD-9 Codes   *fall from hight*

- 825.0 Calcaneal fracture closed
- 825.1 Calcaneal fracture, open

HEEL FAT-PAD SYNDROME

Overview

- The heel pad is made of small compartments containing fat and is surrounded by fibrous connective tissue. Disruptions of the fibrous tissue septa or loss of fat leads to less cushioning, causing pain over the heel pad with weight bearing.

Mechanism

- A direct blow to the bottom of the heel; may also be due to degeneration

Examination/Evaluation

- Tenderness over the weight-bearing portion of the calcaneus

Emergent Treatment

- NSAIDS, modified weight-bearing activities, heel cup

Tests

- AP, lateral, and oblique x-rays to rule out other etiologies
- Consider bone scan or MRI if stress fracture is suspected

Definitive Treatment/Follow-up/ Return to Play

- As in emergent treatment
- Consider corticosteroid injection with care, as it poses a risk for fat atrophy or disruption of the septa, which can worsen the condition
- Well-padded shoes
- Condition is usually self-limited

Complication

- Persistent symptoms

ICD-9 Code

- 924.20 Heel contusion

NAVICULAR STRESS FRACTURE

Overview *track athletes*

- Rare but underappreciated. Most commonly occurs in track athletes.
- Patients complain of vague dorsal midfoot pain

Mechanism

- Repetitive stress injury

Examination/Evaluation

- Tenderness to palpation over the navicular between the anterior tibialis and the extensor hallicus longus tendons

Emergent Treatment

- Non-weight-bearing below-the-knee cast or removable brace with crutches for 4–6 weeks

Tests *Navicular stress fracture*

- AP, lateral, and oblique x-rays of the foot are often normal
- Bone scan typically shows increased uptake throughout the entire navicular
- CT scan with thin-sliced cuts is helpful to determine whether fracture is complete

Definitive Treatment/Follow-up/ Return to Play

- Progress slowly. Average time to return to play is 5–6 months from diagnosis.
- Surgical treatment with internal screw and bone grafting may be necessary for those who fail to respond to conservative treatment

Complications

- Failure to respond to nonoperative treatment

ICD-9 Code

- 825.29 Navicular stress fracture

Bibliography

DeLee JC, Drez D (eds): *Orthopaedic Sports Medicine: Principles and Practice.* Philadelphia: Saunders, 1994.

Eiff M, Hatch R, Calmbach W: *Fracture Management for Primary Care.* Philadelphia: Saunders, 1998.

Rockwood CA, Green DP (eds): *Fractures in Adults and Children.* Philadelphia: Lippincott, 2001.

29

Contusions

Chris McGilmer

SOFT TISSUE CONTUSIONS

Mechanism of Injury/Pathology

- An acute traumatic injury due to direct blunt trauma to soft tissue such as skin, muscle, ligaments, tendons and adipose tissue; prevalent in contact sports
- Contusions can be very painful and are usually associated with significant swelling
- Extravasation of blood into surrounding muscle and soft tissue may worsen swelling
- Eventual formation of heterotropic bone and cartilage—known as myositis ossificans traumatica (MOT)—may develop at intramuscular hematoma sites
- MOT occurs mainly in the quadriceps muscles but may be seen in other muscle groups exposed to direct trauma, such as those of the upper arm and calf

Diagnostic Keys

- Athletes may initially experience minimal pain or discomfort and are usually able to continue sport
- Afterwards, when athlete cools down, pain, swelling, and stiffness rapidly develop
- With a significant blow, the athlete may present with limp, muscle spasm, and a mass
- If there is no improvement with standard therapy or regression, MOT and other complications should be suspected

Examination

- Observe for swelling, ecchymosis, and tenderness of involved muscle
- Increased pain is noted with active muscle contraction and passive muscle stretch

- Restricted range of motion of joint above or below the involved muscle may develop
- Early palpable mass suggests a hematoma and late masses suggest MOT

Emergent Treatment

- Mild contusions can be treated with rest, ice, analgesics, and a compression dressing
- NSAIDs in first 48 h may increase risk of bleeding and exacerbate hematoma formation
- Moderate contusions should be treated as above with immobilization of involved muscle in a stretched position and possibly crutches
- For severe contusions aspiration of a large hematoma—to minimize subsequent recovery time—may be considered
- Some practitioners have even advocated injection of local anesthetic and/or steroids; however, data supporting this practice are sparse and the risk of complications must be considered
- Initial avoidance of heat and other physical therapy modalities is important, as they may exacerbate bleeding and hematoma formation

Tests

- Radiographs are rarely indicated but may be helpful in cases of severe trauma to rule out a fracture
- Radiologic evidence of MOT may take 6–8 weeks after initial injury to become positive
- Ultrasound and bone scan may demonstrate MOT before plain films
- CT may be needed if surgical excision of MOT is indicated
- Significant or recurrent bruising may warrant workup for coagulation disorder
- Intercompartmental catheter pressure readings may be indicated if compartment syndrome is suspected

Definitive Treatment/Follow-up/ Return to Play

- Most athletes are able to return to play with protective padding once swelling is reduced, range of motion has returned, and pain is tolerable
- Rehabilitation to increase range of motion and eventually strength before return to play may be needed
- NSAIDs have been shown to decrease the incidence of progression to MOT
- Light massage and transcutaneous electrical nerve stimulation (TENS) may be helpful after the initial inflammatory phase subsides
- For severe contusions, a much more gradual rehabilitation program is needed to avoid repetitive microtrauma and complication of MOT

- MOT with persistent limited range of motion may require surgical excision of heterotropic bone formation once it has matured, usually 6–12 months after initial injury
- Compartment syndrome warrants emergent surgical release

Complications

- Myositis ossificans traumatica
- Compartment syndrome
- Traumatic pseudoaneurysm
- Thrombophlebitis

ICD-9 Codes

- 728.12 Myositis ossificans traumatica
- 924.00 Quadriceps contusion or hematoma

Bibliography

Anderson K, Strickland S, Warren R: Hip and groin injuries in athletes. *Am J Sports Med* 29(4):521–533, 2001.

Bracker M, Rice L, Yassini P: The 5-Minute Sports Medicine Consult. Philadelphia: Lippincott Williams & Wilkins, 2001.

Gindele A, Schwamborn D, Tsironis K, Benz-Bohm G: Myositis ossificans traumatica in young children: Report of three cases and review of the literature. *Pediatr Radiol* 30:451–459, 2000.

Jespen M, Graham S: Traumatic myositis ossificans of the levator scapulae muscle. *Am J Otolaryngol* 19(5):345–348, 1998.

King J: Post-traumatic ectopic calcification in the muscles of athletes: A review. *Br J Sports Med* 32(4):287–290, 1998.

Part 3

Sports- and Event-Specific Concerns

30

Baseball and Softball

Quincy Wang

INTRODUCTION

- Baseball and softball are generally safe sports. Potential injury comes from being hit by a thrown or batted ball, being hit with a bat, impact with the ground during a slide or dive, and overuse.

SOFT TISSUE INJURIES

Contusions

- Contusions are among the most common although minor injuries suffered in baseball and softball
- Supportive care with icing and protective padding is generally all that is needed for treatment
- Be aware of potential fracture at contusion site
- Common contusion areas
  - Wrist—contusions often to the heel of the glove hand with infielders. Padded extensions to the heel of the glove can be attached to limit further injury.
  - Shin and foot—usually from foul-tipped, batted balls that strike the lower leg. Soccer-style shin guards and those with extensions to protect the medial ankle and foot can be used as a protective measure.
  - Chest and face—usually a result of being hit by a pitched ball. At the level of Little League Baseball, there are advocates for the use of chest protectors by batters to prevent commotio cordis (impact-induced ventricular arrhythmia) as well as the use of face masks on batting helmets to prevent facial injury.

Abrasions and Lacerations

- Abrasions
  - Often occur on the hands, forearms/elbows, knees, thighs, and buttocks. Usually due to sliding or diving.
  - Treatment consists of thorough irrigation, topical antibiotic, and dressing to protect from recontamination. Tetanus status should be reviewed and universal precautions followed.
  - Protective measures include the use of gloves, pads, and sliding shorts, as abrasions can plague the athlete the whole season if reabrasion occurs
- Lacerations (see Chap. 16)
  - Treatment consists of anesthesia, irrigation and debridement, suturing under sterile conditions, and sterile dressings
  - Review tetanus status; universal precautions should be followed

Return to Play

- Return to play is allowed for simple abrasions and superficial lacerations that can be definitively treated quickly on the sidelines
- For more serious abrasions and lacerations, the team physician must decide if temporary wound management with delayed treatment is appropriate. If return to play will worsen the wound—increasing the risk of further tissue damage, wound contamination, or the contamination of others—the athlete should not return to play.

SHOULDER (SEE CHAP. 24)

Rotator Cuff

- The rotator cuff consists of the **S**upraspinatus, **I**nfraspinatus **T**eres minor, and **S**ubscapularis (**SITS** muscles). The rotator cuff abducts and externally rotates the arm.
- Maximal stress occurs during the deceleration and follow-through phases of throwing

Rotator Cuff Tendinitis/ Shoulder Impingement Syndrome

Definition

- Pain and inflammation of the rotator cuff muscles from repetitive throwing

Symptoms

- Painful throwing followed by a progressive decrease in the velocity and distance of throws. Shoulder pain with any overhead motion.

Signs

- Pain to the proximal humerus, near the tip of the acromion. Weakness secondary to pain with external rotation and abduction of the arm. Pain with Neer and Hawkins maneuvers. Night pain. Pain at rest if severe.

Treatment

- Relative rest—limiting repetitions and velocity of throwing below the threshold of pain. Total rest (about 2–4 weeks) if any throwing causes severe pain. Advance throwing as tolerated with a controlled, progressive throwing program.
- Medications—NSAIDs of choice as tolerated. Subacromial steroid injection effective in treating pain and inflammation. One week of rest recommended after injection.
- Ice—two to three times per day
- Rehabilitation program—stretching and strengthening exercises for the rotator cuff muscles. Also include exercises for scapular stabilization, back strength, and leg strength to maintain the "kinetic chain" of body parts involved with throwing.

Complications

- Chronic impingement syndrome that is not responsive to therapy may require surgical acromioplasty if a type II (curved) or III (hooked) acromion is seen on radiographs
- Chronic impingement syndrome may lead to further degeneration of the rotator cuff muscles, resulting in full or partial rotator cuff tears
- Adhesive capsulitis may develop if prolonged immobilization is used and therapy is delayed

Rotator Cuff Tears

Definition

- Full- or partial-thickness tears of the rotator cuff tendons at their attachment to the proximal humerus

Mechanism

- Generally seen in older athletes over 40 years of age due to chronic overuse
- Occurs with acute injury or trauma when seen in younger athletes

Evaluation

- Pain with overhead motion
- Decreased range of motion or inability to raise arm overhead

- Weakness or pain with abduction and/or external rotation
- Rotator cuff atrophy if injury is of long standing
- Positive drop-arm test—from 90 degrees of abduction athlete unable to lower the arm smoothly and slowly. Tapping the arm will cause it to drop to his side.
- Subacromial injection of lidocaine eliminates pain but weakness of or the inability to abduct or externally rotate the arm persists

Imaging Studies

- Plain radiographs may show calcific tendonitis if injury is of long standing. A type II (curved) or III (hooked) acromion may also be seen.
- MRI may be helpful in identifying a rotator cuff tear

Treatment

- NSAIDs and ice to control pain and inflammation
- Partial tears can be responsive to relative rest, physical therapy, and a progressive throwing program
- Subacromial steroid injection effective in treating pain and inflammation. 1 week of rest after injection recommended.
- Orthopedic referral warranted for full thickness tears

Biceps Groove Tendinitis

Definition

- Pain and inflammation of the long head of biceps in the region of the biceps groove of the humerus

Mechanism

- Chronic overuse with repetitive overhand or underhand throwing

Evaluation

- Pain with throwing to the anterior shoulder
- Point tenderness to the biceps groove
- Positive Speed's test
- Pain to the biceps groove with resisted supination of the wrist
- Pain to the biceps groove when stretching arm by extending posteriorly with elbow flexed
- No pain or weakness with abduction or external rotation
- Negative drop-arm test

Treatment

- Relative rest
- NSAIDs and ice
- Physical therapy and progressive throwing program

Glenoid Labrum Tears

- Superior labrum anterior to posterior (SLAP) tears can occur with overhead throwing. The superior labrum is the site of attachment of the long head of the biceps tendon.

Mechanism

- Chronic repetitive traction of the long head of the biceps tendon during overhead throwing can lead to a SLAP lesion
- Acute injury to the glenoid labrum in baseball and softball usually occurs with landing on an outstretched arm, as during head-first sliding. Direct compression of the glenoid labrum or acute traction to the biceps tendon can lead to a glenoid labrum tear.
- Dislocation of the shoulder often results in injury to the glenoid labrum

Evaluation

- Painful throwing with decreased velocity, even after prolonged rest
- Repetitive "click" associated with throwing and with specific shoulder motions
- Pain with abduction and external rotation. Reproducible click with passive motion may be present.
- Physical examination findings may overlap with other shoulder pathology (e.g., rotator cuff injury, shoulder instability), which makes diagnosis difficult.
- Plain radiographs are not helpful but can rule out other pathology
- Saline or contrast-injected MRI of the shoulder is helpful if positive; however, the false-negative rate is high

Treatment

- NSAIDs, ice, and relative rest
- Shoulder rehabilitation with a progressive throwing program
- Orthopedic referral if the problem persists, as definitive diagnosis and treatment may require surgical intervention

ELBOW (SEE CHAP. 23)

Medial Epicondylitis

Definition

- Medial elbow pain from stress applied to the medial epicondyle during repetitive throwing

Mechanism

- Valgus stress to the medial epicondyle during throwing is due to tension applied by the ulnar collateral ligament (UCL) and wrist/finger flexors, which attach to the medial epicondyle
- Avulsion fracture of the medial epicondyle is a possible complication if symptoms are left untreated in the skeletally immature athlete

Evaluation

- History consistent for pain to medial elbow with decreased throwing distance and velocity
- Pain often continues after games and practices
- Constant pain even at rest, lateral elbow pain, and/or numbness radiating to the hand (ulnar nerve distribution) may indicate more serious injury
- Palpation of medial epicondyle resisted wrist/finger flexion, and valgus stress of the elbow in slight flexion creates pain
- Positive laxity with valgus stress and a positive Tinel's sign at the cubital tunnel are signs of more serious injury
- Three-view radiographs are recommended if avulsion fracture is suspected in the skeletally immature athlete. Bilateral comparison views are helpful.
- Medial epicondylar fractures displaced greater than 5 mm warrant orthopedic referral

Treatment

- NSAIDs, ice
- Rest, no throwing activities until pain-free—generally within 2–4 weeks
- Begin progressive throwing program as well as wrist/forearm strengthening exercises
- Avulsion fractures displaced <5 mm: complete rest with sling and posterior splint (long arm cast can also be used) for 2–3 weeks until pain-free with daily activities. Progressive throwing can begin if pain-free and radiographs show healing of the fracture fragment (generally 4–6 weeks).

Ulnar Collateral Ligament Injuries

Definition

- Pain and instability at the medial aspect of the elbow due to sprain/attenuation or rupture of the ulnar collateral ligament
- Injury to the anterior band (specifically the posterior bundle of the anterior band) leads to medial elbow laxity
- Usually seen in skeletally mature athletes 16–40 years of age

Evaluation

- Medial elbow pain with throwing, with decreased velocity and distance of throws
- Sensation of the elbow "opening" during the late cocking and/or acceleration phase of throwing
- Elbow "pop" during a throw is the classic initiating event; however, low-grade medial elbow pain that worsens with throwing is the more common history
- Pain on palpation 2 cm distal to the medial epicondyle at the insertion of the ulnar collateral ligament or the ulna
- Lateral and posterior elbow pain as well as ulnar nerve paresthesia are additional complications of medial elbow laxity
- Valgus stress test positive for laxity. Lock the athlete's hand and wrist between the examiner's elbow and trunk. Bend the elbow 30 degrees to free the olecranon from the olecranon fossa. Gently apply valgus stress to the elbow with the heel of the examiner's hand, noting for laxity at the medial joint line of the elbow. Compare to the opposite side. Increased laxity or no firm end point indicates incompetence of the ulnar collateral ligament.
- Valgus stress radiographs can show laxity. If the distance of the medial joint space of the elbow is larger than the unaffected elbow under valgus stress, injury of the ulnar collateral ligament is suspected.
- MRI—can be helpful if positive. False-negative readings may be encountered with attenuation of the ulnar collateral ligament.

Treatment

- Surgical—indicated for athletes with a complete rupture of the ulnar collateral ligament who wish to return to high-level throwing activities. Surgery is also indicated for persistent medial elbow pain and instability after nonsurgical treatment for 3 months or more.
- Nonsurgical—if evaluation reveals no complete tear of the ulnar collateral ligament, a trial of nonsurgical treatment is warranted. Complete rest for 2–4 weeks is followed by a wrist/elbow-strengthening program. Throwing can begin at 3 months.

Osteochondritis Dissecans of the Elbow

Definitions

- Articular surface degeneration due to repetitive microtrauma
- Osteochondral fracture, loose bodies, and avascular necrosis are potential complications

Mechanism

- Osteochondritis dissecans of the elbow usually occurs at the radiocapitellar joint due to compressive forces across this joint during throwing

Evaluation

- Gradual onset of pain with worsening to the lateral aspect of the elbow
- Pain with palpation to the lateral and anterior aspect of the elbow
- Decreased range of motion with supination and pronation. Flexion contracture can also be present.
- Plain radiographs will be positive for a osteochondral lesion or loose body of the capitellum
- MRI is helpful to assist in staging and determination of a loose fragment
- Bone scans are helpful in identifying vascularity and serving as a prognostic indicator

Treatment

- Complete rest. No throwing or physical stress to the elbow for 2–3 months.
- Physical therapy can begin once pain resolves
- Progressive throwing can resume once evidence of healing is seen via MRI or bone scan
- Surgical treatment is warranted for failed nonsurgical treatment, formation of loose bodies, or if the osteochondral defect is large

ANKLE SPRAIN (SEE CHAP. 27)

KNEE INJURY (SEE CHAP. 26)

HEAT INJURY (SEE CHAP. 17)

EYE INJURY (SEE CHAP. 12)

BASEBALL VS. SOFTBALL

Baseball Phases of Pitching

- Phase I—windup and cocking
- Phase II—acceleration and release
- Phase III—deceleration and follow-through

Softball Phases of Pitching

- Phase I—windup and stride
- Phase II—delivery
- Phase III—follow-through

Delivery Mechanics

- Baseball—humerus positioned perpendicular to the plane of the body
- Softball—humerus positioned parallel to the plane of the body

Power Generation

- Baseball
  - Leg push-off
  - Hip and shoulder rotation from "closed" to "open" position (with reference to home plate)
  - Internal rotation of the humerus
- Softball
  - Leg push-off
  - Hip and shoulder rotation from "open to closed" position (with reference to home plate)
  - Adduction of the humerus across the body

Arm Deceleration

- Baseball—eccentric contraction forces from the rotator cuff
- Softball—contact of the arm to the thigh and torso as well as some forces from the rotator cuff

Peak Shoulder Distraction Forces

- Baseball—peak forces occur in phase III during the deceleration phase
- Softball—peak forces occur in phase II during delivery

Common Baseball Shoulder Injuries

- Rotator cuff impingement or tear
- Glenoid labrum tear

Common Softball Shoulder Injuries

- Biceps groove tendinitis of long head of biceps
- Pectoralis and subscapularis strain

Bibliography

Bryan WJ:. Baseball and softball, in Reider B (ed): *Sports Medicine: The School-Aged Athlete*. Philadelphia: Saunders, 1996, pp 491–541.

Mueller FO, Marshall SW: Injuries in little league baseball from 1987 through 1996. *Phys Sports Med* 29(7):41–48, 2001.

Richards DB: Injuries to the glenoid labrum: A diagnostic and treatment challenge. *Phys Sports Med* 27(6):73, 1999.

Rubin AL: Managing abrasions and lacerations. *Phys Sports Med* 26(5):45, 1998.

Safran MR: Elbow injuries in athletes. *Clin Orthop* 310:257–277, 1995.

Wang QC, Rubin AL, Safran MR: Ulnar collateral ligament injuries of the elbow, in Bracker MD (ed): *The 5-Minute Sports Medicine Consult*. Philadelphia: Lippincott Williams &Wilkins, 2001, pp 320–321.

Wolin PM, Tarbet JA:. Rotator cuff injury: Addressing overhead use. *Phys Sports Med* 25(6):54, 1997.

31

Basketball

Marc R. Safran
Denise M. Romero

ANKLE (MOST COMMON SITE OF BASKETBALL INJURIES)

Common Injuries (See Chap. 27)

- Lateral ankle sprain—most commonly involving the anterior talofibular ligament (ATFL) and the calcaneofibular ligament (CFL)
- Medial ankle sprain—involving the deltoid ligament
  - Must be differentiated from avulsion fracture of medial malleolus
- High ankle sprain—involving the interosseous membrane of the anterior intraosseous talofibular ligament (ATFL, or AITFL

Specialized Equipment Needs

- High-top sports shoes
- Ankle brace (lace-up or stirrup)
- Athletic tape

Treatment

- Rest, ice, compression, and elevation (RICE). Early motion with bracing or taping. Uncommonly, immobilization with cast. Early range-of-motion (ROM) exercises, strengthening, proprioceptive training, and prophylactic bracing/taping. Surgery rarely necessary.

Return to Play

- Demonstrated ability to perform sports-specific activities. Prophylactic ankle stabilization is recommended.

KNEE (SEE CHAP. 26)

- Second most common site for basketball injury
- Common injuries
  - Ligamentous injuries—most commonly involving the anterior cruciate ligament (ACL) and medial collateral ligament (MCL). Laxity in injured ligament may be elicited.
  - Medial or lateral meniscus tears—with joint-line tenderness, swelling, decreased ROM, locking, and giving way of the knee. Lateral more common in basketball than many other sports.
  - Patellar tendinitis or "jumper's knee" and Osgood-Schlatter disease in adolescents. Iliotibial band inflammation, inflamed medial plica, and pes anserinus syndrome.
  - Patellofemoral tracking problems—more common in females

Specialized Equipment Needs

- Knee sleeve may aid in return to play for mild MCL injuries
- Patellar tendon band or knee sleeve may aid in return to play for patellar tendinitis

Treatment

- ACL—for return to competitive play, surgical reconstruction is often required. In adolescents with open growth plates, treatment may be conservative, with activity modification, hamstring strengthening, and knee bracing.
- MCL—conservative treatment with active and passive ROM, strengthening of quadriceps and hamstrings, and hinged bracing if severe
- Meniscus—surgical repair for peripheral tears or partial/total meniscectomy for irreparable tears
- Patellar tendinitis—activity limited by symptom, hamstring and quadriceps stretching and strengthening, RICE, ultrasound, NSAIDs, and patellar tendon taping
- Patellofemoral—quadriceps strengthening (leg press not to exceed 90 degrees flexion), McConnell taping, and patella-restraining brace

Return to Play

- Meniscus (see Chap. 26)
- ACL—typically 6 months following reconstructive surgery or 3–6 months following nonoperative rehabilitation, with full ROM, good strength, and freedom from pain
- MCL—ligament nontender to palpation or stress, minimal ligament laxity, full ROM, and good strength
- Tendinitis—activity limited by symptoms

BACK

Common Injuries

- Lumbosacral sprains, stress fractures to pars interarticularis, and disk injuries

Treatment

- Rest, ice, compression, ROM exercises, strengthening of lumbosacral and abdominal musculature, rehabilitation of deficiencies in lower extremities, and bracing. Epidural injections and surgery may be considered with disk injuries.

Return to Play

- Sprains—activity limited by pain. Stress fracture—typically 3–6 months, occasionally back bracing may be indicated. Back surgery—following 4–6 months of rehabilitation.

LOWER EXTREMITY

Common Injuries

- Overuse injuries are common and may be exacerbated during play, requiring treatment during play
  - Periosteal inflammation (shin splints)
  - Stress fractures including tibial (34 percent), fibular (24 percent), metatarsal (18 percent), and other bones of the foot
    - Proximal fracture of fifth metatarsal (see Chap. 28)
- Tendinitis and tendon ruptures
  - Achilles, quadriceps, patellar, peroneus longus or brevis, anterior or posterior tibialis, or long toe flexor

Treatment

- Inflammation and tendinitis—RICE, stretching, strengthening, NSAIDs, ultrasound, and taping of affected area
- Tendon rupture—requires surgical repair
- Stress fractures—rest. Other fractures—surgery or immobilization by casting.

Return to Play

- Tendon rupture—healing may take up to 1 year following surgery. Inflammation and tendinitis—activity is limited by symptoms. Fracture—varies by degree and site of fracture.

OTHER PROBLEMS

- Shoulder impingement or rotator cuff injuries (see Chap. 24)
- Shoulder dislocation (see Chap. 24)
- Phalangeal dislocation (see Chap. 22)
- Metacarpal interphalangeal dislocation (see Chap. 22)
- Concussion (see Chap. 6)
- Eye trauma (see Chap. 12)
- Facial fracture (see Chap. 10)
- Dental injury (see Chap. 2)
- Sudden cardiac death (see Chaps. 3, 4, and 5)

SPECIALIZED EQUIPMENT NEEDS

- Splint material (see Chap. 19)
- Ophthalmoscope and eye tray (see Chap. 58)

Bibliography

Bassett FH III: Basketball, in Fu FH, Stone DA (eds): *Sports Injuries: Mechanisms, Prevention, and Treatment.* Lippincott Williams & Wilkins, 1994, pp 209–222.

Caborn DNM, Coen MJ: Basketball, in Safran MR, Van Camp SP, McKeag D (eds): *Spiral Manual of Sports Medicine.* Philadelphia: Lippincott-Raven, 1998, pp 544–545.

32

Bicycling (Road and Mountain Biking)

John Martinez

INTRODUCTION

Road Cycling

- International organizations: Union Cycliste Internationale (UCI)
- National organizations: USA Cycling U.S. Cycling Federation (USCF), U.S. Professional Racing Organization (USPRO)

Types of Races

Road (One-Day) or Stage (Multiple-Day) Race

- Mass-start, point-to-point race
- Distances vary from 40 to over 100 mi for elite cyclists
- No aerobars allowed for mass-start events

Criterium

- A short loop (0.5 to 1.5 mi) closed course for a specific amount of time (30–90 min)
- No aerobars allowed for mass-start events

Time Trial

- Individual rider start at specific intervals apart (30 s to 3 min)
- Aerobars and solid-disk wheels allowed

Track

- Races held on banked oval track—include individual and team races
- Single-fixed-gear bikes without brakes

Mountain Biking

- National organization: National Off Road Bike Association (NORBA)

Cross-Country

- Typically 5- to 7-mi loop course with multiple laps

Short-Track

- Criterium-style off-road racecourse—short loop with timed race (30–90 min)

Downhill

- Individual downhill course with speeds in excess of 55 mph on rocky, uneven terrain
- Competitors wear protective gear, including full-face-mask helmet as well as chest, back, and leg protection

Dual and Quad Slalom

- Side-by-side race through slalom course with gates and jumps

Endurance and Team Events

- 24-h and endurance events (e.g., 24 h of Moab, Leadville 100, Race Across America)
- May be individual or team competition

Cyclocross

- Winter cycling season—varied terrain with some sections requiring the bike to be carried
- Short-loop course lasting 30–60 min with modified road bikes (wider tires, smaller gears)

COMMON INJURIES

Evaluation of the Initial Injury

- Priority: prevent further injury to the rider and prevent injury to other riders
- Especially important in criterium-style road races or cross-country mountain bike races, where there is a short-loop course and other racers will be returning to the accident scene

Table 32.1 Supplies for the Medical Cyclist

Finger splint (1)	Tongue blades (4)
Bandage scissors (1)	Tweezers (1)
Sterile 2 × 2 gauze (6)	Sterile 4 × 4 gauze (6)
Tube stretch gauze (Tubigauze)	Vaseline gauze (Adaptic)
Gauze dressing (4 × 4)	1-in. roll tape (1)
3-in. elastic bandage	100 mL sterile 0.9% normal saline (1)
Povidone-iodine scrub brush (4)	Hydrogen peroxide (8 oz)
Epi-pen (2)	Alcohol pads (8)
Neosporin, mupirocin ointment (3)	Nonadherent bandages (1- and 3-in.)
Nonadherent dressings (4)	Acetaminophen 325 or 500 mg (bottle)
Ibuprofen 200 mg (bottle)	Aspirin
Latex gloves (8 pair)	Albuterol inhaler
Diphenhydramine or other antihistamine	Sunscreen SPF 15, waterproof
Viscous lidocaine	Penlight
Prescription pad	Water soluble ointment
Nitroglycerin sublingual	Instant glucose (1 tube)
Moleskin	

Source: Montalto NJ, Janas TB: Medical coverage of recreational cycling events. *Clin Sports Med* 13(1):249–258, 1994.

- Quick trauma survey—airway, breathing, circulation (ABCs), neurologic deficit
- Stabilize c-spine if neck or head injury suspected
- Follow trauma protocol—**DO NOT** *delay emergency transport or treatment!*
- See Table 32.1 for basic supplies

Head Injuries

- Although a relatively rare injury in cycling, head injuries have the greatest potential for a catastrophic outcome
- 1000 bicyclists die in United States each year due to head injuries
- Head injuries account for approximately 62 percent of cycling deaths
- Most common cause of death is from subdural or epidural hematoma
- Concussions and skull fractures are also common head injuries

Prevention

- Helmet—should meet American National Standards Institute (ANSI) or Snell Memorial Foundation (SNELL) standards
- Helmet should be replaced after one impact even if no significant visible damage is evident

Treatment (See Chap. 6)

Dental Emergencies and Treatment (See Chap. 11)

Ocular Trauma/Emergencies (See Chap. 12)

- Most common ocular injuries are due to foreign bodies and corneal abrasions
- Prevention: encourage use of protective eyewear

Musculoskeletal Injuries

Shoulder Injuries (See Chap. 24)

Clavicular Fracture (See Chap. 24)

- Common injury, usually due to fall onto shoulder

Treatment/Return to Competition

- Athlete may continue to compete if pain tolerable
- Stationary trainer in 48 h if pain allows; easy road riding in 2–3 weeks if pain allows
- Return to road racing in 6–8 weeks, mountain-bike riding in 6–12 weeks

AC Joint Separations (See Chap. 24)

- Athlete may continue to compete if pain is tolerable

Shoulder Dislocation

- Uncommon injury but may occur with downhill racing
- Return to racing—as above

Hand/Arm/Elbow Injuries/ Trauma (See Chap. 22)

Gamekeeper's Thumb (Ulnar Collateral Ligament Sprain)

- More common in mountain bikers due to fall and abduction of thumb
- Complete disruption of ulnar collateral ligament requires surgical repair

Treatment

- Thumb spica splint initially. May use gauntlet or thumbster splint for competitions.

Radial Head Fractures

- Common due to falls on outstretched hand

Treatment

- Use of sling for comfort

Return to Competition

- Athlete may return to riding when pain is tolerable. Time-trial position may be more uncomfortable.

Ulnar Nerve Palsy

- Due to compression at elbow ulnar tunnel in time-trial position or prolonged pressure on handlebars

Prevention/ Treatment

- Evaluate and consider changing time-trial or riding position
- Gloves with extra padding or extra-thick handlebar tape may help prevent symptoms

Medial Nerve Palsy (Carpal Tunnel Syndrome)

- Due to compression of the medial nerve through the carpal tunnel of the wrist
- Common injury with longer-distance cycling due to wrist extension while holding top of handlebars

Prevention/Treatment

- Frequent adjustment of hand position while riding

Chest/Back Injuries (See Chap. 21)

Acute Back Injury/Trauma

- Due to fall or trauma. Injuries more common in downhill racing, where falls are more frequent.

Prevention—Specialized Equipment

- Use of protective chest and back pads—hard outer shell with soft foam liner to protect chest and spine from direct trauma

Neck or Low Back Spasm or Strain

- Common overuse injuries in road and time-trial cyclist

Prevention

- Assess bike frame for proper fit. Incorrect frame size can result in a riding position that is uncomfortable.
- Adjust riding position to more upright position
- Adjust elbows in time-trial position so that humerus is perpendicular to ground. This places more of the body weight on the skeletal structures, not muscular system.

Genitourinary Injury

Bicycle Seat Injuries

- Acute trauma (see Chap 15)
- Pudendal (bicycle seat) neuropathy
- Caused by compression of pudendal nerve or localized ischemia
- Usually resolves upon stopping biking, although resolution may take days or weeks if condition is chronic. May cause temporary paresthesia and, in men, impotence or prostatitis. Also common in women.

Prevention—Specialized Equipment

- Change to bicycle seat with cutaway center seat portion to alleviate pressure
- Alter angle of bicycle seat—slight drop of nose of seat may relieve pressure
- Have cyclist stand occasionally to relieve pressure

Saddle Sores/Folliculitus

- Due to combination of pressure, infection, and friction
- Blocked glands may allow infection to develop

Prevention—Specialized Equipment

- Use of synthetic, padded bicycle shorts and padded bicycle seat
- Keep area clean, dry, and protected. Wash and air-dry cycling shorts after rides
- Mild topical steroid creams for localized irritation, antibiotics if infection suspected

Hip and Pelvic injuries

Common Injuries

- Greater trochanteric bursitis (see Iliotibial Band Syndrome, below)

Knee Injuries and Trauma (See Chap. 26)

Patellar Tendinitis

- Pain below patella due to overuse and poor bike fit. Also due to excessive, repetitive force across patellar tendon or excessive side-to-side movement of knee during pedal stroke.

Prevention/Treatment

- Raise bicycle seat to decrease knee flexion (<1 cm per adjustment)
- Avoid steep climbs at low cadence; higher cadence relieves stress across tendon

Biceps Femoris Tendinitis

- Caused by overextension of knee at bottom of pedal stroke

Prevention/Treatment

- Proper bike fit. Lower bicycle seat (<1 cm per adjustment).

Iliotibial Band Syndrome

- Usually a chronic injury but may present with acute sharp pain at lateral knee or greater tuberosity

- Caused by medial rotation of tibia and foot on pedal or lateral motion of knee on pedal upstroke
- Excessive pronation of foot on pedal may also be a factor

Prevention/Treatment

- Recommend floating cleat system if cyclist is using fixed cleat
- Adjust pedal cleat to prevent significant medial rotation of foot
- Shims between cleat and pedal to correct pronation if present
- Raise bicycle seat if lateral knee motion present

Foot/Ankle Injuries and Trauma

Acute Trauma

- Common in downhill and slalom

Prevention

- Use of shin/leg protectors and pads

Metatarsalgias, Morton's Neuroma, and Foot Numbness

- Due to tight toe box and rigid sole of cycling shoe, causing compression of digital nerves in foot
- Pressure on foot from small pedal platform may also contribute

Prevention/Treatment

- Use of metatarsal pads. Move pedal cleat position to relieve pressure.
- Adjust or loosen shoes or change to wider pedal platform

Skin Injuries and Trauma (See Chap. 16)

Road Rash (Superficial Abrasions)

- Superficial skin abrasions due to falls

Treatment

- Scrub clean with disinfectant
- Topical lidocaine for anesthesia if extensive
- Antibiotic ointment, nonstick bandage, and tube gauze to hold in place
- Consider tetanus prophylaxis

Lacerations

- Evaluate need for immediate versus delayed (postrace) closure
- If bleeding can be controlled, athlete may continue with race

Sunburn

- Common on face, back of neck, arms, and thighs

Prevention/Treatment

- Use of long-acting sunblock on exposed areas

Bibliography

Gregor RJ, Conconi F: *Handbook of Sports Medicine and Science: Road Cycling.* Oxford, UK: Blackwell Science, 2000.

Mellion MB, Burke E: *Clinics in Sports Medicine: Bicycling Injuries.* Philadelphia: Saunders, 1994.

Montalto NJ, Janas TB: Medical coverage of recreational cycling events. *Clin Sports Med* 13(1):249–258, 1994.

Pfeiffer RP: Off-road bicycle racing injuries—the NORBA pro/elite category. *Clin Sports Med* 13:207–218, 1994.

Weiss BD: Clinical syndromes associated with bicycle seats. *Clin Sports Med* 13:175–186, 1994.

33

Boxing

Brian A. Davis
Tony Alamo

REQUIREMENTS OF THE BOXING PHYSICIAN

- To be a fan of boxing
- To be a good doctor
  - There is no substitute for experience
  - Boxing is a contact sport; injuries are part of it. The physician must differentiate serious injuries from others.

COMMON INJURIES

Neurologic

- Concussions (mild confusion to severe loss of consciousness) (see Chap. 6)
  - In the ring, quick mental status and physical examinations are required. In a quick 15 s, the physician must ascertain whether a boxer can continue or must be withdrawn from the fight.
  - Each physician at ringside should focus primarily on one boxer yet also keep an eye on the general flow of the match. Boxers who cannot protect themselves are at risk of serious injury and should be watched closely for a few moments after a head blow to see whether it has been sustained without causing disorientation or disability.
    - Professional matches are frequently stopped by the referee in the ring. They may have to be stopped by physician if the referee does not recognize the seriousness of the boxer's injury.
  - Professional vs. Amateur: Suspensions for Head Injuries
  - Amateur boxing (USA Boxing rules): Referee provides initial decision of RSCH 30 (referee stops contest due to head blows), whereas all others are determined by the physician. Physician can add additional restriction time as required.
    - RSC (referee stops contest): Referee may stop contest due to "outclassing of opponent." No restriction given.

- RSCH 30: Referee stops contest due to too frequent head blows in a round, a severe head blow without loss of consciousness causing standing eight count, three standing eight counts in a round, or four standing eight counts in a match. Automatic 30-day restriction from contact.
- RSCH 90 (referee stops contest due to head blows): Referee stops contest due to boxer being knocked unconscious for less than 2 min. Automatic 90-day restriction from contact.
- RSCH 180 (referee stops contest due to head blows): Referee stops contest due to boxer being knocked unconscious for more than two minutes. Automatic 180-day restriction from contact.
- Restrictions levied after prior restrictions are compounded (e.g. a 30-day restriction after a 30-day restriction will result in a 90-day restriction)
- Professional boxing: Varies based on the state. Match stopped secondary to head blows often given a 45-day minimum restriction of contact. More severe injuries restricted for longer time periods. Often determined by physician experience and severity of head injury sustained during match. Some states require advance brain imaging at regular intervals and may require EEG and advance imaging after some head injuries. Most states require evaluation by a neurologist, neurosurgeon, or occasionally by physiatrist.
- Subdural hematomas and other types of cerebral injury
  - Life-threatening event. Typically presents with slow progression of neurologic changes due to venous bleeding. Boxer may not be aware of neurologic problems until after leaving a match venue. If such injury is suspected, the athlete should receive immediate transfer to a trauma center with a neurosurgical team.
- Headaches
  - Fighters rarely complain of headaches during or after a bout. If they do, they should be watched closely and and given options of follow-up depending on symptoms and serial examinations. Headaches can indicate an impending catastrophic event.

Orthopedics

- Points of contact:
  - Metacarpal fractures, scaphoid fracture (see Chap. 18)
  - Nasal and orbital fracture (see Chap. 10)
- Shoulder dislocation (see Chap. 24)
- Knee injury (see Chap. 26)
- Ankle sprains (see Chap. 27)
- Ulnar collateral ligament (UCL) injuries (thumb) (see Chap. 22)
- Elbow dislocation (see Chap. 23)

Cut Management

- Soft tissue swelling and cuts (rarely life-threatening)

- Cuts: the most common reason for stopping a fight
- Match may be stopped for poor "sight through blood"—not "sight of blood" (the boxer cannot see through the blood for adequate self-defense—*correct* reason to stop a fight; ring doctors and/or referees do not like the "sight of blood"—*incorrect* reason to stop a fight)
- Common areas of cuts are sharp bony ridges such as the supraorbital rim, zygomatic areas
- Open laceration of the eyelid itself can indicate that moderate to severe forces could have been transferred to the globe. Remember the eye without its eyelid is now unprotected from further trauma.
- Professional vs. Amateur
  - Amateur boxing (USA Boxing rules): Fight stoppage depends on cut location and potential for further injury, not on severity of bleeding. Initial restriction is determined by ringside physician with follow-up required prior to next match.
    - Cuts are rarely seen due to headgear. Most common cuts occur below the headgear. Improperly fitting headgear may be responsible for cuts either by lack of protection or from contusion/laceration caused by headgear rubbing.
    - Cut locations and recommendations:
      - Cuts lateral and perpendicular to the eye: Match usually does not need to be stopped
      - Cuts over eyebrow: If cut could lead to supraorbital nerve injury, match should be stopped
      - Cuts inferior to the eye: Match usually does not need to be stopped. Cuts that could lead to damage of the lacrimal duct (superior) should lead to match stoppage.
      - Cuts through the lip: Should stop the match
  - Professional boxing: Each state typically mandates minimum restriction times. Frequently a boxer is banned from contact for 60 days or more, with follow-up required prior to next match.
    - Headgear is not worn
    - Many cuts due to head butting
    - Cut locations and recommendations:
    - As above for amateur boxing; cut locations that can lead to further serious injury should lead to match stoppage

Pulmonary Injury

- Reactive airway disease: More likely to occur at outdoor boxing events or in arenas that allow cigarette/cigar smoking
- Pneumothorax: May be *very* difficult to detect early in presentation due to patient reporting only chest pain from body blow. Arena noise often makes auscultation difficult as well. Patient should receive emergent transport if pneumothorax is suspected. Placement of large-bore intravenous catheter for tension pneumothorax may be lifesaving.

Ophthalmologic Injury

- Hyphema, retinal detachments, corneal abrasions, open globes, orbital fractures
  - With the exception of orbital fractures, the other mentioned injuries are found by the fighter's subjective complaint "Doc, I can't see." It does not matter how normal the physical examination appears to the physician. The boxer's chief complaint is reason to stop the fight. Some boxers may not admit to loss of vision, but a good referee will notice a boxer receiving undue punishment to a particular side without proper self-defense, so that the match should be stopped.

Facial Injury

- Nosebleeds
  - Amateur: Match stoppage when:
    - Bleeding impairs boxer's vision
    - Bleeding impairs boxer's respiratory status, most likely with posterior nasal bleeds. Physician should evaluate degree of posterior pharyngeal blood. Brisk posterior bleeding should lead to match stoppage.
    - If both boxers are bleeding briskly. Risk reportedly due to possible passage of HIV or other blood-borne pathogen.
  - Professional: Match stoppage typically only if respiratory status or vision is impaired
- Mandibular fracture: Look for malocclusion of the upper and lower teeth or ecchymosis within the oral cavity as a sign of trauma. Clicking of the temporomandibular joint (TMJ) is also suggestive.
- Tracheal fracture: Potentially life-threatening emergency. Look for subcutaneous emphysema and signs of trauma. Any signs of extremis should prompt attempt at intubation. If intubation fails, immediate cricothyroidotomy or tracheostomy should be performed.

BASIC PRINCIPLES

- When in doubt, obtain a CT scan and arrange for follow-up care
  - Ring physician must keep in mind that once he or she is working in an official capacity, the boxer becomes a patient. The physician is obligated to become the boxer's advocate and to care for the boxer with all of the responsibility that would normally be involved in the physician's own practice. Being a ring physician requires knowledge of the patient (boxer), including the patient's history and physical examination. It also involves responsibility for good follow-up care.

THE DAY BEFORE THE EVENT

- The first exposure to the fighter occurs the day before, during a weigh-in
  - Get to know the fighter
  - Obtain a history
  - Perform physical examination
  - Know the fighter's capabilities
    - Elicit any medical worries that may have to be dealt with the next day at the boxing event. Boxer's record is very insightful. Ask questions. What was weight two weeks ago? Ever been knocked out? When? For how long?
    - It is the ring physician's responsibility to elicit this information for the safety of the fighter. The boxer may be resistant because he or she wants the fight to occur, but the doctor must always remember the health and safety of the boxer is paramount and of most importance.

THE DAY OF THE EVENT

- Determine requirement for medical personal and equipment
  - Sufficient number of physicians so if two boxers are injured and currently undergoing evaluation in their dressing rooms there are still one or two physicians available at ringside to continue the card
  - ACLS equipment: *Must be at ringside* with ability to move an unconscious fighter through the arena. Such bulky equipment can be kept under the ring itself. At least two paramedic-level (EMT-P) transports available. In the event a transport happens, no further cards should continue unless another physician is present. Two available transports can ensure continued uninterrupted cards.
  - Recommend that all physicians assure availability of oxygen, bag-valve-mask, intubation equipment, cricothyroidotomy equipment, intravenous fluids, and large-bore intravenous needles (for intravenous line placement or tension pneumothorax treatment)

THE ROLE OF FOLLOW-UP AND REEVALUATION

- In boxing, it is somewhat easier to identify potential serious injuries during the initiation of the fight. For example, when a fighter is knocked out, it is obvious that that he or she can no longer continue; therefore the fight is stopped.
- The more dangerous injuries are those that go undiagnosed. As in all medical practice, the less obvious injuries pose the greatest risk of being missed by medical personnel and thus are more likely to have deleterious effects.

- Therefore, by evaluating and examining the fighter postbout in the dressing room, many injuries will come to light; thus a more prudent follow-up plan can be developed
- For boxers who have suffered either a significant beating or who have any neurologic compromise in the form of loss of consciousness, whether transient or more profound, suspension should be mandated, ranging from a number of days of no fighting and/or no contact whatsoever to a complete suspension of licensure until the fighter is cleared by another physician

DRUG TESTING

- Some form of random or mandatory toxicology and steroid testing must be considered
- The ring physician may need to establish the drug-testing policy
- Each state determines its own policy on banned substances and testing

SUGGESTED PHYSICAL EXAMINATION

- The physical examinations for boxers preceding a bout should be brief but address the most important areas of the body. This is *not* a mandatory checklist, as each physician will be using his or her own clinical judgment and placing his or her own license "on the line." It is strongly recommended that the physician use the following physical examination at the minimum. Any evidence on examination of a problem should warrant a more focused examination.
- General questionnaire: Ask if the boxer has had any of the following:
  - Headaches, dizziness, chest pain, shortness of breath, wheezing, seizures, palpitations, blackouts, knockout in last 3 months, recent illnesses
  - Any treatments being provided by a physician
  - Any medications being taken and indications
  - Focus on any positive history
- Boxing log (amateur): Look at boxing record book and see if any restrictions were placed on the boxer at the last fight he or she had

PREBOUT PHYSICAL EXAMINATION

- Blood pressure, heart rate, respiratory rate, temperature (often done by assisting personnel)
- Cardiac: Look for murmurs, especially diastolic
- Check murmurs with deep inspiration and Valsalva maneuver
- Pulmonary: Especially wheezing or decreased inspiratory capacity If decreased capacity, look to occult rib fractures
- Face (including zygoma, mandible, maxilla, and supraorbital ridge)
  - Check for loose teeth
- Chest/ribs: brief palpation

- Musculoskeletal: Brief evaluation of elbow, wrist, and hands—palpate
- Neurologic
  - Cranial nerves
  - Extraocular muscles—specifically looking for nystagmus
  - Masseter strength
  - Eye closing (tight)
  - Sternocleidomastoid strength
- Upper/lower extremities
  - Biceps strength
  - Triceps strength
  - Intrinsics or grip strength
  - Hip flexion strength
  - Knee extension strength
  - Ankle dorsiflexion strength
- Coordination
  - Index finger to nose from each hand alternating as rapidly as possible
  - One-legged stance for 10 s
- Abdominal: Brief palpation for tenderness and more advanced to check for organomegaly if an athlete has signs/symptoms of mononucleosis
- Remember to evaluate further if necessary to rule out any neurologic or medical issue

POSTBOUT QUESTIONNAIRE

- Ask about any problems during the fight. Specifically ask about:
  - Headache
  - Light-headedness
  - Dizziness
- Pain in any location
- Focus on any positive responses

POSTBOUT PHYSICAL EXAMINATION

- Neurologic
  - Look for general awareness
  - Any boxer who has received a standing eight count or appeared dazed in the ring at any time should receive the following:
    - A mental status examination
    - Cranial nerve examination
    - Test for coordination
    - Test general strength
    - Focus on any abnormality and test as needed
- Facial bones—palpate orbital ridge, zygoma, maxilla, mandible
- Neck—palpate for pain
- Chest/ribs—palpate for pain and auscultate

- Musculoskeletal—brief evaluation of elbow, wrist, and hands
- Abdomen—palpate for pain
- Any athlete who appears unstable in any way should be transferred via ambulance/911 as soon as possible. Any athlete who does not clear cognitively within 20–30 min should be transferred for further evaluation. Any athlete who has not recovered from mild headache, dizziness, nausea, or other findings consistent with mild head injury must be observed by family or coach, provided with information on head injuries, and given appropriate follow-up instructions.
- Use your best judgment in evaluating these athletes. If there is ever any question, err on the side of conservatism. Consulting physicians should always be available by pager for consultation.

Bibliography

American College of Surgeons Committee on Trauma: *Advanced Trauma Life Support for Doctors, Student Course Manual*, 6th ed. Chicago: American College of Surgeons, 1997.

Bakre S, Neuendorf K, Postma I, Vanlandingham A (eds): *USA Boxing Official Rules.* Colorado Springs, CO, 2000.

Cantu R: *Boxing and Medicine.* Champaign, IL: Human Kinetics, 1995.

Estwanik J: *Sports Medicine for the Combat Arts.* Boxergenics Press, Charlotte, NC: 1996.

Jordan BD: Boxing, in Safran MR, Van Camp SP, McKeag D (eds): *Spiral Manual of Sports Medicine.* Philadelphia: Lippincott-Raven, 1998, pp 546–549.

34

Extreme Sports

John Martinez

INTRODUCTION

- *Extreme sports* is a broad term that can cover many different athletic pursuits but may best describe adventure racing. Adventure racing and other "extreme" sports have been more popular as individuals search for new challenges. Many of these events take place in remote or wilderness areas that may pose significant logistic problems for the medical team in the event of a medical emergency. Proper planning, training, and communication among all medical and race staff can prevent serious or catastrophic outcomes.
- Many of these events involve teams of athletes and require them to travel from checkpoint to checkpoint by various means of transportation such as hiking, rapelling, or canoeing/kayaking. These races may cover a variety of terrains from the desert to high-altitude mountains.

Adventure Racing

- Eco-challenge and other multi-sport or multiple segmented races

Ultraendurance Events

- Ultramarathons (Leadville 100)
- Open-water distance swimming (Manhattan Island)
- Endurance mountain biking events (24 h of Moab)

Mountaineering and Climbing Expeditions

- Requires massive planning and staging of medical supplies.
- Rapid extraction is not often available, so medical staff must be prepared.

Medical Organization and Planning for Events

- In addition to organizing a centralized medical command center, the medical staff should have the following resources:

Medical Director

- Oversees overall function and structure of medical staff.
- Should have familiarity with wilderness medical emergencies.
- Should have ability to communicate with competitors and medical staff.
  - May require short-wave (HAM) radios or other communication setup.
- Acts as contact person with outside medical personnel—i.e., EMS and hospital emergency department.
- Should have access to up-to-date weather conditions as well as ocean and tide reports if applicable.

Medical Tent/Area

- Designated area for triage and treatment of competitors.
- Should have easy access to EMS vehicles and competitors from course.

Mobile Medical

- Should be available at transition areas and ready to respond to emergencies on the racecourse.
- Staff can consist of first responders—EMTs or wilderness medicine–trained individuals.

Search and Rescue (See Chap. 45)

- SAR teams need to have the ability to operate in a variety of conditions and climates, from whitewater to high-altitude mountainous terrain.
- Local SAR teams should be notified of event and on call for potential emergencies.

COMMON INJURIES AND MEDICAL CONDITIONS

- Injuries seen by medical personnel are dependent upon the sport or activities required by the competitors.
- Skin (see Chap. 16)
  - Abrasions and lacerations
  - Blisters
  - Sunburn

- Musculoskeletal injuries and trauma
  - Acute trauma—fractures and dislocations
  - Soft tissue injuries
- Heat injuries (see Chap. 17)
  - Heat cramps, exhaustion, and heat stroke.
- Cold injuries (see Chap. 17)
  - Frostbite and hypothermia
- Cold-water immersion and near drowning
- Altitude illnesses (see Chap. 17)
  - Acute mountain sickness (AMS)
  - High-altitude cerebral edema (HACE)
  - High-altitude pulmonary edema (HAPE)
- Infectious Diseases
  - Be aware of endemic diseases in local areas. Many outbreaks can be prevented by immunizations, prophylactic antibiotics, proper hygiene, and ensuring clean, drinkable water.
  - The Centers for Disease Control and Prevention maintain up-to-date information for travel medicine at www.cdc.gov
  - Vaccinations—routine
    - Tetanus and diphtheria vaccine (Td)
    - Inactivated poliomyelitis vaccine (IPV)
    - Measles, mumps, rubella vaccine (MMR)
    - Hepatitis A and B vaccine
    - Influenza vaccine
    - Pneumococcal vaccine
  - Vaccinations—destination-dependent
    - Consult CDC or WHO for current recommendations
- Traveler's Diarrhea
  - Acute episode of watery diarrhea, commonly with abdominal cramping and pain.
  - Prevention
    - Bottled or treated water and ice or canned beverages.
    - Cooked foods or fruits with outer skin that require peeling.
    - Avoid raw, undercooked meats, fish, vegetables, and ice from untreated water.
  - Water filters and purifiers
    - 0.2-μm filter removes most enteric bacteria and protozoan cysts.
    - 5-μm filter for protozoan cysts.
  - Bottled or pretreated water or canned beverages.
  - Medication
    - Bismuth subsalicylate—two tablets four times a day
  - Antibiotics for Prevention
    - Doxycycline 100 mg once a day
    - Trimethoprim 160 mg/sulfamethoxazole 800 mg once a day
    - Ciprofloxacin 500 mg once a day
    - Norfloxacin 400 mg once a day
  - Treatment
    - Fluid replacement to avoid significant dehydration.
    - Bismuth subsalicylate—30 mL every 30–60 min up to eight doses
    - Loperamide (Imodium)—or Diphenoxylate (Lomotil)

- Antibiotics for Treatment
  - Doxycycline 100 mg bid for 3 days
  - Trimethoprim 160 mg/sulfamethoxazole 800 mg bid for 3 days
  - Ciprofloxin 500 mg bid for 3 days or 750 mg once at start of symptoms
  - Levofloxacin 500 mg once a day for 3 days

Malaria

- Caused by *Plasmodium vivax, P. falciparum, P. malariae, P. ovale.*
- Endemic in most tropical locations.
- Incubation period is about 7 days.

Prevention/Treatment

- Chemoprophylaxis based on chloroquine-resistant *P. falciparum.*
- Check with CDC for latest chloroquine-resistant areas and recommended chemoprophylaxis.
- Start at least 1 week before travel to endemic area.
- Continue for 4 weeks after return.
- Use of pants, long-sleeved clothing insect repellent (DEET or permethrim), and sleeping nets advisable.

Giardia

- Caused by *Giardia lamblia*—flagellate protozoan.
- Most common intestinal protozoan worldwide.
- Typically water-borne.
- Endemic in western United States—Cascades, Rockies, and Sierra Mountains.
- Incubation period of 1–3 weeks.
- Presents with watery diarrhea, severe abdominal cramping, fever, malaise, and vomiting.

Prevention/Treatment

- Avoid contaminated water sources.
- Metronidazole 250 mg tid for 5 days.

Leptospirosis

- *Leptospira interrogans*—spirochete.
- Outbreak in Eco-Challenge-Boreno 2000 due to contaminated fresh water.
- Presents as febrile, flu-like illness with malaise, myalgia, headache.

Prevention

- Doxycycline 200 mg once a week
- Avoidance of freshwater ponds and streams near endemic areas.

Treatment

- First-line: doxycycline 100 mg PO bid for 7 days
- Second-line: tetracycline 500 mg PO tid/qid for 7 days or penicillin G, 3 million U/day
  - Patients may have Jarisch-Herxheimer reaction after treatment due to endotoxin release.

Bibliography

Auerbach PS: *Wilderness Medicine,* 4th ed. St Louis: Mosby, 2001.

35

Football

Joseph P. Luftman

COMMON INJURIES

- Concussion (see Chap. 6)
- Cervical spine injuries (see Chap. 20)
- Clavicular fracture
  - Mid-third most common: assess for skin tenting, neurovascular compromise.
  - Distal and proximal third less common but more complications.
- Acromioclavicular (AC) joint sprain or shoulder separation
- Anterior shoulder dislocation and subluxation
- Jersey finger (see Chap. 22)
  - Avulsion of flexor digitorum profundus tendon
  - Tenderness, swelling, ecchymosis at base of DIP joint
- Hip pointer (see Chap. 25)
  - Contusion or muscular avulsion at border of the iliac crest
  - Pain often very severe with minimal signs of injury on examination
- Hip dislocation (see Chap. 25)
- Thigh/quadriceps contusion (see Chap. 29)
- Knee (see Chap. 26)
  - Ligamentous injury
  - Cartilage injury
  - Dislocation—significant neurovascular injury must be ruled out.
- Ankle (see Chap. 27)
  - Lateral
  - "High" or syndesmotic
- Turf toe (see Chap. 28)
- Physeal injuries in children
  - Distal femoral physeal injuries can mimic injuries to the medial collateral ligament.
    - Laxity on valgus stress testing of the knee.
    - Tender over distal physis at proximal aspect of femoral condyle.
  - Ankle fractures: distal fibular physis, Tillaux, triplane.

SPECIALIZED EQUIPMENT NEEDS

- Head and Neck Injuries
  - Cellular phone
  - Cervical collar and spine board with sand bags
  - "Trainer's Angel" to cut grommets on the helmet (see Fig. 20.1)
  - Cricothyroidotomy kit/needle
  - Ophthalmoscope/penlight
  - Pocket mental status exam guide
  - Methylprednisolone (Solu-Medrol) injectable for catastrophic neck injury if intravenous access obtained.
- Fractures
  - Splint material, knee immobilizer, ice pack
- Allergies/anaphylaxis
  - Epi-pen, albuterol metered-dose inhaler
- Dehydration
  - Intravenous fluids (NS or LR) with angiocatheter (16–20 gauge) and tubing

TREATMENT

- Cervical spine immobilization (see Chap. 20)
  - Methylprednisolone (Solu-Medrol) 30 mg/kg IV loading dose, then 5.4 mg/kg/h infusion.
- Concussion management (see Chap. 6)
- AC joint sprain
  - Rest, ice, compression, elevation (RICE) and physical therapy for shoulder range of motion (ROM), strengthening.
- Shoulder reduction after dislocation, immediately after injury (see Chap. 24)
  - Gentle axial traction in seated position with arm internally rotated or in prone position on the bench with arm dangling.
  - Sling for comfort 1–2 weeks, then rehabilitation program.
  - Surgery often necessary, especially for linebackers and defensive backs.
- Jersey finger (see Chap. 22)
- Hip pointer
  - Ice and NSAIDs
- Hip dislocation (see Chap. 25)
- Quadriceps contusion
  - Ice and NSAIDs [consider a cyclooxygenase-2 (COX-2) inhibitor—less antiplatelet effect].
  - Splint knee in hyperflexed position for 24–48 h.
- Knee
  - Collateral ligament injuries usually treated nonoperatively.
    - Protected weight bearing, gentle ROM, RICE.
    - Bracing with medial/lateral support.
  - Cruciate ligament injuries often treated operatively.
    - RICE, and protected weight bearing for comfort.

- Early ROM to prepare for surgical procedure.
- Acute knee dislocation with vascular injury (orthopedic emergency) must be ruled out.
- Fractures (see Chap. 18)
  - For obvious deformity, splint for stability and transport to nearest ER.
- Dislocation
  - Attempt to reduce manually, especially if there is neurovascular compromise, and then place in a splint.
  - Transport immediately.
- Cartilage injury
  - Meniscal injuries managed with RICE and NSAIDs.
  - "Locked" knee with minimal to no ROM is an orthopedic emergency.
- Ankle (see Chap. 27)
  - Lateral talocrural ligament sprain (ATFL most common)
    - Control swelling
    - X-ray to rule out fracture, based on Ottowa Ankle Rules
  - "High" ankle sprain (syndesmotic injury)
    - Often only minimal swelling
    - X-ray to rule out tibiofibular widening distally
    - Protected weight bearing with cam walker and/or short leg walking cast with crutches
- Turf toe (see Chap. 28)
  - Mild-to-moderate dorsal capsular injury: ice, taping to restrict dorsiflexion, rigid metal insole
  - Suspected chondral injury or dislocation: remove from contest, x-rays, cam-walker boot, immobilization with taping/splint

RETURN TO PLAY

- Players with the following injuries may return to play immediately:
  - Glenohumeral subluxation, stinger, or AC sprain with minimal to no pain plus full ROM and protective strength
  - Jersey finger, protected with tape or splint
  - Mild hip pointer with full trunk and hip ROM
  - Quadriceps contusion if knee/hip has full ROM, no early swelling, essentially full knee extension strength, and minimal to no limp
  - Mild turf toe
- May return to play after further evaluation/treatment
  - Neck paraspinal muscle injury with full ROM, minimal to no tenderness
  - Grade I concussion with symptom resolution <20 min
  - Proximal interphalangeal (PIP) or distal interphalangeal (DIP) joint dislocation—postreduction with full ROM, minimal pain, and protective taping
  - Collateral ligament knee injuries and mild ankle and midfoot sprains with full stability/strength on testing position-specific running and cutting maneuvers

- Asthma exacerbation—after treatment with albuterol inhaler, no wheezing or respiratory distress on examination
- Return to play is delayed or contraindicated with the following:
  - Any significant cervical spine injury
  - Grade II concussion or higher
  - Shoulder, elbow, wrist, hip, knee, midfoot, and ankle dislocations
  - All suspected fractures
  - Cruciate ligament injury to the knee
  - All suspected tendon ruptures (except jersey finger—see above)
  - Suspected physeal injury in a child (especially distal femoral physis)

Bibliography

Bracken MB, Shepard MJ, Collins WF, et al: A randomized, controlled trial of methylprednisolone or naloxone in the treatment of acute spinal-cord injury. Results of the Second National Acute Spinal Cord Injury Study. *N Engl J Med* 322(20):1405–1411, 1990.

McCrea M, Kelly JP, Kluge J, et al: Standardized assessment of concussion in football players. *Neurology* 48(3):586–588, 1997.

Putukian M, Stansbury N, Sebastianelli W: Football, in Mellion MB, Walsh WM, Shelton GL (eds): *The Team Physician's Handbook,* 2d ed. Philadelphia: Hanley & Belfus, 1997, pp 639–663.

Waninger KN, Lombardo JA: Football, in Mellion MB (ed): *Sports Medicine Secrets,* 2d ed. Philadelphia: Hanley & Belfus, 1999, pp 369–377.

36

Golf

Evan Bass
Bernadette Pendergraph

GENERAL

- Incidence of injury
  - >40 percent of amateurs sustain injuries that prevent play >5 weeks.
  - >50 percent of professionals sustain injuries that prevent play >5 weeks.
  - <40 percent of injuries resolve within 4 weeks.
  - 70–75 percent of injuries resolve within 6 months.
  - ~10 percent of injuries persist >1 year.

COMMON INJURIES

Listed in order of frequency for male amateur golfers:

Lower Back (See Chap. 21)

- Four multidirectional forces on lumbar spine with swing
  - Lateral flexion, anteroposterior traction, rotation, compression
- Frequent error of amateurs: swinging harder with poor technique
- Carrying golf bag (20–25 lb) over one shoulder
- Special considerations in treatment
  - Equipment changes (extra-long putter)
  - Pull cart or backpack style straps to even out weight distribution
  - Have swing technique adjusted by professional instructor

Elbow (See Chap. 23)

- Epicondylitis
  - Lateral (5:1 occurrence vs. medial)
    - Occurs most in leading arm of swing.
    - Generally due to overuse.

- Medial (less common yet known as "golfer's elbow").
  - Occurs most in trailing arm of swing.
  - More commonly caused by divoting with shots.
- Special treatment considerations
  - Consider more flexible club shaft.
  - Use club with shock-absorbing material in shaft at grip.
  - Reduce divoting with shot.
  - Reduce elbow lock with swing.
  - Use golf glove and new club grips to reduce grip force.

Wrist (See Chap. 22)

- Overuse sprains/strains.
- Ganglion cysts.
- Traumatic and stress fractures of the hook of the hamate.
  - Important to look for this injury.
  - Need carpal tunnel view or CT to diagnose.
  - Consider surgical excision, especially in professionals.

Shoulder (See Chap. 24)

- Represent about 10 percent of injuries to golfers.
- Most commonly due to overuse.
- Also due to overrotation of shoulder on back swing and follow-through.
- Injuries usually involve lead arm in swing (nondominant in most cases)
- Common Injuries
  - Bursitis with impingement
  - Instability
    - Posterior subluxation at the top of the back swing
  - Acromioclavicular joint injury
    - Osteolysis often requires surgical correction
  - Degenerative joint disease

Lower Extremities

- Rare injuries (less than 10 percent)

COMMON ETIOLOGIES OF INJURY

- Amateur golfers
  - Flaws in swing technique
  - Spine injuries most common, followed by elbow, hand, and wrist
  - Generally overuse injuries
    - Poor warmup practices
    - Practice range allowing high volume in little time

- Infrequent and "seasonal" play
    - One-third of injuries occur in early-"season"
    - One-half of injuries occur in mid-"season"
  - Uneven and muddy terrain
  - Cartless golfers walk about 6 mi during a round, carrying about 25 lb.
- Acute traumatic injuries
  - Poor judgment on hazard shots
    - Ground impact on swing
    - Tree impact on swing
- Club- or ball-impact trauma
  - Crowded course conditions
  - Impatient and inconsiderate players
  - Poor accuracy and judgment
- Golf cart trauma
  - Unexpectedly uneven terrain
  - Grass often slick, even if dry and especially if wet
  - No seat belts
  - Rare safety instruction prior to use
  - Poor judgment, horseplay
- Female golfers
  - Less prone to spine injuries than male golfers
- Older golfers (~25 percent of golfers over age 50)
  - Degenerative joint disease
  - Loss of flexibility requiring technique adjustment
- Professional golfers
  - More prone to wrist and hand injuries, elbow injury less common
  - More often overuse-related, less often technique-related
  - More aggressive play and attempts at hazard shots

PREVENTION OF INJURY

- Warmup is essential.
  - Stretching routine focusing on lower back, upper extremities
  - Half-strength and short-distance shots to start
- Evaluation of technique by certified professional instructor
  - Can significantly reduce musculoskeletal stress yet improve performance

OTHER MEDICAL CONSIDERATIONS

Environmental Exposure

- Usual round of golf is 4–5 h
  - Significant sun exposure, often little shade
    - Hyperthermia
    - Sunburn

- Little protection from wind and rain
  - Hypothermia
- Lightning strikes
  - Play often suspended with lightning threat

Head Trauma to Other Golfers and Spectators

- Ball speed with hard strike—130 mph
  - Focused point of impact
  - Skull fractures
  - Intracranial bleeds, sometimes delayed in onset
  - Seizures

Very Large Area of Play

- Spectators often walk great distances to follow favorite golfers.
- Generally older crowd.
- No roads on course, emergency access can be a concern.

TREATMENT (ACUTE ON-SITE CARE)

- Emergency access plan for course
  - Cell phone
  - Automated electronic defibrillator
  - Basic life support equipment
  - Ambulance access to course
- Be prepared for trauma
  - Be aware of slippery grass or uneven terrain.
  - Monitor golfball–impact injuries closely.
    - Intracranial bleeding can be delayed in onset.
    - Posttraumatic seizures reported more than 4 h postinjury.
  - Many injuries reported from falls off golf carts.
    - Poor safety instruction on use.
    - Poor judgment in slick, uneven conditions.
    - No seat belts.
- Provide access to timely weather reports.
- Be prepared for exposure injuries.
  - Hypothermia.
  - Hyperthermia.
  - Sun, wind exposure.
  - Extended duration of exposure, often all day for spectators.
    - Need easy access to hydration throughout course.

Other Considerations

- Ice for acute strain injuries
- First aid kit for minor injuries
- Bronchodilator for cold weather and allergen exposure
- Epinephrine anaphylaxis kit
- Counterforce and other braces

RETURN TO PLAY

- Varies by injury
- Most injuries due to overuse.
  - Require significant rest.
  - Technique or equipment changes may help hasten return and prevent re-injury.
  - Use of golf carts can hasten return from certain injuries.

PHASES OF GOLF SWING AND ASSOCIATED INJURIES

- Ball address and back swing
  - Forward flexion of spine instead of hips increases vertebral hypermobility and back tension.
  - Overextended arms and locked elbows increase forearm stress and elbow and wrist injuries.
  - Too wide of a stance increases stress on the spine by limiting trunk rotation.
  - Improper or too loose a grip leads to impact injuries (elbow and wrist) due to club rotation and ground impact.
  - Excessive back swing causes spine overrotation and loss of balance, leading to ground-impact injuries, thumb and wrist strain, and lead shoulder impingement.
  - Excessive weight shift can lead to strain and sprain of nonlead ankle.
- Forward acceleration and ball impact
  - Thoracic and abdominal muscle strain from overly forceful rotation.
  - Forward weight shift creates substantial forces on lead hip, knee, ankle, and foot, especially problematic in those with osteoarthritis.
  - Too tight of a grip and hyperextended elbows is a significant factor in epicondylitis.
  - Ground impact can cause traumatic hand and wrist injury.
- Follow-through
  - Overly vigorous activity causes significant rotator cuff stress.
  - Hip and lumbar spine injury from overdeceleration.
  - Hyperextension of spine with forceful shot
  - Loss of balance causing lead ankle, knee, and foot injury

Bibliography

Booher J, Amundson M: Golf, in Mellion MB, Walsh WM, Madden C, et al (eds): *Team Physician's Handbook,* 3d ed. Philadelphia: Hanley & Belfus, 2002, pp 695–702.

Lindsay DM, Horton JF, Vandervoort AA: A review of injury characteristics, aging factors, and prevention programmes for the older golfer. *Sports Med* 30(2):89–103, 2000.

Mallon W: Golf, in Safran MR, McKeag DB, Van Camp SP (eds): *Manual of Sports Medicine.* Philadelphia: Lippincott-Raven, 1998, pp 571–572.

Stockard AR: Elbow injuries in golf. *J Am Osteopath Assoc* 101(9):509–516, 2001.

Theriault G, Lachance P: Golf injuries: An overview. *Sports Med* 26(1):43–57, 1998.

37

Gymnastics

Kimberly Harmon

EPIDEMIOLOGY

- 600,000 participants in school or club-level gymnastic competitions
- 86,000 gymnastics related injuries treated by health care providers annually
- National Collegiate Athletic Association (NCAA) data
  - Athletes are over twice as likely to get injured at matches than practices.
  - Gymnastic practice injuries in college athletes are second only to spring football injuries in rate of incidence (7.6 per 1000 athlete exposures).
  - Gymnastic match injury rate in college athletes is in the top four (18.8 per 1000 athlete exposures).
  - Half of match injuries result in a time loss of more than a week.
  - 20–36 percent of match injuries required surgery.
- The rate of catastrophic injury in high school and college gymnastics is 3 per 100,000 athletes.
- Injuries most frequently occur when landing in a routine or when landing after a dismount.
- Floor exercises are the most common cause of injury.

COMMON INJURIES

- Sprains
  - Ankle sprain most common (see Chap. 27).
  - Knee (see Chap. 26)
    - Anterior cruciate ligament (ACL)
    - Medial collateral ligament (MCL)
    - Meniscus
- Strains
  - Common in hamstrings, groin, quadriceps
- Concussions (see Chap. 6)
  - When landing on head or hitting a piece of equipment
- Fractures (see Chap. 18)
  - Potential for serious injury given force of impact when landing.

- If impact occurs when gymnast is inverted, there is potential for serious neck and head injury.
- Dislocations
  - Elbow/shoulder (see Chaps. 23 and 24)
    - Hand position required to complete certain maneuvers, particularly on uneven bars, may place the shoulder or elbow at risk for dislocation.

SPECIALIZED MEDICAL EQUIPMENT

- Splint set
- Backboard and cervical spine collar
- Emergency plan to facilitate and coordinate access to EMS (see Chap. 63).

TREATMENT

- Concussion (see Chap. 6)
  - Consider restricting gymnast from further competition even with mild injury, as proprioception is often affected in concussion and premature return to play may increase chances of catastrophic injury.

RETURN TO PLAY

- Ankle sprain
  - When able to jump on one foot, land, cut, and run pain-free
  - Tape or ankle brace recommended initially
- ACL
  - After surgery (9–12 months)
  - With demands of sport, conservative treatment unlikely to be successful and a failed trial of conservative treatment places the knee at risk for additional damage.
- MCL
  - When knee has full ROM, strength is 90 percent of opposite knee, there is no tenderness over the ligament and no pain with valgus stress testing or functional movements
- Mensicus
  - When patient has functional ROM, strength is full, and patient can land from jumps
- Muscle strains/contusions
  - When 90 percent strength of opposite leg is restored and there is no pain with functional activities after adequate warmup
- Concussion
  - When athlete is asymptomatic and symptoms do not recur with exertion

- Consider restricting gymnast from further competition even with mild injury, as proprioception is often affected in concussion and premature return to play may increase chances of catastrophic injury.
- Fractures
  - Dependent on type of fracture and required treatment
- Shoulder dislocation
  - When there is full range of motion, muscle strength is 100 percent, and there is no apprehension in abduction and external rotation, athlete may begin supervised guarded return to activity.
  - As this injury is likely to recur, particularly in young athletes, surgical stabilization after first-time dislocation should be considered, given the demands of the sport.
- Elbow dislocation
  - Athlete needs full ROM and stability of elbow ligaments.
  - This is often a career-ending injury for a gymnast.

Bibliography

Daly RM, Bass SL, Finch CF: Balancing the risk of injury to gymnastics: How effective are the counter measures? *Br J Sports Med* 35:8–20, 2001.

Mandelbaum BR, Nattiv A: Gymnastics, in Safran MR, McKeag DB, Van Camp SP (eds): *Manual of Sports Medicine.* Philadelphia: Lippincott-Raven, 1998.

Sands WA: Injury prevention in women's gymnastics. *Sports Med* 30(5): 359–373, 2000.

Weber J: Gymnastics, in Mellion MB, Walsh WM, Shelton GL (eds): *The Team Physician's Handbook,* 2d ed. Philadelphia: Hanley & Belfus, 1997.

38

Hockey

Greg Maletis
Ray Tufts

COMMON INJURIES

Head and Neck

- Facial lacerations—usually due to contact with another player, the puck, or a hockey stick.
  - Malar, zygomatic, mandibular, and orbital fractures may coexist with facial laceration.
  - Check for pain, crepitus, and malocclusion, which may signify an associated fracture.
  - Rule out a concussion.
- Eye injury (see Chap. 12)
  - Corneal abrasion
  - Laceration—pain, decreased visual acuity
  - Orbital blowout fracture—fracture of floor and medial wall of orbit
- Concussion (see Chap. 6)
  - Assume c-spine injury in unconscious player.
  - Protect cervical spine in the unconscious player until it can be cleared.
- Cervical spine injury—axial load through the head, usually with the neck in a slightly flexed position (see Chap. 20).
  - Leave helmet on until c-spine is cleared.
  - Stabilize helmet to backboard for transport.
- Nasal fracture (see Chap. 10)
  - Pain, epistaxis, and nasal congestion
- Dental injuries (see Chap. 11)
  - Luxation—tooth loosened within socket
  - Avulsion—tooth completely displaced from socket
- Laryngeal fracture (see Chap. 3)
  - Due to puck or stick across front of neck.
  - Hemoptysis, stridor, loss of Adam's apple, subcutaneous emphysema.
  - May be life-threatening if airway is disrupted.

Upper Extremity

- Shoulder (see Chap. 24)
  - Acromioclavicular (AC) separation—most common shoulder injury, usually from hitting the acromion on the boards or the ice.
    - Clavicular fracture is more common in young athletes.
  - Glenohumeral dislocation—usually from a fall onto an outstretched arm.
  - Rotator cuff strain or tear—due to impact with the boards.
- Elbow (see Chap. 23)
  - Olecranon bursitis—due to falls on the ice.
- Wrist and hand (see Chap. 22)
  - Wrist fractures—falls onto a hand may cause wrist or scaphoid fractures.
  - Hand fractures—usually due to being slashed by an opponent's stick or the result of fighting.
  - Gamekeeper's thumb—thumb is forcibly abducted by the hockey stick or occasionally during a fight.

Trunk

- Sternum and rib contusions—as a result of being checked from behind and hitting the boards chest-first.
- Back injuries—very common, usually due to muscle strain.

Abdomen (See Chap. 14)

- Viscera—splenic and kidney injuries may occur from being cross-checked.
- Abdominal wall—rectus avulsion from pubic symphysis.
- Sports hernia—disruption of the inguinal canal without detectable hernia; may be caused by rapid acceleration with skating.
- Hockey player's syndrome (slap-shot gut)—tear of the external oblique aponeurosis with inguinal nerve entrapment due to trunk rotation during shooting and acceleration while skating.

Lower Extremity

- Hip/groin—among the most common injuries
  - Adductor muscle/tendon strain—the skating motion relies heavily on the adductors and quadriceps; rapid acceleration may lead to adductor strains.
  - Hip pointer—contusion of the anterior superior iliac spine or the iliac crest.
- Thigh contusion
  - Usually due to a blow from an opponent's knee or stick directly to the thigh.

- • May lose knee ROM with increasing severity of contusion.
- • Knee—the most commonly injured area (see Chap. 26).
  - • MCL—most common knee injury, due to a blow to the lateral knee with the skate caught on the ice or the boards.
  - • ACL—fairly uncommon, may be a result of a hyperextension or twisting injury.
  - • Meniscus and articular cartilage—occasionally injured in a twisting fall.
- • Ankle (see Chap. 27)
  - • Syndesmotic rupture (high ankle sprain)—foot is forcefully pronated and externally rotated when skate gets caught on the boards or ice.
  - • Fractures and sprains—uncommon with the rigid skates that lace up above the ankle.
- • Foot (see Chap. 28)
  - • Contusion and fracture—usually a direct blow from the puck, often occurs when trying to block a shot with the foot.
  - • Blisters and swelling over malleoli and calcaneus are common from constant rubbing on tight, stiff skates.

EQUIPMENT

- • Face mask removal equipment is usually not needed.
  - • Full face masks can be released and flipped up to gain airway access.
  - • Face shields cover only the upper face; therefore airway access is still possible. A screwdriver is required to remove the face shield and is not practical in an emergency situation.
- • Laceration repair
  - • 5.0 or 6.0 nylon or prolene suture for facial lacerations.
  - • Dermabond glue may be used for more superficial lacerations but is not as secure if the player is going to return to play immediately.
- • Airway management (see Chap. 3)
  - • 14-gauge angiocatheter or crichothyrotomy kit for emergency cricothyrotomy, Ambu bag
  - • Albuterol inhaler—for exercise-induced asthma, which may be exacerbated by cold temperatures.

TREATMENT

Head and Neck

- • Facial lacerations (see Chap. 16)
  - • If superficial, can be anesthetized, cleaned and primarily closed with 5.0 or 6.0 suture.
  - • Deep lacerations and those involving the ocular muscles or nasolacrimal duct need specialized care by a plastic surgeon or ophthalmologist.

- Eye injuries—check visual acuity, pupil reactivity, and extraocular eye motion.
  - Lacerations to the globe and orbital blowout fractures
    - Patch and immediately refer to an ophthalmologist.
- Nasal fracture
  - Pack to stop bleeding.
  - Reduction within 1 week if needed.
- Dental injuries (see Chap. 11)
  - Luxation—displaced tooth should be guided back into position.
  - Avulsion—rinse with milk or sterile saline, replant into socket if possible; if not possible, then place tooth in Hank's solution or milk and transport as soon as possible.
    - Success of replantation is dependent on length of time tooth is out of socket.
- Cervical spine injuries (see Chap. 20)
  - Head and neck must be stabilized as player is transferred to backboard.
  - Helmet and shoulder pads should be left on and helmet taped to backboard; sandbags can be used to stabilize the head.
  - Backboard should be lifted onto gurney, which has been rolled out onto the ice.
    - Medical personnel should enlist the help of a player or official to help them skate out onto the ice to get to an injured player. Trying to run on the ice may lead to an injury.
- Laryngeal injuries—if severe airway obstruction, may require intubation or cricothyrotomy.

Extremity Injuries

- Sprains and contusions should be treated with rest, ice, compression, and elevation (RICE).
- Dislocated joints must be reduced as soon as possible.
- Fractures should be splinted until definitive treatment can be rendered.

Abdominal Injuries

- Splenic or liver injuries—intravenous fluids and immediate transport to the hospital if signs of hypovolemia or internal bleeding (tender or rigid abdomen).
- Sports hernia—surgery indicated if activity-related pain persists.

RETURN TO PLAY

General Requirements

- When pain-free ROM has been reestablished.
- No functional instability.

- Good strength.
- Able to perform sport-specific tasks.

Head and Neck

- Facial laceration—may return to play after superficial laceration is closed.
- Facial fracture—4–6 weeks depending on severity, with face mask for protection.
- Eye injury—may not return to game if there is pain, blurred vision, or blood in the anterior chamber.
- Nasal fracture—may return to game if there is no deviation of septum or septal hematoma; face shield or mask to be used for protection.
- Concussion (see Chap. 6)
  - Should not return to game if there was any loss of consciousness or signs and symptoms of concussion.
    - Headache, nausea, vomiting, dizziness, memory loss, blurred vision, problems with concentration
  - Professionals required to take neuropsychological test, which is compared to preseason test before athlete is allowed to return to play.

Upper Extremity

- AC separation
  - Grades 1 and 2—return in 1–2 weeks with donut pad over AC joint
  - Grade 3—return in 3–6 weeks with donut pad over AC joint
- Glenohumeral subluxation—return in 1–2 weeks depending on severity
  - Dislocation—may require surgery
- Hand and wrist fracture—return in 4–6 weeks
  - May require surgery if displaced
  - Return limited by ability to grasp stick
- Gamekeeper's thumb—if mild sprain, may return in 1–2 weeks with thumb braced or taped.

Lower Extremity

- Hip pointer—may return with extra hip padding
- Knee
  - MCL grade 1—return in 1–3 weeks, usually with a knee brace
  - MCL grade 2—return in 3–6 weeks with a knee brace
  - MCL grade 3—return in 4–8 weeks with brace if no other associated injuries
  - ACL—usually requires surgery, return in approximately 6 months
- Ankle and foot
  - Fractures—if nondisplaced, may return when able to skate pain-free
  - Syndesmotic sprain—return in 4–6 weeks with ankle brace

Bibliography

Bartolozzi AR, Palmeri M, DeLuca PF: Ice hockey, in Safran MR, McKeag DB, Van Camp SP (eds): *Manual of Sports Medicine.* Philadelphia: Lippincott-Raven, 1998, pp575–577.

Minkoff J, Stecker S, Varlotta GP, Simonson BG: Ice hockey, in Fu FH, Stone DA (eds): *Sports Injuries,* 2d ed. Philadelphia: Lippincott-Raven, 2001, pp 483–532.

39

Marathon

Carrie Jaworski

INTRODUCTION

- The popularity of marathons is increasing among recreational athletes.
- Approximately 2–12 percent of entrants will utilize a medical aid station, depending on the event.
- LaSalle Bank's Chicago Marathon now limits registration to 37,500 participants.
- These events are popular with spectators as well. There were >950,000 spectators for the 2001 Chicago Marathon.

EVENT PLANNING

- Primary goal of medical team is to ensure safety of competitors.
- Secondary goal is to prevent emergency room overload.
- Mass participation events also have risk of mass casualty/disaster.
- Medical director needs to oversee disaster plan in the event of such an emergency.
- Managing the medical care of a large road race/marathon requires the cooperation of many individuals within a community.
  - Financial support for supplies
  - Local hospitals, physicians, nurses, EMTs, and other allied health professionals to work as medical team
  - Police and fire departments to assist medical team
- Preevent planning
  - Primary prevention strategies to minimize risk to competitors and spectators
- Event day
  - Secondary prevention strategies to stop progression of injury/illness
- Postevent planning
  - Gather statistics on injuries/outcomes for future strategies.
- "Good Samaritan" laws do not always cover event physicians.
  - Medical team members should inform insurance carriers.
  - Event insurance should extend coverage to include medical team.

INJURY PREVENTION AND PLANNING

- Predetermine hazardous conditions that will warrant cancellation, alteration, or postponement of the event.
  - Examples include lightning, cold stress, combined heat and humidity, and air pollution.
  - Publish protocols in advance.
  - Announce risks under current conditions at start of event.
- Schedule to avoid extremes in weather.
  - Avoid hot, humid months and very cold months.
  - Summer races should be scheduled for early morning or evening.
  - Winter races should be midday.
- Measure heat-stress index at the site of the race prior to start and during event.
  - Ambient temperatures reported by weather channels are only one component of environmental heat or cold stress.
  - The wet bulb globe temperature (WBGT) index is widely used to account for all factors (humidity, wind speed, and radiant heat).
  - Recommended by the American College of Sports Medicine for use in running endurance events.
  - WBGT = (0.7 twb) + (0.2 tg) + (0.1 tdb)
  - twb = wet-bulb temperature = water-saturated cloth wick over dry-bulb thermometer measured in direct sunlight.
  - tg = black-globe temperature = dry bulb in black metal globe measured in direct sunlight.
  - tdb = shaded dry-bulb temperature = air temperature with standard dry-bulb thermometer not in direct sunlight.
  - A WBGT thermometer can be purchased from Quest Technologies, Oconomowoc, WI (1-800-245-0779).
- Use of colored-flag system to visually signal the thermal injury risk to participants.
  - Display at start (and along the course if changes expected).
  - Black flag = extreme risk
    - WBGT >28°C (82°F)
    - Event should be canceled, postponed, or modified.
  - Red flag = high risk
    - WBGT = 23°–28°C (73°–82°F)
    - Advise participants to slow pace and increase hydration.
    - Persons sensitive to heat or humidity should not run.
  - Yellow flag = moderate risk
    - WBGT = 18°–23°C (65° to 73°F)
    - Heat-sensitive participants should slow pace.
  - Green flag = low risk
    - WBGT = 10°–18°C (50°–65°F)
    - No restrictions
    - Hyperthermia and hypothermia can still occur in this range.
  - White flag = lower risk for hyperthermia but increased for hypothermia.
    - WBGT <10°C (50°F)

  - Slow runners during long races most susceptible.
  - Worse if wet or windy
- Blue flag = increased risk for hypothermia and frostbite.
  - Ambient temperature <20°C (−4°F)
  - Consider canceling or postponing.
- Anticipate and prepare for common problems and uncommon catastrophes.
- Use of *predicted incidence of injury* to project supply, staff, and equipment needs until event-specific data are available (usually 2–3 years).
  - (Anticipated number of participants) × (casualty incidence).
  - Ranges from the literature
    - Running (41 km) = 1–20%
    - Running (<21 km) = 1–5%
    - Triathlon (225 km) = 15–30%
    - Triathlon (51 km) = 2–5%
  - Risk of sudden cardiac death during marathoning ranges in the literature from 1:50,000 to 1:100,000 entrants.

TYPES OF CASUALTIES

- Establish medical protocols for common casualties and emergencies, such as the following:
  - Exercise-associated collapse
    - Hypothermic
    - Normothermic
    - Hyperthermic
  - Dehydration
  - Hyponatremia
  - Gastrointestinal bleeding
  - Hematuria
  - Trauma
    - Macrotrauma—fractures, dislocations, sprains, strains, contusions.
    - Microtrauma—usually overuse. Medial tibial stress syndrome, stress fractures, plantar fasciitis.
    - Skin trauma in areas of friction—nipples, groin, feet.
  - Random life-threatening medical emergencies
    - Cardiac arrest
    - Asthma and anaphylaxis
    - Insulin shock
    - Low incidence, high public visibility
- Predetermine *impaired competitor policy*
  - Decide how to handle athlete who is injured or ill during event.
  - Do not disqualify for medical evaluation (as was done in the past).
  - Use clinical criteria to proceed.
    - Oriented to person, place, and time.
    - Demonstrates appropriate competitive posture.
    - Is able to proceed in straight line toward finish.
    - Appears clinically fit.

- Publish in advance.
- Predetermine transfer protocol.
  - Not responding to usual treatment.
  - Severe casualties not responding rapidly.
  - Suggested automatic transfers—cardiac arrest, respiratory arrest, shock, hyperthermia with seizure, or rectal temperature <94°F.
- Notify local emergency rooms of time, location, and expected casualties.

MEDICAL SUPPORT

Medical Director

- Sports medicine–trained physician.
- Works with race director regarding policies, liability and competitor education.
- Acts as spokesperson in the event of a medical problem.

Medical Personnel

- Medical assistance should be available if race is 10 km or longer.
- Consider ratio of the following health providers per 1000 runners:
  - 1–2 physicians
  - 4–6 podiatrists
  - 1–4 emergency medical technicians
  - 2–4 nurses (at least 1 trained in intravenous therapy)
  - 3–6 physical therapists
  - 3–6 athletic trainers
  - 1–3 assistants
- 75 percent of these personnel are stationed at the finish line.
- Consider 1–2 physicians and 2–4 nurses trained in the care of wheelchair athletes.
- 1 physician and 10–15 medical assistants to triage at finish line/chute.
- Designate medical volunteers with easily identifiable hats, shirts, etc.

Medical Aid Stations

Main Medical Tent

- Located near finish.
- Triage at finish line/chute with transport to main tent.
- No public access; security guards at entryways.
- Areas within tent
  - Triage area
  - Medical records
  - Intensive medical area

- Intensive trauma area
- Minor medical area
- Minor trauma area
- Medications
  - ACLS drugs (see Chaps. 5 and 61)
  - D50%W
  - Albuterol nebulizer and MDI
  - Epi-pens
  - Antihistamines
  - Diazepam
  - Acetaminophen
- Intravenous fluids
  - Event <4 h: D5 ½ NS or D5NS
  - Event >4 h: D5NS
  - Avoid fluids containing K^+ until a serum K^+ has been measured.
- See Table 39.1 for recommended supplies.

Table 39.1 Main Medical Tent Supplies*

Equipment
ACLS kits
Adhesive and paper tape
Air conditioner/heater
Alcohol wipes
ALS ambulance
Automatic external defibrillator/defibrillator
Bacitracin ointment
Bandage scissors
Band-Aids
Batteries for equipment
Biohazard bags
Blankets (cloth and mylar)
Blood glucose monitor and strips, lancets
Cots
Cotton tip applicators
Cups
Elastic bandages (2″, 4″ and 6″)
Elastic wrap for securing ice bags
Emesis bags/basins
Endotracheal tubes (3mm, 5mm, 7mm)
Examination gloves
Eye kits (blue light, eye pads, fluorescence stain strips, saline solution)
Face masks/shields for CPR
Fans for cooling
Flashlights
Gauze pads (4 × 4 inch)
Laryngoscope (adult and pediatric size)
Measuring tape
Medical record forms
Moleskin
Nasal pharyngeal airway/oropharyngeal airway (3 sizes each)
Oto/ophthalmoscope
Oxygen tanks with masks
Paper
Pens
Petroleum jelly
Plug strips
Portable clothes dryer
Portable telephone/radios
Rapid serum electrolyte/chemistry panel machine
Rectal thermometers—High and low temperature
Reflex hammer

Table 39.1 (*Continued*)

Equipment

Safety pins
Scalpels (#11 blade)
Sharps containers
Skin disinfectant
Slings/inflatable splints
Sphygmomanometers
Stethoscopes
Stretchers
Tables for supplies
Tampons
Thermometer covers
Tin snips
Tongue blades
Urinals
Ventilation bags/mask
Wading pool for immersion
Water jug
Wheelchairs
Wound care kits (sterile fields, dressings and gloves, steristrips, benzoin, sutures)

Trauma Needs

Back boards
Cervical collars
Cricothyrotomy kit
Crushed ice in bags
Crutches
Knee immobilizers
Nasal packing
Wound care equipment such as sterile gloves, sterile fields, dressings, saline/syringes for
irrigation, steri-strips, and suture materials

Medication and Intravenous Fluid Needs

Acetaminophen
Albuterol nebs and metered-dose inhalers (MDIs)
Atropine
Demerol
D50%W
D5% ½ NS or D5% NS
Diazepam
Diphenhydramine
Epinephrine 1:10,000 and 1:1000
IV tubing kits
Lidocaine (local)
Morphine
Naloxone
Nitroglycerin (sublingual)
Ophthaine
Propranolol
Sodium bicarbonate
Tourniquet
Vein catheters (16, 18, 22 gauge)

*These are general recommendations only. Some items depend on environmental conditions and established policies of particular event regarding what to treat in the medical tent and what to transport. Quantities should be determined based on previous years or established standards for event size.

Secondary Aid Stations

- Position at 2- to 3-km (1.2- to 1.9-mi) intervals for races >10 km.
- Position at halfway point for shorter races.
- See Table 39.2 for recommended supplies.

Table 39.2 Secondary Aid Station Supplies*

Adhesive tape
Albuterol MDIs
Alcohol pads
Automatic defibrillator
Bacitracin
Band-Aids
Cots
Elastic wrap for securing ice bags
Emesis bags/basins
Facial tissue
Garbage bags (cut arm and head openings to use as windbreaker)
Gauze pads (4 × 4 inch)
Ice and bags
Medical record forms, clipboards, pens
Moleskin
Mylar blankets
Penlights/flashlight
Pocket masks
Rectal thermometer
Scalpels (#11 Blade)
Tampons
Tongue blades
Vaseline

*These are general recommendations. Determine quantities based on previous years or established standards for event size.

Transport Support/Mobile Medical

- One ambulance per 3000 runners at finish for hospital transports.
- Ambulance or mobile medical van support along the course.
- Transportation for well runners who drop out along the course (10 to 40 percent average).

FLUID STATIONS (BASED ON ACSM POSITION STAND)

- Provide equal volumes of water and carbohydrate-electrolyte solution.
- Water should suffice for shorter races.
- Start and finish
    - 12–16 ozs of fluid per runner
    - High carbohydrate–type foods and fruits at finish as well as along course for longer events.
- Racecourse
    - 10–12 oz of fluid per runner
    - Fluid stations every 2–3 km
- Number of cups ($\geq$10 oz) per fluid station on course = number of entrants × 25 percent additional for spillage and double use (double the number for out-and-back course).
- Number of cups at start and finish = (2 × number of entrants) + 25 percent.
- In cool or cold weather, equivalent amounts of warm fluid should be available.
- Runners drink larger volumes if volunteers hand them filled cups.

COMMUNICATION/SURVEILLANCE

- Two-way radios or telephone communication between medical director, aid stations, mobile medical vans, and receiving emergency rooms.
- Have radio-equipped vehicles ahead of and behind participants to monitor for impaired runners.

COURSE CONSIDERATIONS

- Avoid steep downhill starts.
- Use variations in start such as split starts to avoid overcrowding.
- Be aware of potential course hazards—immovable objects, altitude changes, traffic.
- Have shelter available for well finishers in case of inclement weather.
- Consider dry-clothes shuttle from start to finish to ensure warm clothing at finish.
  - Portable clothes dryer can be used in medical tent so that casualties may have access to dry clothes.

PARTICIPANT EDUCATION

- Provide preevent seminars or information on topics such as training, fluids, clothing selection, and signs/symptoms of heat/cold illness.
- Provide participants with race policy regarding impaired runners.
- Provide participants with names of fluid and food types so they can use same types in training.
- Provide participants with locations of aid stations and fluid stations prior to event.
- Advise participants to place name, address, telephone number, and medical problems on back of race bib prior to race.
- Announce weather conditions and location of aid stations at start of race.

COMMON INJURIES/MEDICAL PROBLEMS
Exercise-Associated Collapse (EAC)

- Athlete requires assistance or collapses during or after endurance event.
- Commonly seen at finish, more ominous if occurs prior to finish.
- Etiology—several hypotheses:
  - Vasovagal response
  - Dehydration
  - Energy-store depletion
  - CNS failure
  - Internal fluid shifts
  - Temporary malfunction in thermoregulation

- EAC can include:
  - Heatstroke
  - Heat exhaustion
  - Heat cramps
  - Heat syncope
  - Exhaustion
  - Exertion leg cramps
  - Hypothermia
- Keys to diagnosis
  - Body temperature—*rectal temperature required*
    - Hypothermic—core temperature ≤97°F (36°C)
    - Normothermic—core temperature between 97°F and 103°F
    - Hyperthermic—core temperature ≥103°F (39.5°C)
  - Mental status
  - Ability to ambulate
- Clinical signs and symptoms
  - Exhaustion, fatigue, inability to walk unassisted
  - Stomach cramps, nausea, vomiting, diarrhea
  - Light-headed, headache, altered mental status, CNS changes
  - Leg cramps, muscle spasms
  - Palpitations, tachycardia
  - Abnormal body temperature
- Severity rating
  - Mild
    - Nonspecific signs or symptoms
    - Walks with or without assist
  - Moderate
    - Unable to walk
    - Severe muscle spasm
    - Extra fluid losses/inadequate intake
    - Temperature ≥105°F (40.5°C) or ≤95°F (36°C)
  - Severe
    - CNS changes
    - Temperature ≥106°F (41°C) or ≤90°F (32°C)
- Treatment
  - Have athlete lie down with legs elevated.
  - Oral fluids preferred if athlete can tolerate them.
  - Intravenous fluids if athlete cannot take oral or if no response with oral hydration.
    - Follow fluid guidelines above.
    - Chicago Marathon requires serum electrolytes prior to intravenous fluid administration.
    - Consider D50%W if slow response to hydration and/or temperature correction.
  - Temperature correction—hypothermic EAC
    - Handle gently.
    - Place in warm area and insulate with warmed blankets.
    - Remove wet clothing and dry the athlete's skin.
    - Place warm packs (intravenous bags) behind neck, in axillae, and in groin area.

- Prewarm intravenous fluids.
- If temperature >95°F, have athlete walk, if able, to generate heat.
- Warm, humidified air if available.
- Monitor at regular intervals.
- Hyperthermic EAC
  - Place in cool, shaded area.
  - Remove excess clothing.
  - Active cooling for temperature >105°F.
    - Ice packs
    - Ice-water tub immersion
    - Fan with cooling mist spray.
    - End when temperature 5 102°F.
  - Precool intravenous fluids
  - Control continued muscle contractions.
    - Diazepam 1–5 mg slow IV push, repeat as needed.
  - Leg cramps
    - Fluid replacement
    - Assisted walking
    - No massage until hydrated
    - Consider diazepam 1–5 mg IV push
    - Consider magnesium sulfate 5 g IV loading dose.
  - Monitor at regular intervals, watch for delayed temperature rise and overcooling.
- Normothermic EAC
  - Maintain temperature.
  - Monitor for delayed hyperthermia and postrace hypothermia.

Hyponatremia

- Serum sodium <135 mg/dL
- Low reported incidence in marathons, consider with ultradistance events.
- Can be caused by excessive free water intake during race.
- More common in slower runners.
  - More time to drink at aid stations
  - Less sweating
- Presents with confusion, seizures, or no symptoms.
- Consider in EAC patient with slow response to treatment.
- Transport for altered mental status or seizure.
- No intravenous fluids for normovolemic or hypervolemic athletes.

Gastrointestinal Bleeding

- Commonly seen after distance running.
- Rare occurrences of acute hemorrhage.
- Rarely presents to event medical tent; athlete discovers later.
- Studies report range of 8–22 percent incidence of clinically detectable bleeding in marathoners after a race

- Possible etiologies include NSAID use, bowel ischemia, traumatic shearing from running, or underlying pathology.
- Must first rule out underlying pathology.
- Usually self-limited, resolving in 72 h.
- Monitor for iron deficiency.

Musculoskeletal Injuries and Other Running Issues

- See Chap. 51.

Random Medical Emergencies

Cardiac Arrest

- Follow ACLS protocols (see Chap. 4 and appendix).
- Consider following modifications:
  - D50%W, since glucose depleted by physical activity.
  - High-dose epinephrine (5–10 mg IV push), as activity depletes catecholamines.
  - Sodium bicarbonate to reverse metabolic acidosis of activity.
- Use these modifications under the guidance of a cardiologist or critical care physician.

Asthma and Anaphylaxis (See Chaps. 7 and 8)

Insulin Shock

- D50%W
- Glucagon

POSTRACE EVALUATION

- Review medical records for trends.
- Review adverse events.
- Make changes and plan for following year using collected data.

Bibliography

American College of Sports Medicine: Position stand on heat and cold illness during distance running. *Med Sci Sports Exerc,* pp. i–ix, 1996.

Roberts WO: Administration and medical management of mass participation endurance events, in Mellion MB, Walsh WM, Shelton GL (eds): *The Team Physician's Handbook,* 2d ed. Philadelphia: Hanley & Belfus, 1997.

Roberts WO: Event coverage, in Safran MR, McKeag DB, Van Camp SP (eds): *Manual of Sports Medicine.* Philadelphia: Lippincott-Raven, 1998.

40

Martial Arts

John Cheng

INTRODUCTION

- The term *martial arts* refers to the collective disciplines of hand-to-hand combat developed and practiced in Asia.
- These disciplines were originally designed for use in military combat.
- Their popularity in the twentieth century has now evolved into a form of personal discipline and for some a sport aimed at developing self-esteem and self-confidence.
- The martial arts also include the use of weapons—such as staffs, swords, spears, and large knives.
- An estimated 1.5–2 million Americans participate in martial arts disciplines.
- The male:female ratio is 5:1.
- Different types and forms of martial arts exist.
- These include kung fu/wushu, karate, tae kwon do, judo, jiujitsu, kickboxing, muy thai, and others.
- The following are mechanisms of injury common to these combat arts:
  - Direct trauma from punching, kicking, elbow strikes, and head butts.
  - Indirect injuries resulting from rotational forces.
  - Injuries from choke holds to the neck and joint locks to the wrist, elbow, and shoulders.

PROTECTIVE GEAR

- This is required by some disciplines while being disregarded in others because of organizational rules or simply personal tastes and martial arts traditions.
  - Headgear
  - Eye protection
  - Mouthpiece
  - Chest protector
  - Gloves
  - Boots
  - Groin protector
  - Shin protectors

COMMON INJURIES

Classification of Injuries

- Injuries to head and face
- Injuries to abdomen and ribs
- Injuries to extremities
- Most common injuries
  - Contusions
  - Bruises
  - Sprains
  - Strains

Mechanisms of Injury

- Direct impact from fists, elbows, knees, feet, head butts
- Repetitive trauma (ballistic and torsional motions)

Serious Injuries

- Concussions
- Paralysis
- Abdominal injuries from visceral rupture

Facial Injuries (See Chap. 10)

- Facial cuts (eyebrow, nasal area, cheeks, lips)
  - Result from direct contact with fists or fingernails.

Treatment

- Direct pressure with gauze for 1–2 min to control bleeding.
- Superficial cuts can be cleaned and approximated with butterfly Band-Aids or covered with a Band-Aid.
- If cuts are deep and involve jagged edges, they may require suturing.
- Often such injuries can be prevented by the use of regulation padded gloves and headgear.
- Return to play depends on the event's rules. Some competitions disqualify the opponent for drawing blood, while others may continue provided that there is no active bleeding.

Eye Injuries (See Chap. 12)

- "Black eye"—results from a direct strike to the eye.
  - Evaluate ROM and vision to rule out ocular fracture.

- If there is bleeding, determine whether the bleeding is from the lid or from within the eye. May require immediate ophthalmology referral.
- Corneal abrasion—results from a scratch (fingernails) from an eye poke or (toenails) from a kick.

Treatment

- If there is a simple periorbital contusion application of ice should be sufficient.

Prevention

- Finger attacks to the eyes should be avoided.
- Participants may consider using protective goggles.
- Participants with previous eye injury or decreased vision should wear eye protection.

Nasal Injuries (See Chap. 10)

- The nose is a common target.
  - Nasal contusion—inspect nasal bridge for any deformity or deviation and for possible fracture. Suspect nasal fracture if there is obvious deformity, deviation, or difficulty breathing from one side of the nose. Check for septal hematoma, which requires urgent treatment.

Treatment

- Apply ice to decrease swelling and tenderness.
- Epistaxis (nosebleed)—inspect nose for deviation or deformity. Anterior nosebleed usually reponds to direct pressure with a cold cloth or ice pack over the side that is bleeding. If bleeding does not respond, consider posterior nosebleed; this requires emergent nasal packing in an emergency setting.

Ear Injuries (See Chap. 10)

- External ear injuries result from direct blows to the ear.

Treatment

- Ice to decrease swelling and bleeding.
- Poorly treated external ear injuries may result in cauliflower ear.
- Eardrum injury results from slaps to the ear with a palm or cupped hand.
  - There may be immediate pain and decrease in hearing.
  - Avoid putting ear drops into the canal at this time so as to avoid middle ear infection.
  - Avoid blowing the nose, as this may cause further damage to the inner ear.

Tongue Injuries

- These occur when the tongue is crushed or cut between the teeth as a blow strikes a partially opened jaw.

Treatment

- Mild bleeding usually resolves with ice and direct pressure.
- If the cut goes through the tongue, it may require suturing.
- Mouth guards usually prevent this injury; also, participants should be taught to keeping their jaw closed.

Head and Neck

- Concussion—results from repetitive head trauma or direct blow with punch or kick (see Chap. 6).
- Consider possible c-spine injury in unconscious athlete or if there is neck pain (see Chap. 20).
- Carotid sinus injury—a choke hold can render a competitor unconscious.
- Carotid artery—external compression decreases blood flow to the brain.
  - Revival techniques—elevate legs with patient in supine position to increase blood flow to the brain. Prepare for possible CPR if patient does not revive after the choke hold is released and with leg elevation of 1–2 ft.

Injuries to Extremities

- Sprains, strains, fractures, dislocations, contusions, hematomas, and tendon avulsions

Fingers (See Chap. 22)

- Dislocations of proximal interphalangeal (PIP)—if there is an obvious dorsal dislocation, it can be reduced on the spot; however, be aware of possible fracture.
- Avulsions of extensor tendons.
- Arthritis from repetitive trauma.

Elbow (See Chap. 23)

- Olecranon fossitis—due to repetitive hyperextension from improper punching technique; remedied by instruction in proper technique of not fully extending the elbow upon punching.
- Tendinitis—medial and lateral epicondylitis: treat with ice, relative rest, bracing.

Shoulder (See Chap. 24)

- Dislocation—95 percent anterior, 5 percent posterior
- Tendinitis
- Rotator cuff strains
- Subluxations
- Acromioclavicular sprains—from poorly executed rolls or falls

Knee (See Chap. 26)

- Hyperextension
- Rotation
- Flexion
- Varus or valgus forces—result from application of these forces by opponent
- Meniscal tears
- Ligament sprains
- Patellar tendinitis—from repetitive kicking practice
- Dislocation—rare

Thigh

- Contusion—usually due to direct trauma from opponent's shin, knee or elbow.
- Hematoma—can lead to myositis ossificans; pain-causing, pulls martial artist out of competition.

Ankle Sprains and Fractures (See Chap. 27)

- Inversion and eversion forces
- Ankle locks

Toes (See Chap. 28)

- Sprains, strains, fractures

Injuries to the Trunk (See Chap. 13)

- Strike to solar plexus
- Costochondritis
- Rib fractures
- Pneumothorax

Abdominal Trauma (See Chap. 14)

- Injury to liver, spleen, kidney, pancreas

Testicular Trauma

- Can be prevented by using groin protector

Skin Conditions

- Impetigo
- Herpes simplex
- Boils
- Scabies
    - No contact permitted until there are no longer any contagious or oozing lesions. Can attempt to cover lesions as long as dressing does not rub or come off.

RETURN TO PLAY

- Disqualifying conditions: noncontact areas are usually considered to be the head, back of the neck, groin, and knee joints.
- However, depending on the style and organization, such attacks may be permitted with appropriate headgear, groin protector, and shin padding.

Bibliography

Estwanik JJ: *Sports Medicine for the Combat Arts.* Charlotte, NC: Boxergenics Press, 1996.

Mellion MB: *Sports Medicine Secrets,* 2d ed. Philadelphia: Hanley & Belfus, 1998.

Wilkerson LA: Martial arts injuries, in Mellion MB, Walsh WM, Shelton GL (eds): *The Team Physician's Handbook*, 2d ed. Philadelphia: Hanley & Belfus, 1997, pp 855–866.

41

Motorsports Medicine

Jeff T. Grange

BACKGROUND

- There are many types of racing—stock cars, open-wheel cars (Championship Auto Racing Teams, Indy Racing League, Formula 1), drag cars, off-road trucks and buggies, go-karts, motorcycles (on-road and off-road), mud racing, boats, planes, etc. Each form has specialized fire, safety, and rescue techniques and specialized equipment. This chapter deals primarily with the most common form of motorsports—auto racing.
- There are multiple types of venues—permanent oval or road-course facilities, temporary street circuits, dirt tracks, stadiums, deserts, etc.
- Auto racing deaths: an average 14 drivers per year die, many others are paralyzed or seriously injured.
- 27 percent of those killed at auto-racing events are track workers, spectators, and journalists.
- Common misconception: motorsports medicine is analogous to routine EMS practice. Experts agree that motorsports medicine requires a well-planned and more complex response.
- There is very little in the medical literature regarding motorsports and there are also few standards.

COMMON INJURIES

- Most driver deaths are caused by head and neck injuries.
  - Head injuries
  - Neck injuries
- Many drivers also die from heart attacks and thus may injure other drivers or spectators.
  - Driving 2 h on a road course is equivalent to running 15 mi in the same time.
  - Medical providers should consider medical screening prior to competition and exclude anyone with significant heart problems from competition.
- Drivers are also at risk for burns, blunt chest trauma, and blunt abdominal trauma.

- Consider carbon monoxide poisoning in drivers who develop symptoms after racing in closed vehicles.

SPECIALIZED EQUIPMENT NEEDS

- Fire suppression/rescue/extrication equipment and personnel (Reference NFPA 1610 Standard)
- Fire suits and other personal protective equipment
  - Methanol burns invisibly and rescue personnel could walk into fire without noticing until they feel burning. Must use extreme caution.
- Specialized airway equipment/techniques for in-car airway management
  - Combitubes
  - Digital intubation
  - Surgical cricothyrotomy kits
  - Other (Per-Trache, Quick Trache, etc.)
- Cervical collars
- The head and neck support (HANS) device (Fig. 41.1)
  - If HANS left in place during extrication, consider front half of Philadelphia collar with straps or duct tape to stabilize neck.
  - HANS and Philadelphia collar combination provide better neck immobilization than standard (controversial) cervical collars due to continued alignment with torso.
  - HANS device is radiolucent so initial c-spine x-rays can be completed with HANS device in place.
- Other head/neck restraint devices

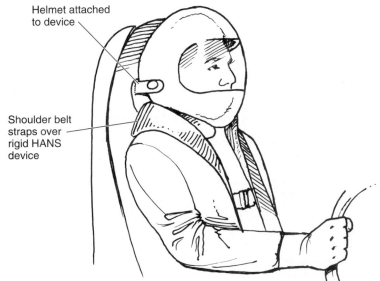

Helmet attached to device

Shoulder belt straps over rigid HANS device

Figure 41.1 HANS device.

- Backboards/litters/cots
  - Should fit in all potential transport vehicles (ambulance, helicopter, etc.).
- Kendrick extrication device (KED)
  - Most commonly available extrication device.
- Most open-wheel race cars need special equipment due to space constraints.
- Ground ambulance—most experts agree ambulance should have advanced life support (ALS) capability for advanced airway management due to high risk.
- Air ambulance—recommended for venues with traffic congestion concerns and prolonged distances to a trauma center.
- Communications
  - Consider head sets.
  - Recommend dedicated on-track emergency channel.
  - Test system prior to event.
- Other equipment/supplies (see Chap. 61)

TREATMENT

- Have a medical action *plan prior to event—most important* (see Chap. 55)
  - Track access
  - Response vehicle and transport planning
  - Level of care providers—minimum level (when available in the community) should be a paramedic with advanced airway capabilities. Ideally, a physician competent in dealing with both minor problems and with advanced airway management, resuscitation, and EMS issues.
  - A locally licensed/accredited medical authority responsible for all care should be established.
  - Race control via pace car, lights, flags, etc.
  - Multiple casualty incident/disaster plan (see Chaps. 55, 61, and 62)
  - Know your local medical facilities (trauma centers, burn centers, closest emergency departments, hyperbaric chambers etc.).
- Scene safety—number-one priority
  - Never turn your back on race traffic.
  - Stop the event if necessary.
  - Consider parking rescue vehicles/ambulance to help protect scene.
  - Do not park directly below crash scene on banked tracks due to fuel runoff and fire risk.
- Triage—most major incidents involve more than one driver.
  - Consider checking drivers with their "nets up" or "not moving" first. Drivers are instructed to lower window nets if they are OK.
  - Could there be other injured patients? Look for debris into grandstands, infield, pits, and other areas.
- *Airway with c-spine* immobilization, breathing, circulation (ABCs).
- All unconscious or altered drivers should be extricated with full spinal precautions.

- Remember that even though they have unstable broken necks, drivers may not initially have neck pain due to adrenaline, lack of time for swelling to take place, and other distracting injuries.
- Initial in-car assessment of driver should include the following:
  - Driver's mental status
  - Ability to move arms and legs
  - Grip strength
  - Question regarding pain, numbness, parasthesias or stiffness in neck, back, extremities, etc. Be conservative regarding possible cervical fractures.
  - "If in doubt, cut them out"—refers to cutting car apart in order to maintain proper cervical immobilization throughout extrication.
- Full-face helmets should be removed.
- While on the track, do only what you have to do to stabilize the patient (ABCs and c-spine).
- A more thorough evaluation can be done in the ambulance or on-site medical facility. Try to prevent public spectacles. Although patient care is your primary responsibility, remember that "The show must go on"—and medical care is not the show.
- Consider methylprednisolone for spinal cord injury—initially a 30-mg/kg bolus followed by a continuous infusion of 5.4 mg/kg/h for 23 h. Although not strongly supported by the medical literature, many still consider this the "standard of care."
- In general, do not pronounce a patient dead at the racetrack.
  - Initiate transportation and resuscitation in the ambulance.
    - Better control of situation
    - Prevent public spectacle
    - Better public relations for venue

RETURN TO PLAY

- All drivers with no injuries or complaints should be observed for at least 15 min following a crash. It takes time for swelling to increase and adrenaline to decrease.
- Follow head injury guidelines (see Chap. 6)
- Drivers are at high risk for leaving "against medical advice" (AMA)
  - Consider Mini-Mental Status exam to confirm that driver is capable of signing out against medical advice.
  - Consider a policy that requires all drivers who are unable to drive their cars away from an accident to be checked out by medical providers.
- Stable cervical fractures should be treated in an orthosis until asymptomatic, then reassessed for stability with flexion/extension x-rays. Consider HANS or other head/neck support device for those returning to racing.
- Drivers with unstable cervical fractures status postoperative repair should not be allowed to race for a minimum of 6 months postoperatively
- Be conservative—an unsafe driver can hurt other drivers as well as spectators.

Bibliography

Chesser TJ, Norton SA, Nolan JP, Baskett PJ: What are the requirements for medical cover at motor racing events? *Injury* 30(4):293–297, 1999.

Grange JT, Baumann G: The California 500: Medical care at a NASCAR Winston Cup Race. *Prehosp Emerg Care* 6 315–318, 2002.

National Fire Protection Agency: NFPA 610—Safety at Motorsports Venues. www.nfpa.org

Trammel TR, Reed DB: Spinal injuries in motorsports *Sports Med Arthrosc Rev* 5:194–197, 1997.

Tremayne D: *The Science of Safety: The Battle Against Unacceptable Risk in Motor Racing*. London: Haynes, 2000.

42

Performing Arts

Lauren M. Simon

OVERVIEW

- Performing artists present with a full spectrum of medical disorders plus injuries more specifically seen in their particular art form.
- Awareness of these disorders can expedite treatment and facilitate a return to performing.

PERFORMING ARTISTS

- Musicians, vocalists/singers, actors, dancers.
- Often exposed to infectious diseases such as upper respiratory infection (URI); work in close quarters with frequent exposure.

ENVIRONMENTAL INJURIES

- May be seen across all groups of performing artists.
- Risk of trauma on set or stage: falling objects, slip and fall injuries.
- Weather-related injuries:
  - Sunburn—outdoor stage
  - Heat injuries/cold related injuries
- Exposures to allergens, cigarette smoke, pollutants.

MUSICIANS

Acute Musculoskeletal Injuries

- Neck pain, temporomandibular pain, facial pain after intense performance
  - Seen in violinists, violists, string players, and wind instrumentalists

Treatment

- Anti-inflammatories, stretching, icing
- Correction of technique

Overuse Syndromes/Musculoskeletal Pain

- Arthritis, ganglion cyst, contractures, tendinitis
- Peripheral nerve compression syndrome
  - Ulnar neuropathy, median neuropathy (carpal tunnel syndrome)
- Tenosynovitis of the wrist and hand
  - Seen particularly in pianists
- Focal dystonia syndrome
  - Cramping pain in forearm and hand with activity

Treatment

- Conservative, symptomatic

VOCALISTS/SINGERS

Voice Injuries

- Hoarseness: coarse, scratchy sound from vocal cord abnormalities (i.e., viral or reflux laryngitis)
- Breathiness: excessive loss of air during vocalization
  - Prevents approximation of vocal cords
  - Mechanism of injury
    - Vocal cord paralysis, vocal fold atrophy, arthritis affecting cricoarytenoids
- Voice fatigue: inability to sing extensively without loss of voice quality
  - Mechanism of injury
    - Oversinging, medical illness, medications
    - Tickling or choking sensation
      - Often from reflux laryngitis or allergies
    - Misuse of abdominal, neck musculature
    - Temporomandibular joint disorder transmits tension to mandible and hyoid bone, resulting in voice fatigue
- Volume disturbance: inability to sing loudly or softly
  - Mechanism of injury
    - URI, hormone changes, neurologic disease
  - Medical problems
    - Allergens, sinusitis, postnasal drip, viral infections
      - Attempts to compensate for this, causing laryngeal strain
  - Environmental exposures
    - Allergies, pollutants, heat, cold, cigarette smoke
  - Musculoskeletal: cervical, lumbar, abdominal strain can affect voice technique

Treatment

- Symptomatic; extend warmup, rest from singing if hoarse
- Treat allergies and infections
- Follow-up: may require fiberoptic laryngoscopy for dysarthria, dysphonia

ACTORS

- Environmental exposures, musculoskeletal disorders, medical problems
  - Similar to vocalists (see above)

DANCERS

Acute Musculoskeletal Trauma

- Ankle sprains (see Chap. 27)
- Knee ligament or meniscal tears (see Chap. 26)
- Subluxation of cuboid
  - From repetitive plantar/dorsiflexion.
  - Can occur along with ankle sprain; presents with lateral midfoot pain.
  - Medial cuboid subluxes medially, displacing fourth metatarsal.
  - Unable to weight bear or go en pointe.

Treatment

- Mobilize rear and midfoot, adduct forefoot and reduce cuboid.

Midfoot Sprain

Lisfranc Joint

- From landing from a jump or loss of balance en pointe
- Midfoot swelling, ecchymosis, tenderness
- Pain on passive pronation/supination of foot
- X-ray—standing foot

Treatment

- Non-weight-bearing cast, immobilization

Fractured Fifth Metatarsal

- Dancer's fracture from inversion injury on toes
- Oblique or spiral fracture mid to distal fifth metatarsal

Treatment

- Immobilization followed by taping: may need open reduction and internal fixation (ORIF)

Avulsion Fracture (See Fig. 28.5)

- Proximal fracture of fifth metatarsal

Treatment

- Conservative

Jones Fracture (See Fig. 28.4)

- Fracture of metaphyseal diaphyseal joint

Treatment

- Non-weight-bearing cast or ORIF

Achilles Tendon Rupture (See Chap. 27)

Blisters

Treatment

- Pressure removal with surrounding padding
- Drain if excessively painful
- Cover with lubricant or synthetic skin/blister coverings

Overuse Conditions

- Patellofemoral pain (see Chap. 26)
- Low back pain (see Chap. 21)
  - Musculoligamentous
  - Spondylolysis
- Snapping hip
  - Iliopsoas tendinitis, sartorius tendinitis
- Piriformis syndrome
  - Posterior hip, gluteal pain, possible sciatic nerve irritation
- Tibial/fibular stress fracture
- Achilles tendinitis (see Chap. 27)
- Flexor hallucis longus tendinitis (see Chap. 28)
  - From extensive plantar flexion/dorsiflexon ankle
  - Pain behind medial malleolus

Os Trigonum Impingement Syndrome

- Compressed between posterior tibia and calcaneus
- Spur formation restricts plantar flexion

Treatment

- Rest, restrict plantar flexion, contrast baths, possible surgery

Sesamoid Fracture vs. Sesamoiditis

- Sesamoids in base first metatarsal
- Injury from jumping on hard surface
- Bone scan helpful in diagnosis

Treatment

- Doughnut pad, rigid-soled shoes, NSAIDs

Hallux Rigidus

- Inability to dorsiflex great toe, metatarsophalangeal (MTP) joint

Treatment

- Conservative, may require surgery

Overuse Syndromes

- Dancers may complain of acute pain exacerbation from overuse injuries

Treatment

- NSAIDS, icing, stretching, strengthening.
- Correction of technique or biomechanics plus above specifications.
- Return to activity is symptom-dependent.

ESSENTIAL MEDICAL EQUIPMENT

- Otoscope/penlight for inspection of upper airway and head
- Elastic bandages, skin lubricant, tape, artificial skin for blisters

Bibliography

Kovero O, Könönen M: Signs and symptoms of temporomandibular disorders and radiologically observed abnormalities in the condyles of the temporomandibular joints of professional violin and viola players. *Acta Odontol Scand* 53:81–84, 1995.

Rettig AC: Wrist and hand overuse syndromes. *Clin Sports Med* 20(3): 591–611, 2001.

Sataloff RT: Evaluation of professional singers. *Otolaryngol Clin North Am* 33(5):923–956, 2000.

Solomon R, Brown T, Gerbino PG, et al: The young dancer. *Clin Sports Med* 19(4):717–739, 2000.

Macintyre J, Joy E: Foot and ankle injuries in dance. *Clin Sports Med* 19(2):351–368, 2000.

43

Rugby

Aaron Rubin

INTRODUCTION

- Rugby is an international contact/collision sport played by both men and women, with 15, 13, 10, or 7 players on a side.
- The goal is to move the rugby ball (which looks like a fat football with rounded ends) down the field to score a "try" by carrying the ball past the opponent's goal line and touching it down to the ground in a controlled manner. A try is worth 5 points. A "conversion" after a goal is kicked through the goal posts from a point in line with where the ball is touched down. A conversion is worth 2 points.
- The ball is moved by running with it down the 100- by 69-m field, called a "pitch." All players must remain "onside" or behind the ball. The ball may not be passed forward but only to the side and backward. Blocking is not allowed.
- Once the player is tackled, he or she must release the ball. The tackler must immediately release the player. Anyone who is standing may then pick up the ball and continue.
- There are variations of "touch" rugby, with rules that keep the contact and collision to a minimum. As soon as the player is touched, he or she must release the ball.
- The ball may also be kicked forward but not dropped forward and picked up by the same team. This is called a "knock-on."
- A "ruck" occurs when the ball carrier is tackled to the ground and a pileup of players struggle for possession.
- A "maul" occurs when the ball carrier is stopped but not gone to the ground and players struggle for possession.
- A "scrum" is the formal lineup that occurs after minor penalties or if the ball becomes tied up.
- Injury potential is present in rucks, mauls, and scrums as well as tackles. "Noncontact" injuries also occur, as in other field sports.

COMMON INJURIES

Head, Face, and Neck

- Lacerations—relatively common (see Chap. 16).
- Concussions—due to contact with another player or with ground. Helmets are generally not worn (see Chap. 6).
- Facial fractures (see Chap. 10).
- Eye injuries (see Chap. 12).
- Cervical spine (see Chap. 20).
  - Players must be taught appropriate tackling techniques and be prepared for the scrum.

Shoulder (See Chap. 24)

- Acromioclavicular injury
- Clavicle fractures
- Shoulder dislocation
- Rotator cuff tears

Hand (See Chap. 22)

- "Jersey" finger (this term originated in rugby.)
- Finger dislocations [interphalangeal (IP) and metacarpophalangeal (MCP)]
- Fractures

Chest, Thorax and Lumbar Spine

- Rib contusions and fractures (see Chap. 13)
- Thoracic and lumbar strains (see Chap. 20)
- Disk pathology

Abdomen (See Chap. 14)

- Blunt trauma of spleen, liver, other internal organs
- Abdominal wall strain
- Hernia

Lower Extremity

- Hip "pointer" (see Chap. 25)
- Adductor strain
- Quadriceps contusion and myositis ossificans (see Chap. 29)

- Quadriceps and hamstring strains
- Knee injuries (see Chap. 26)
  - Anterior cruciate ligament (ACL), medial collateral ligament (MCL), meniscus, posterior collateral ligament (PCL)
  - Patellar dislocation
- Calf contusions and strain
- Achilles tendon injury (see Chap. 27)
- Ankle sprains

SPECIALIZED EQUIPMENT NEEDS

- Helmets are rarely worn.
- Mouth guards.
- "Electrical" tape over the ears to keep the ears from being pulled by other players.
- Medical gear
  - Suture, skin staples
  - Wound–care supplies
  - Backboard, supplies for cervical spine immobilization
  - Concussion guidelines

TREATMENT

- The referee will call medical team to the pitch to treat minor injuries. Play may be allowed to continue while treatment is occurring. Play should be stopped for more serious injury.
  - The referee will send players to be treated off the pitch if they are actively bleeding. A temporary substitute may be used. Player may return once bleeding is controlled and permission from the referee obtained. Blood-soaked equipment should be replaced.

RETURN TO PLAY

- An injured player may rejoin the match after evaluation by the medical staff and with permission of the referee.
- As always, the health and well-being of the player is of the utmost importance.
- Various concussion guidelines have been developed (see Chap. 6).

Bibliography

Bruckner P: Rugby, in Safran MR, McKeag DB, VanCamp SP: *Manual of Sports Medicine.* Philadelphia: Lippincott-Raven, 1998.

Marshall SW, Waller AE, Loomis DP, et al: Use of protective equipment in a cohort of rugby players. *Med Sci Sports Exerc* 33(12):2131–2138, 2001.

44

Scuba Diving

Timothy R. McCurry

OVERVIEW
Preparticipation Checklist and Preventive Measures

- Meticulous preparticipation preparations can prevent most problems.
- Divers Alert Network (DAN) is available for consultation for accidents: 24-h emergency hotline 919-684-8111.
- Know where the closest hyperbaric chamber is that deals with diving accidents (dive operators can assist you, usually local hospitals).
- Plan diving so air travel is at least 12 h after the last dive and preferably 24 h to prevent decompression sickness induced by altitude.
- All divers should be certified by recognized agencies [Professional Association of Diving Instructors (PADI), National Association of Underwater Instructors (NAUI), Young Men's Christian Association (YMCA), Confédération Mondiale des Activités Subaquatiques (CMAS), Scuba Schools International (SSI, and others] and show certification card or be with a certified instructor.
- Diver attestation (signed waiver) that:
  - Diver is healthy as well as physically and mentally prepared to dive in current conditions (water temperature current, type of dive).
  - Diver has no additional problems or diseases since original medical dive clearance. Women divers are not pregnant. (The many disqualifying diseases or special evaluations are beyond the scope of this chapter.)
  - Diver is not drinking alcohol or taking consciousness-altering substances no matter whether over-the-counter, legal, illegal, or prescription.
  - Diver's personal diving equipment has been checked and serviced per manufacturer (an annual inspection is usual).
  - Diver will dive with a buddy and within the published dive tables. If a dive computer is being used, the dive profile should be double checked with these tables.
  - Diver will follow dive plan set forth by dive master, including depths, return tank pressure, and time in the water.

- Dive operator
  - Boat or buoy should fly U.S. or international dive flag to mark dive area.
  - Should have 100% oxygen breathing system on board (or shoreside if not boat diving) for initial dive accident treatment (not universally accepted by dive operators). Someone on board should know CPR.
  - Dive tanks should be freshly filled. If oxygen-enriched mixtures (Nitrox) are used, oxygen content should be checked by analyzer.
  - Certified dive master must be familiar with location and currents as well as dangerous animals and plants.
  - All rental equipment must be serviced and checked regularly.
  - All divers are to check in at boat loading and at the end of each dive.
  - Depths within sport-diving guidelines to be enforced (130 ft deep in salt water).
  - Safety stop on all dives at 10 to 15 ft to be encouraged.

SERIOUS AND POSSIBLY LIFE-THREATENING CONDITIONS

Any aches, pains, itching, neuralgias, shortness of breath, weakness, loss of consciousness, headache, personality changes, or psychiatric symptoms that occur within 48 h of compressed-air diving, regardless of depth, should be referred to a qualified dive physician, and Divers Alert Network should be notified. Common age-appropriate nondiving related diagnoses should be considered in treating diving conditions.

Nonbarotrauma Gas Effects

- Nitrogen narcosis—nitrogen under the pressure of increasing depth can cause alcohol-like intoxication sensations, often compared to drinking on an empty stomach; it worsens with further depth of the dive.
  - Prevention: self-perception and buddy system; since individuals have different susceptibilities, buddy can initiate surfacing.
  - Consequences: disorientation, confusion, running out of air, and drowning have all been described.
  - Treatment: none needed, resolves during ascent; if symptoms persist, consider decompression sickness.
- Oxygen toxicity—neurologic symptoms of seizure do not occur at usual sport-diving depths when using compressed air. When oxygen-enriched mixtures (Nitrox) are used, risk increases as depth increases to maximum sport limit.
  - Consequences: in water drowning due to seizure.
  - Treatment: ascent, airway, breathing, circulation (ABCs).
- Carbon dioxide toxicity—excessive buildup of this gas.

- Prevention: breathing normally and not trying to save air by holding breath during dive ("skip" breathing.)
- Consequences: acidosis, which can lead to shortness of breath, headache, confusion, and drowning.
- Treatment: treat presenting symptoms, but hypercapnea resolves on its own.

- Decompression sickness type I (DCS I)—prolonged time at depth followed by surfacing can cause saturated nitrogen to precipitate bubbles in joints (bends), causing pain and stiffness, or under the skin, causing itching or inflammation.
  - Prevention: follow diving tables as conservatively as possible, ascend slowly. Most experts recommend a safety stop at 10 to 15 ft of water to allow more nitrogen to dissipate from the tissues.
  - Consequences: joint damage; can progress to DCS II (see below).
  - Treatment: immediate use of 100% oxygen, immediate dive physician evaluation even if symptoms have resolved. Hyperbaric chamber treatment.

- DCS II—prolonged time at depth time followed by surfacing can cause saturated nitrogen to precipitate bubbles in the cardiovascular, pulmonary, nervous, or other vital organ systems causing symptoms that may include fatigue, paresthesias, shortness of breath, chest pain, and paralysis. Symptoms typically appear after the diver has returned to the boat or shore and has removed his or her diving equipment.
  - Prevention: same as DCS I above.
  - Consequences: permanent neurologic deficit, critical tissue damage, death.
  - Treatment: ABCs if needed, 100% oxygen, supportive treatment and immediate dive physician evaluation even if symptoms have resolved. Hyperbaric chamber treatment.

Ascent Barotrauma

- Air gas embolism (AGE)—breath-holding during ascent can cause air from the lungs to enter the arterial system, causing embolic disease—specifically neurologic syndromes resembling serious strokes. Such emboli involve larger volumes of air than those seen in DCS, and the air continues to expand on ascent. Symptoms typically appear while the diver is in the water or just as the diver is getting out of the water. They include cardiovascular collapse, confusion, syncope, and signs of cerebral infarction. Additionally, pneumothorax or other signs of air leakage may be present.
  - Prevention: no breath-holding while diving, especially on ascent.
  - Consequences: death, permanent neurologic defects, seizures.
  - Treatment: ABCs if needed, 100% oxygen, supportive treatment, and immediate evaluation by dive physician even if symptoms resolve. Hyperbaric chamber treatment.

NON-LIFE-THREATENING INJURIES

Descent Barotrauma

- Middle ear squeeze—diver is unable to put air into the middle ear from upper airway using equalization techniques.
  - Prevention: if there is trouble equalizing, diver should go back up to the surface and descend feet-first with head tilted back, prefilling middle ear with air before pressure on the ears is felt.
  - Consequences: inability to dive due to ear pain; afterward tympanic membranes (TMs) appear reddened and possibly hemorrhagic, precluding further diving until healed. Rarely, round window rupture.
  - Treatment: time; rarely, anesthetic drops.
- Sinus squeeze—pain in maxillary or frontal sinuses from blockage/swelling of affected sinus.
  - Prevention: avoidance of diving with nasal congestion.
  - Consequences: inability to dive unless air can be put into affected sinuses. Hemorrhage in sinus or epistaxis possible. Epistaxis is rarely severe but can look enormous when mixed with water in mask.
  - Treatment: nasal decongestant drops, but awaiting resolution of congestion is best. If persistent, ENT evaluation of sinuses and meatal complexes.
- Mask squeeze—bloodshot eyes, subconjunctival hemorrhage, or skin petechia from not equalizing pressure in mask.
  - Prevention: periodically exhaling through nose.
  - Consequences: none usually.
  - Treatment: reassurance.
- Alternobaric vertigo—vertigo probably caused by unequal ear pressures, possibly in association with ear-squeeze problems.
  - Prevention: good ear pressure equalization.
  - Consequences: nausea, vomiting, disequilibrium.
  - Treatment: leaving the water, ENT evaluation if no resolution; rupture of round window can occur with significant middle ear squeeze.
- Tooth squeeze (barodontalgia)—pain in filled or cracked tooth, air pocket with negative pressure on descent.
  - Prevention: good dental care.
  - Consequence: pain.
  - Treatment: see dentist regarding particular tooth or filling.

Ascent Barotrauma

- Reverse middle ear or sinus squeeze—edema of eustachian tube or osteomeatal complex (rarely significant) not allowing release of expanding air.
  - Consequences: pain of affected sinus or ear; TM rupture possible if eustachian tube is blocked.
  - Treatment: supportive, no further diving in either case until causative edema has resolved. No diving with TM rupture.

- Alternobaric vertigo—as above
- Gastrointestinal gaseous distress—probably caused by aerophagia while diving or gas production in gut during dive.
  - Prevention: conscious prevention of aerophagia.
  - Consequences: gaseous distention, belching, flatus, and distress; rarely intestinal perforation.
  - Treatment: successful belching and passage of flatus. Referral if symptoms unresolved.
- Reverse tooth squeeze (barodontalgia)—as with tooth squeeze, but in ascent an air pocket has equalized pressure at depth and is now expanding, causing pain.
- Hazardous marine life is beyond the scope of this chapter (see Chap. 48).

SUGGESTED EQUIPMENT

- Otoscope with insufflator
- Stethoscope and basic CPR equipment (buddy breather) if not available
- 100% oxygen breathing equipment (encouraged)
- Listing of radio or phone contact for Coast Guard or other rescue services, Divers Alert Network (DAN), and nearest hyperbaric chamber
- Dive tables

Bibliography

Martin L: *SCUBA Diving Explained: Questions and Answers on Physiology and Medical Aspects of SCUBA Diving.* Flagstaff, AZ: Best Publications, 1997. Electronic version available at ⟨http://www.mtsinai.org/pulmonary/books/scuba/contents.html⟩

Rodale's scuba diving: Training and safety: Dive medicine. *Rodale's SCUBA Diving Magazine.* Feb. 5, 2002. ⟨http://www.scubadiving.com/training/medicine/⟩

Weisman S: University of Maryland, Kinesiology 147N, Introduction to SCUBA Diving, SCUBA Diving Physiology. Feb. 5, 2002. ⟨http://rtsx-109.umd.edu/UMd/Physics&Phys/physiology.h ml⟩

45

Search and Rescue/ Wilderness Medicine

R. Tucker Thole

OVERVIEW

- Search and rescue (SAR)/wilderness medicine involves practicing medicine in a wilderness environment.
  - Areas uninhabited or untouched by humans (alpine, desert, forest, rivers, lakes, ocean, tropics, high altitude)
  - Isolated from definitive medical care and reliable communication
- Unique aspects of SAR/wilderness medicine
  - SAR staff exposed to same environment and potential injury as victim.
  - Requires experience and knowledge in medicine as well as wilderness survival.
  - First necessity may be to locate patient.
  - Ability to improvise is essential.
  - Difficult to transport and utilize standard medical center resources.
  - Urban protocols difficult to apply to back-country setting.
  - Emergency care and stabilization of patient can be prolonged because of transportation challenges.
- Sports medicine event coverage in wilderness setting
  - Be familiar with local SAR resources if covering an event where the participants can become lost or injured in a wilderness setting.
  - Be familiar with incident command system (ICS) (see Chap. 62).

COMMON INJURIES

- Dependent on environment of victim (alpine, water, desert, etc.)
- Factors contributing to requiring an SAR mission
  - Inadequate planning, improper clothing, fatigue, dehydration, hypothermia, hyperthermia, inadequate skills (excessive ambition), poor physical condition or motivation, inadequate nutrition

- Most injuries are due to inexperience or lack of preparation and are magnified by environmental or medical conditions.
- The cause of morbidity and mortality is usually multifactorial.
  - For example, an alpine rock climber who overestimates his ability gets stuck on rock route at night—becoming fatigued from inadequate nutrition as well as hypothermia—leading to poor decision making and ultimately a fall.

Traumatic Injuries

- Musculoskeletal injuries
  - Fractures, sprains, strains, soft tissue injuries
- Lacerations, blisters, drowning, suicide, motor vehicle accidents, wild animal attacks
- Environmentally related
  - Hypothermia, frostbite, altitude illness, heat illness, dehydration
- Medically related
  - Cardiac events, anaphylaxis, diabetes, dementia, infection, diarrhea, viral illness
- More injuries involving substance abuse and assaults than rock climbing and wild animal attacks

SPECIALIZED EQUIPMENT

- Dependent on victim's environment
  - Personal gear for rescuers
    - Appropriate footwear, clothing, gloves, helmets, eye protection
    - Specialized gear dependent on rescue environment (personal flotation devices, fire-resistant clothing, climbing harness and gear, flashlight, etc.)
  - Rescue equipment
    - Specialized gear dependent on rescue environment; for example, high-angle rescue on ice in alpine environment or white-water rescue in remote desert canyon
  - Radio and radio communication equipment
  - Helicopters
    - Knowledge of basic operation around helicopters (see below under transport)

Medical Equipment (See Chap. 61)

- Ability to improvise with available resources is essential.
- Medications and equipment vary depending on specific rescue situation.

TREATMENT

- Determination of need for an SAR operation
  - Victim is reported or suspected to be lost or injured in a wilderness environment.
  - Key information
    - Name and age of victim(s), number of victims, and remaining group members
    - Victim's vital signs, level of consciousness, mechanism and time of injuries and/or nature of illness, medical care already performed
    - Remaining groups' equipment and level of preparedness

ORGANIZATION OF SAR

- Key element of search-and-rescue operation is coordination of available resources.
- Local protocols will determine sequence of events after establishing the necessity of a SAR operation.

Four Phases: Locate, Access, Stabilize, Transport (LAST)

Locate

- If victim is lost, searching can become a significant challenge.
  - Not all victims are found.
- Involves coordination of resources.
  - SAR teams, local authorities (Police, Fire, Sheriff, Forest Service), volunteers, local specialists, aircraft, tracking dogs, etc.
- Lost subject's behavior is important in providing clues as to where he or she might be found.
  - Based on epidemiologic studies of past victims.
  - Characterized by age, sex, level of preparedness, personality, concomitant medical problems of lost subject.
    - For example, lost hikers travel two to three times farther than lost campers.

Access

- Involves getting rescuers and supplies to victims after they are located.
- Analyzing potential dangers to rescuers and victims and creating a plan to minimize those dangers.

Stabilize

- Ensure safety of rescuers and victim.
- Provide "extended emergency care."

- Stabilization and medical care performed will likely go beyond first "golden hour" of trauma care.
  - Requires skills in assessment and prolonged care and monitoring.
- Key medical skills in victim stabilization
  - Airway and shock, use of medications and oxygen, back-country field management of environmental and medical emergencies, reduction of fractures, packaging patient for transport, protecting patient from environmental dangers

Transport

- Transport to definitive medical care.
- 90 percent of SAR evacuations are performed on foot.
- Process is slow and requires many personnel if patient is unable to walk.
  - Pace may be 1–2 h per mile.
  - Requires six rested litter bearers per mile.

Helicopters

- 90 percent of rescues in French Alps utilize helicopters.
- Effective in optimal situations.
- Use limited by availability, weather, altitude, range, cost.

Helicopter Safety

- Approach only after making visual contact with pilot and being signaled to move toward the helicopter. Approach and depart downhill in a crouched position, toward the front or side of helicopter. *Never approach a helicopter from the rear unless it is shut down and air crew gives instructions to do so.* Watch for flying debris and loose equipment.

IMPORTANT DECISIONS IN WILDERNESS MEDICINE

- What is wrong? What is the diagnosis?
- How serious is it?
- Can it be treated in the field or is evacuation to definitive medical care necessary?
- If evacuation is necessary, are adequate resources available to the party or will outside resources be required?
- If field treatment is necessary, are the knowledge, skills, resources, and equipment available on site?

Bibliography

Accidents in North American Mountaineering. Golden, CO: The American Alpine Club, 2001.

Auerbach PS: *Wilderness Medicine,* 4th ed. St Louis: Mosby, 2001.

Bowman W:. Perspectives on being a wilderness physician: Is wilderness medicine more than a special body of knowledge? *Wild Environ Med* 12:165–167. 2001.

Johnson L. *Wilderness Medicine Conference Syllabus.* Snowbird, UT: Mountain Medical Seminars, 2000, pp 169–196.

46

Soccer

Daniel V. Vigil

THE RULES OF THE GAME

- 11 players per team
  - 10 field players, 1 goalkeeper
- Players may make contact with the ball with any part of the body except the hands or upper extremity.
  - Typically, the ball is moved by kicking or by heading.
  - The goalkeeper may use hands within the goalkeeper's box.
- Continuous action
  - Two 45-min halves with one half-time break.
  - Clock does not stop and teams may not call time out, but referee may stop play for injuries or penalties. Referee may add time so that total playing time of 45 min per half is achieved.
- On field injuries
  - Play is allowed to continue until the ball is out of play if, in the opinion of the referee, a player is only slightly injured.
  - Play is stopped if, in the referee's opinion, a player is seriously injured.
  - After questioning the injured player, the referee may request medical personnel to enter the field to evaluate the injury and to arrange the player's safe and swift removal from the field.
  - A player may not be treated on the field.
  - A player with a bleeding wound must leave the field of play. Once the bleeding is controlled and the wound properly dressed, the player may be cleared to return to play.

COMMON INJURIES

- Injuries related to kicking technique: for precision dribbling and passing, a player most often strikes the ball with the medial midfoot. This technique results in foot pronation, eversion, and plantarflexion. Concomitantly, the knee assumes a valgus posture. In more powerful kicks, the ball is struck with the dorsal fore- and midfoot. In this instance, ankle plantarflexion plus toe flexion is a more typical posture.
- Repetitive/overuse injuries

Medial Collateral Ligament (MCL) Knee Sprain

- A traction injury of the MCL due to valgus knee stress during repetitive medial foot kicking. Physical examination shows tenderness over the medial knee and medial knee pain when a valgus stress is applied. Treatment for this chronic sprain emphasizes modified activity to allow ligament remodeling and healing. Taping and bracing can give some relief, but ultimately the soft tissues must be allowed to remodel and adapt to the stresses of the sport.

Peroneal Tendinitis

- An overuse injury of the peroneal muscles (usually the peroneus brevis) in positioning the foot in eversion for medial foot kicking. Lateral foot and/or ankle pain is elicited by asking the athlete to plantarflex and evert the foot against resistance. This is an overuse injury that requires modified activity while the injury heals. Focused rehabilitation and strengthening of the peroneals helps prevent recurrence. If the retinaculum has been damaged, resulting in subluxation of the peroneal tendon, a period of immobilization may be required. More severe cases require surgical reconstruction.

Posterior Tibialis Tendinitis

- A traction injury of the posterior tibialis due to the hyperpronation foot posture of medial foot kicking. May also be related to poor arch support of supple soccer shoes. Arch tenderness and pain on plantarflexion plus inversion characterize the injury. Like the chronic ligamentous sprains, this is an overload injury that requires relative rest to allow remodeling of the damaged soft tissue. Unlike ligamentous static stabilizers, this muscle is a dynamic ankle and foot stabilizer that can be strengthened and retrained. Rehabilitation that emphasizes these points helps prevent recurrence.

Flexor Hallucis Longus (FHL) Tendinitis

- An overuse injury of the FHL due to repetitive toe flexion in positioning the foot for kicking. With resisted ankle and great toe MTP plantarflexion, pain is noted behind the medial malleolus and may course along the plantar foot to the plantar MTP joint. Relative rest, great toe and ankle taping, along with a semirigid shoe insert may aid in recovery.

First Metatarsophalangeal (MTP) Joint Capsular Sprain

- Turf toe: higher incidence associated with greater traction on artificial turf. This injury is due to excessive dorsiflexion of the first MTP joint, resulting in sprain of the plantar capsule. Plantar joint pain with passive MTP dorsiflexion is the hallmark finding. Treatment focuses on limiting MTP flexion/extension. Taping can help during the healing phase. For more acute or painful cases, a rigid shoe insert or rigid cast shoe is effective.
- Reverse turf toe: injury to the dorsal first MTP may occur as a result of acute or chronic excessive great toe plantarflexion. This injury may accompany or be an extension of FHL tendinitis. Pain and tenderness over the dorsal MTP joint is characteristic. Treatment is similar to that for turf toe.

ACUTE LIGAMENT SPRAINS AND MUSCLE STRAINS

- Ankle sprain: the most common acute soft tissue injury resulting in lost participation time (see Chap. 27).

Muscle Strain

- In the skeletally mature athlete, most acute muscle strains may be managed with the principles of rest, ice, compression, and elevation (RICE), followed by recovery of range of motion and then by strengthening.
- In the skeletally immature, acute soft tissue injury near musculotendinous junctions must raise the question of apophyseal bone injury rather than muscle/tendon injury.
  - Common sites include:
    - The anterior superior iliac spine
    - Patella (Sindig-Larsen-Johansen apophysitis)
    - Tibial tubercle (Osgood-Schlatter apophysitis)
    - Calcaneus (Sever's apophysitis)
    - Fifth metatarsal base (Iselin's apophysitis)
  - Acute cases may be complicated by partial or complete avulsion through apophysis. Surgery may be indicated for grossly displaced avulsions, but most cases are chronic or subacute and respond to the principles of RICE. When pain has diminished, gradual return to play coupled with rehabilitation emphasizing flexibility and strengthening of associated muscle groups can be advised.

GROIN PAIN

- Common ailment among higher-level players thought to be related to high degree of lateral movement inherent to the sport.
  - Etiology: chronic adductor strain often related to strength imbalance between adductors and abductors. With fatigue or forceful contraction, acute-on-chronic adductor muscle strain may result in inability to run, especially laterally, due to pain. Inguinal hernia and hip joint pathology should not be overlooked.
  - Injured muscles: the adductor magnus, adductor longus, adductor brevis, sartorius, rectus femoris, and rectus abdominis have been implicated. Injury may occur at the musculotendinous junction, muscle belly, or enthesis (tendon-bone junction). Once thought to be a problem of inflexibility, recent literature suggests relative muscle weakness is a greater risk factor for injury.
  - Treatment: acute treatment employs RICE. Rehabilitation focuses on pain-free range of motion and strengthening. Strength balance between adductors and abductors must be achieved or risk of re-injury remains high.
  - Return to play: when pain subsides, simple drills may be allowed. Straight-line running and then sprinting follow. When healing is complete, lateral running and 90-degree cuts at high-speed running should be pain-free.

FRACTURES

Stress Fractures

- Overuse injury of load-bearing bones resulting in microtraumatic injury. Early injury is often dismissed as soft tissue strain, resulting in further injury from continued loading.
  - Clinical diagnosis: a history of repetitive activity and recent increase in intensity and/or volume of training are typical. Physical findings commonly include focal bone tenderness and localized pain on weight bearing.
  - Imaging: plain radiographs may show periosteal thickening but are often normal. Bone scan is much more sensitive and specific and currently viewed as the "gold standard." According to recent literature, MRI has shown great promise owing to its ability to show grade of injury.
  - Sites of injury: involved sites commonly include metatarsals, navicula, calcaneus, tibia, and fibula.

Treatment: cornerstone is rest. A period of immobilization and avoidance of weight bearing is sometimes necessary. In contrast to many acute fractures, stress fractures take longer to heal. Healing times of 8–12 weeks are not uncommon. Gradual return to play may begin when player is completely pain-free.

Acute Fractures (See Chap. 18)

- Fall on outstretched hand (FOOSH): common fractures include distal radius, scaphoid, phalanges
- Kick to leg or foot: despite shin guards, a forceful kick to the leg may result in tibial or fibular fracture. Similarly, metatarsal and phalangeal fractures may occur after a kick or after being stepped on.
- Avulsion fracture: forceful foot inversion, as occurs in lateral ankle sprain, may result in avulsion of the styloid process (Dancer's fracture) from the base of the fifth metatarsa. Alternatively, the fracture may occur through the fifth metatarsa diaphysis (Jones fracture).
- Casts and braces: players with such protective equipment (e.g., short arm cast, wrist brace) are allowed to participate as long as the cast is well padded and covered and the referee is notified.

HEAT ILLNESS (SEE CHAP. 17)

- By some estimates, a soccer player may run up to 10 km during a single match. Aside from the half-time break, no scheduled breaks or time-outs are allotted for rest or rehydration. Therefore, consequences of dehydration and heat stress must be considered, especially in extreme conditions. If a match is to be held at a time of high heat, high humidity, or high wet–bulb globe temperature, precautions against dehydration should be taken.
  - Encourage players to hydrate adequately during the pregame period.
  - During every stoppage of play, encourage players to hydrate, especially at half time.
- In certain competitions, rules of the game may be modified to decrease the risks of dehydration and heat illness:
  - Add rehydration breaks.
  - Allow more player substitutions.
  - Shorten playing time.

INJURIES DUE TO COLLISION/CONTACT

Concussion

- Soccer is a contact/collision sport.
  - Blunt head trauma can occur through various mechanisms.
  - Head vs. head (two players simultaneously trying to head the ball).
  - Head vs. extremity (elbow, knee, foot).
  - Head vs. fixed object (ground, goalpost).
  - Head vs. ball may result in concussion when a ball moving at high speed strikes the head of a player who is unprepared to head the ball. Improper heading technique has been thought to contribute to mild traumatic brain injury and cervical spine injury, but data are not conclusive. Regarding proper heading technique and the resulting repet-

itive head-ball impacts integral to the game, current evidence does not suggest that brain injury or neuropsychological deficits are significant consequences.

- Diagnosis, management, and return-to-play criteria are similar to those in other contact sports (see Chap. 6).

Contusions

Muscle Contusions

- One player's knee vs. another's thigh commonly results in quadriceps contusion. More severe injury may result in deep contusion and hematoma formation. Acute treatment conforms to the principles of RICE. In addition to RICE, wrapping the injured extremity with the knee in flexion will help limit hematoma formation and prevent contracture of the quadriceps. Most small hematomas resolve with this noninvasive treatment. Larger hematomas may be aspirated. Nonsteroidal anti-inflammatory drugs should be avoided acutely, as they may contribute to hematoma formation; however, they may be used in the subacute phase of the injury.

Myositis Ossificans

- An undesirable consequence of muscle contusion is calcification within the injured muscle, known as myositis ossificans (MO). This may lead to chronic pain and tenderness as well as decreased strength and range of motion. Risk of MO is greater with more severe muscle injury and hematoma formation. Therefore, prevention of MO assumes great importance (see Chap. 29).

Bone Contusions

- With the exception of shin guards, no specific pads are required in soccer. Bony prominences are vulnerable to blunt trauma. The most commonly contused sites include the anterior superior iliac spine (ASIS), greater trochanter, and patella. Hematoma formation over the ASIS has been termed a *hip pointer*. This painful injury is usually not serious but can significantly limit function and performance. Treatment includes hematoma aspiration followed by RICE. Sequelae of greater trochanteric and patellar contusions may include effusion in the overlying bursae. These usually respond well to RICE, but aspiration can speed recovery. Occult fractures with these injuries are rare but should be considered in more severe cases.

SOCCER ORGANIZATIONS

- More information about soccer at various levels of play and competition is available through the organizations listed below.

American Youth Soccer Organization (AYSO)

- AYSO is a nationwide non-profit organization that develops and delivers quality youth soccer programs in a fun, family environment. Website: www.soccer.org.

United States Soccer Federation (USSF)

- The USSF is the national governing body of soccer in the United States. Its mission statement includes "to make soccer, in all its forms, a preeminent sport in the United States and to continue the development of soccer at all recreational and competitive levels." Website: www.ussoccer.com.

Federation Internationale de Football Association (FIFA)

- The international governing body of soccer, FIFA's aim is to see that the game is played by one unified set of rules all over the world. Through the sponsorship of development programs and supervision of international competitions, including the World Cup, FIFA strives for the positive promotion of soccer throughout the world. Website: www.fifa.com.

Bibliography

Kirkendall DT, Jordan SE, Garrett WE: Heading and head injuries in soccer. *Sports Med* 31(5):369–386, 2001.

Mellion MB, Walsh WM, Shelton GL (eds): *The Team Physician's Handbook*, 2d ed. Philadelphia: Hanley & Belfus, 1997.

Puffer JC (ed): *20 Common Problems: Sports Medicine*. New York: McGraw-Hill, 2002.

47

Skiing and Snowboarding

Todd Jorgenson

SNOWBOARDING

- Fastest-growing winter sport in the United States.
- Aerial maneuvers, often inverted, are inherent to the sport.
- Approximately 50 percent of injuries involve the upper extremities.
- Nearly 50 percent of injuries occur in *beginners*, often within the first half day.

COMMON INJURIES

Upper Extremity

- Wrist (usually distal radius) fractures (see Chap. 22)
  - Most common snowboarding injury.
  - Fractures are often severe; 50 percent may require surgery.
  - Mechanism: fall on outstretched hand.
  - Prevention:
    - "Closed-fist" fall may decrease fracture risk.
    - Wrist guards decrease risk by 50–75 percent
- Elbow, shoulder injuries (see Chaps. 23 and 24)
  - Dislocations, fracture/dislocations reported.

Lower Extremity

- Ankle
  - "Snowboarder's ankle"—fracture of lateral talar process.
    - May represent 15 percent of ankle injuries presenting.
    - Often involves lead leg, when landing a jump.
    - Mechanism: dorsiflexion, inversion.
    - Examination findings are similar to those of simple lateral sprain.
    - Diagnosis: plain x-ray or CT.
    - Prevention: "hard boots" to protect ankle.

Cervical Spine (See Chap. 20)

- Serious spinal injury is four times more common than in skiing.
- Jumping (intentional jump > 2 m) is the primary cause of spinal injury.

Head (See Chap. 6)

- Severe intracranial injury may represent up to 10 percent of snowboarding injuries presenting to a trauma center.
- Mechanism: blow to the back of the head on snow, or high-speed collision.
- Prevention:
  - Helmet use is becoming more socially acceptable and probably advisable.
  - Helmets may prevent mild concussion.
  - No data to prove that helmets protect against severe head injury.
  - Helmets may increase risk taking (false sense of security).

Chest and Abdomen (See Chaps. 13 and 14)

- Spleen, liver, and renal injuries reported.
- Risk increases with higher speeds and with aerial maneuvers.

ALPINE SKIING

- Improved boot/binding technology has greatly reduced ankle and lower leg injuries.
- Unfortunately, stiffer boots concentrate forces on the knee.

Common Injuries

Knee

- 20–36 percent of all skiing injuries (see Chap. 26).
  - Anterior cruciate ligament (ACL) injury
    - Threefold rise in incidence since early 1970s
    - Incidence of 50–70 per 100,000 skier-days
      - Similar to college football rate
      - Same incidence in women as in men
    - Mechanisms of injury different than in other sports and usually involve less injury to other knee structures.
      - Valgus-external rotation
        - Catching inside edge and falling forward

- Boot-induced
  - Landing on back of ski with knee extended
- "Phantom foot"
  - Falling backward between skis, catching inside edge
- Prevention
  - Good ski instruction
  - Properly adjusted bindings
  - "Self-test" daily (test for binding release with controlled mechanism)
  - Education
    - Training program may decrease risk (i.e., learning how to avoid mechanisms of ACL injury).
- Medial collateral ligament (MCL) injury
  - Mechanism: valgus stress
  - Milder (grades I and II) MCL sprains more common in women.
- Tibial plateau fracture
  - Mechanism: valgus stress causing compression of lateral compartment.

Thumb

- 8–10 percent of skiing injuries
  - "Skier's thumb"—acute rupture of ulnar collateral ligament (UCL) of thumb
    - Skiing is the most common cause of UCL injury.
    - Mechanism
      - Fall with ski pole in hand, which forces abduction/extension of thumb
    - Examination/management
      - Tenderness over ulnar metacarpophalangeal joint of thumb, laxity of UCL
      - If UCL injury suspected, obtain x-ray before stress testing.
      - 52–78 percent incidence of Stener lesion—soft tissue interposition preventing healing; requires surgical treatment.
      - Return to skiing 1–2 days with thumb spica gauntlet cast.
    - Prevention: allow for easy release of pole in a fall.
      - Use of "quick-release" straps.
      - Use pole without straps.

Shoulder

- 4–11 percent of skiing injuries
  - Anterior dislocation (25–50 percent of shoulder injuries)
    - Mechanism
      - Fall on outstretched arm
      - "Skiing past pole plant," causing abduction/external rotation
  - Rotator cuff strains
  - Acromioclavicular sprains

- Clavicular fracture
  - Treatment as in general athletic population

Head and Spine

- 7 percent of ski injuries
  - Simple falls are the most common mechanism.
  - High-speed collisions with immovable objects are most severe.
    - "Typical" victim is male, 25–35 years old, accomplished skier.
    - Helmets have not proven effective in high-energy accidents.

Altitude Illness (See Chap. 17)
Sunburn

- Ultraviolet B (UVB) intensity increases exponentially with altitude.
- Reflectivity of snow is significant factor (up to 40 percent) increasing risk of sun exposure.

EQUIPMENT

- Communication equipment that functions on the mountain
- Rescue sled
- Splints
- Snowmobile
- Blankets

TREATMENT

- Splint.
- Prevent hypothermia.
- Evacuate.
- Cardiac problems need to be treated on the mountain, early defibrillation is lifesaving.

RETURN TO PLAY

- See individual injury chapters.
- Knee bracing may facilitate return to activity and may be worn under ski clothing or fitted to wear outside of clothing.
- Gauntlet thumb spica cast molded to fit around ski pole will aid return to skiing with UCL injury. Skier may have to wear oversize mitten over cast to prevent cold injury.

Bibliography

Ettlinger CF, Johnson RJ, Shealy JE: A method to help reduce the risk of serious knee sprains incurred in alpine skiing. *Am J Sports Med* 23(5): 531–537, 1995.

Hunter RE: Skiing injuries. *Am J Sports Med* 27(3):381–389, 1999.

Thordardson DB: Talar body fractures. *Orthop Clin North Am* 32(1):65–77, 2001.

Young CC: Snowboarding injuries. *Am Fam Physician* 59(1):131–136, 141, 1999.

48

Surfing

Sam Sunshine

OVERVIEW

- In a 1996 estimate, nearly 2 million people surf in the United States, and there are over 18 million surfers worldwide. Relatively speaking, surfing is a safe sport, with estimated 2.7–4.0 injuries per 1000 surfing days. Contact with the surfboard causes most injuries.

COMMON INJURIES

Traumatic Skin Injuries

- Lacerations
  - The most common surfing injury overall and most common injury resulting in a surfer seeking medical attention and resulting in the temporary inability to surf.
  - Most lacerations are caused by the sharp fins, tail or nose of surfboard.
  - The head (skull), face (chin), and extremities (feet and legs) are the most commonly affected sites.
- Coral reef cuts
  - High propensity for infection
  - Increased infection rates in warmer climates
  - Avoid suturing puncture wounds
- Sea ulcer
  - Result from under- or untreated lacerations, abrasions, and puncture wounds.
  - Most common on the backs of hands, feet, and ankles—areas of diminished circulation.
  - High incidence among daily recreational and professional surfers. The ocean water exposure erodes the scab and lessens the body's healing ability.
- Soft tissue injuries
  - Focal contusions and hematomas
  - 35–45 percent of surfing injuries that require medical attention

- Extremities and the head are the most vulnerable areas to trauma
- Contact with the surfboard is the most common cause of soft tissue injuries.

Treatment (See Chap. 16)

Specialized Equipment

- Rubber surfboard nose covers, e.g., Nose Guards, Diamond Tips—aid in mitigating injuries induced by contact with nose of the surfboard.
- Urethane bordered fins, e.g., Pro Teck performance fins (www.surfcohawaii.com) softens the fin's sharp edge to protect the body from lacerations.
- Safety helmets, e.g., Gath Headgear (www.murrays.com) is made of a shatterproof plastic and lined with foam. It is designed to provide some protection against impact injury and the elements, such as wind and water chill, and the sun's rays. Helmets also help to minimize the risk of chronic damage to eyes, ears and skin, such as surfer's ear (exostosis), soft tissue growth over the eyes (pterygium), and head and neck skin cancers.

Return to Sport

- For simple lacerations, a minimum of 2 days out of the water should be allowed for initial wound healing.
- For more significant lacerations with associated soft tissue injury, allow 7–10 days for the wounds to heal and sutures to be removed.

Skin Infections/Rashes

- Folliculitis.
- Most commonly occurs about the neck and shoulders.
- An acne-like skin reaction where hair follicles are irritated by the neoprene wet suit.
- Most commonly caused by *Staphylococcus aureus.*
- Surfer's dermatitis—caused by irritant, mechanical and allergic factors.
- Chest knobbies—irritation of the lower anterior rib cage as it rubs against the board during paddling.
- Neck, nipple and axillary rash—irritation of the skin as it rubs against the wetsuit.

Treatment

- Staph infections respond well to topical (Bacitracin, Bactroban) and oral (cephalexin, erythromycin) antibiotics.

- Showering immediately after surfing and rinsing the wetsuit will limit outbreaks of skin infections.
- Wearing a rash guard made of 80 percent nylon and 20 percent spandex protects the neck and chest areas from friction and can help limit the occurrence of folliculitis.
- Headhunter rash guard (www.headhuntersurf.com) is a waterless hypoallergenic gel designed to help prevent and heal wetsuit rash.

ENVIRONMENTAL EXPOSURE

- Sunburn and windburn
  - Most commonly first- and second-degree burns.
  - The water intensifies the sun's ultraviolet light.
  - Fair-skinned surfers burn more easily.
  - Wind intensifies the effects of the sun.
- Cold-induced angioedema
  - Similar to cold-induced urticaria.
  - Characterized by swelling, erythema, and itching of the involved body part.
  - Usually affects the distal extremities fingers and toes.
  - Can be associated with nausea, lightheadedness and even syncope.

Prevention

- Apply a water resistant sunscreen with sun protection factor (SPF) of at least 15 or greater 30 min prior to sun exposure.
- Reapply sunscreen every 3–6 h.
- Use lip balm with SPF.
- Preferred sunscreens contain titanium dioxide or zinc oxide for improved ultraviolet A and B (UVA and UVB) protection.
- Wearing a hat can reduce sun exposure to the head and face but can be problematic in large, challenging surf.
- Wearing a wetsuit with appropriate thickness and fit can prevent cold-induced angioedema.

Treatment

- First-degree sunburn responds well to aloe vera–containing lotions and gels. Cold compresses and nonsteroical anti-inflammatory medications can also help calm the pain and swelling.
- Avoid hot water (e.g., Jacuzzi or hot shower) and further sun exposure for 24–48 h after sustaining a sunburn.
- Second-degree sunburn may benefit from a short course of prednisone in addition to the therapy outlined above.

HEAD AND NECK INJURIES

- Constitute up to 45 percent of all acute surfing injuries.
- Most are due to minor superficial trauma.
- Skull and maxillofacial fractures are most commonly due to being struck by the surfboard.
- Cervical spine injuries are far more common in body surfers than in board surfers.

Prevention

- Avoid shallow surf breaks.
- If you fall, try to stay behind your board. If you are submerged after a wipeout or lose your board, cover your head with both arms as you surface.
- Gath helmets are designed to provide some protection against impact injury and lacerations (www.murrays.com).

Treatment (See Chaps. 6, 20)

DENTAL EMERGENCIES AND TREATMENT (SEE CHAP. 11)

OCULAR TRAUMA/EMERGENCIES (SEE CHAP. 12)

- Most commonly caused by direct trauma from the nose of the surfboard after a wipeout

Prevention

- Rubber surfboard nose covers—e.g., Nose Guards, Diamond Tips—can aid in protecting the surfer from injury caused by the sharp nose of the board.
- Blunting the nose of the surfboard has been advocated.
- Surf goggles are made of polycarbonate, a lightweight, shatterproof, and scratch-resistant material and can be worn to protect the eyes from sand, sun, and wind—also to reduce risk of eye trauma (Barz sport goggles www.murrays.com or Spex amphibious eyewear www.spexusa.com).
- Provide 100 percent UVA and UVB protection.
- Surf goggles are more commonly used by contact lens wearers to prevent lens loss.

CONDITIONS AFFECTING THE EAR

Surfer's Ear (External Auditory Canal Exostosis)

- A benign malady that affects 80 percent of avid surfers who have surfed more than 10 years (uncommon in surfers who have surfed less than 5 years).
- Most surfers with exostosis are asymptomatic.
- Surgery is rarely indicated.

Swimmer's Ear (Acute Otitis Externa)

- Caused by prolonged water exposure which leads to reduced ear wax and local skin maceration.

Prevention

- Ear plugs can be used to reduce wind and water irritation (Doc's Pro Plugs, Seals custom ear plugs).
- Use of a neoprene hood.
- Routine use of a 50/50 mixture of vinegar and isopropyl alcohol instilled into the ear canal will reduce its recurrence by evaporating excess water and disinfecting the epithelium.

Treatment/Return to Activity

- Ciprofloxacin otic drops used twice daily for 7 days (hydrocortisone/polymixin/neomycin otic is a treatment alternative).
- Avoid use if tympanic membrane is perforated.
- Surfer should remain out of the water during the week of treatment.

Perforated Ear Drum

- Causes include compression on hitting the water, submerging after a wipeout, or diving under a wave while paddling out.
- Usually involves the pars tensa, below the umbo and malleolus.

Treatment/Return to Activity

- Allow 2 weeks to heal. Repeat otologic exam in 1–2 weeks.
- Keep the external auditory canal dry, wear earplugs in the shower. The majority will heal spontaneously.
- May require tympanoplasty if spontaneous closure does not occur.
- If surgery is required, refrain from surfing for at least 6–8 weeks to allow the tympanic membrane to heal.

MUSCULOSKELETAL INJURIES

Shoulder Injury (See Chap. 24)

Back Injury (See Chap. 21)

Back Spasm

- The most common cause of disability among surfers.
- Potentiated by the isometric hyperextension position of the surfer's trunk during paddling.
- Injury can also occur during high-intensity, rapid movement of certain standing surfing maneuvers—e.g., cutbacks and tail slides.
- Spondylolysis pain should be suspected in young athletes who complain of pain that localizes to the low back.

Prevention/Return to Activity

- Routine stretching and warm-up.
- Abdominal muscle conditioning.
- Ice, NSAIDs and rest should be used in the first 48 hours.
- Surfing can be safely resumed once the pain has resolved, usually 1–4 weeks.

Knee Injury (See Chap. 26)

- Ligamentous strains
    - Medial collateral ligament strain is not an uncommon injury.
    - The knee of the back leg (right leg in regular-stance surfers) is flexed and assumes the more stressful genuralgum position while surfing.
    - The injury can also be precipitated by the back foot slipping off the tail or the front foot slipping forward on the board, placing the back, support knee in an accentuated valgus position.
- Meniscal and anterior cruciate ligament tears
    - Uncommon injuries
    - Caused by the weight-bearing, knee-flexed position of most forceful twisting surfing maneuvers.

Prevention/Return to Activity

- Ample use of surfboard wax or deck traction pads (www.stickybumps.com) help prevent foot slippage.
- Routine stretching and presurf warmups improve flexibility.

- Surfing can be resumed when the athlete can perform a duck walk without discomfort and strength is symmetric with the uninvolved side.
- Continued use of a neoprene knee sleeve may provide comfort.

BITES AND STINGS

- Constitute 3 percent of all acute surfing injuries.
- See Table 48.1.

Table 48.1 Marine Animal Bites and Stings

Marine Animal	Common Facts	Type of Injury/ Symptoms	Treatment
Sharks (Angel, white, and black reef, great white, bull, white-tip and tiger)	Attacks are rare. Only 10% result in death. Many attacks are provoked.	Mild to severe soft tissue injury and dismembering injuries. Can result in significant blood loss.	Press dry towels against the wound, avoid tourniquets, keep the person warm. IV fluids and supportive measures if symptoms of shock develop. Get immediate medical attention.
Sea snakes	Found throughout the tropical and subtropical ocean waters. Hundreds of reported deaths annually, but few among surfers.	Injection of highly toxic venom. Can cause severe muscle pain, flaccid paralysis and ultimately respiratory paralysis.	Antivenom is available. Apply a firm bandage and immobilize the limb. Do not use a tourniquet or attempt to suck out the venom.
Stingrays and fish	A common worldwide hazard. Stingrays have a tail that contains venom.	Immediate, severe pain, erythema, swelling and numbness Systemic symptoms can include syncope, nausea, weakness and anxiety.	Hot water immersion for 30–90 min. Debride and suture larger wounds. Attempt to remove integumentary sheath left behind by stingrays. Analgesia—IM ketorolac Consider prophylactic antibiotics with *S. aureus* coverage.
Coelenterates (Cnidarians) Corals, sea anemones, jellyfish and hydroids (e.g., Portuguese man-of-war)	Many possess a stinging unit that penetrates the skin. A single tentacle may release thousands of nematocysts.	Papular and linear skin eruptions. Pain may be severe, itching is common Systemic symptoms include weakness, nausea, headache muscle pain and spasms, lacrimation and nasal discharge, increased perspiration, changes in pulse rate, and chest pain.	Immediately rinse off area with saltwater (avoid fresh water). Remove tentacles with an instrument or gloved hand Apply 50/50 mix of vinegar and isopropyl alcohol to disinfect the wound. Sawyer Itch Balm Plus (www.sawyerproducts.com) a topical antihistamine-analgesic-corticosteroid can soothe the skin. IM ketorolac for more severe pain. IV fluids and supportive measures in cases where signs of shock develop.

(continued)

Table 48.1 (*Continued*)

Marine Animal	Common Facts	Type of Injury/ Symptoms	Treatment
Echinoderms (Sea urchins)	Several classes are venomous but injuries are rare. Far more common are injuries due to sea urchin spines.	Sea urchin spines break off into the skin and cause local reactions. Most commonly seen on the palms and soles. If not removed, can migrate deeper and cause a granulomatous nodular reaction. Joint and muscle pain has been reported.	Remove spines immediately. Difficult due to brittle nature of the spines. Clean the area with 50/50 mix of vinegar and isopropyl alcohol. Soak the affected area in vinegar several times daily (vinegar dissolves the spines). Surgery is seldom necessary.

SURFING SAFELY

- Surfers should have a strong ability to swim and basic knowledge of water safety.
- Never surf alone. Always surf with a buddy.
- Avoid alcohol consumption prior to surfing. Alcohol increases the risk of fatal drowning and reduces response time in emergency situations.
- Choose the right board. Consider using one with a more rounded nose or apply a plastic or rubber tip to the nose. Use a soft-foam surfboard to learn on.
- If you fall, try to stay behind your board. If you are submerged after a fall, cover your head with both arms as you surface.
- Wear a leash. This will prevent the board from striking other surfers (but will increase the risk of being struck by your board) and provides you with a floatation and rescue device.
- Wear the right wetsuit. Make sure it fits properly and is thick enough to prevent hypothermia. In warm-water climates, wear at least a wetsuit vest to avoid wind chill.
- Respect warning signs that have been posted during dangerous surf conditions.
- Avoid shallow breaks and exposed reefs.
- When traveling in tropical and subtropical climates, be aware of venomous marine animals, e.g., man-of-war and jellyfish.

Bibliography

Allen RH, Eiseman B, Streckley CJ: Surfing injuries at Waikiki. *JAMA* 237:668–670, 1977.

Fenner P: Dangers in the ocean: The traveler and marine enveromation. II. Marine vetebrates. *J Travel Med* 5:213–216, 1998.

Hartung GH, Goebert DA, Taniguchi RM: Epidemiology of ocean sports-related injuries in Hawaii. *Hawaii Med J* 49:52–56, 1990.

Lowdon BJ, Pateman NA, Pitman AJ: Surfboard-riding injuries. *Med J Aust* 2:613–616, 1983.

Lowdon BJ, Pitman AJ, Pateman NA: Injuries to international competitive surfboard riders. *J Sports Med* 27:57–63, 1987.

Renneker M, Starr K, Booth G: Sick surfers ask the surf docs and Dr Geoff. Palo Alto, CA: Bull Publishing, 1983.

49

Swimming and Diving

C. Mark Chassay

INJURIES

Orthopedic

- Shoulder: overuse—most commonly affected joint injury in swimmers. Traumatic injury more common in divers, especially platform divers due to the force hitting the water.
- Knee: collateral ligament sprains more common in breaststrokers due to valgus kicking.
- Back: usually from overuse in swimmers, especially butterfly participants. Usually due to trauma in divers.

Traumatic

- Lacerations: more common in divers if poor dive results in contact with the springboard or platform. Occasionally can occur in backstrokers if inattentive to pool markers before turns.
- Neck: diving into unknown and/or shallow water is the number-one reason for catastrophic damage to the cervical spine.
- Fractures/sprains of the hand, finger, foot, or toe: more common in swimmers making improper turns during events or practice.
- Wrist sprains: more common in divers on water entry. Can occur in swimmer when touching wall.

MEDICAL CONCERNS

- Eyes: conjunctivitis—more likely to be from chlorine or other irritants than bacterial.
- Ears: otitis externa (swimmer's ear)—secondary to prolonged exposure to water. Pain can be incapacitating. Barotrauma/perforated tympanic membrane—due to pressures under water. Usually at least 3 ft below water level.

- Asthma: common in swimmers due to activity selection. Reason: aquatic sports are less asthmagenic than running and cycling (and other outside) activities.

Infections

- Infectious mononucleosis. Common medical illness among adolescent swimmers. Possibility of traumatic spleen rupture indicates caution (though spleen can rupture spontaneously without trauma).
- *Cryptosporidium*:—more commonly encountered in open swims. Likely to be diagnosed in retrospect due to incubation period. Symptoms usually develop 4–6 days after infection but may appear between 2 and 10 days after infection. Symptoms: watery diarrhea (most common), abdominal cramps, nausea. Signs: low-grade fever, dehydration, and weight loss.

Environmental

- Hypothermia: open swims becoming more popular, probably due to events such as triathlons.
- Hypoxia: more likely to be seen in synchronized swimming due to prolonged underwater maneuvers that require breath-holding. Symptoms: dizziness, fainting. Signs: confusion, disorientation, and convulsions.

Training

- Dehydration: swimmers frequently cannot monitor and appreciate the loss of fluids (i.e., sweat) due to prolonged times in the water.
- Overtraining syndrome: very common in swimmers. All good swimming coaches push their athletes to maximum training before they taper into competition.
  - Symptoms: altered sleep patterns, appetite changes, fatigue, inability to concentrate, irritability, loss of motivation, change in bowel habits, chronic muscle soreness, frequent medical and musculoskeletal disorders. Signs: increased resting heart rate and weight change.

Congenital

- Down's syndrome: increased atlantoaxial instability is associated with this genetic syndrome. Individuals with Down's should be excluded from participation in diving and swimming dive starts until plain-film radiographs have excluded this disorder.

SPECIALIZED PREPARATIONS AND EQUIPMENT

- Pool/body-of-water monitoring
  - Environmental: temperature, acidity, and chlorine
  - Configurations: lane lines, wall markings, and starting blocks
  - Diving: water depth, spring boards.
- Lifeguards and recovery contingency plan: assistance by Red Cross, YMCA, etc.
- Wet suits: for open-water swims and prevention of hypothermia.
- Goggles: protect from chlorine (though more pools are using chlorine less).
- Ear molds (i.e., Silly-Putty or customized molds) or ear plugs for baro-trauma/perforated tympanic membrane, otitis externa, or otitis media. swim caps may also be helpful.
- Shower shoes: prevent transmission of fungal and viral infections to the feet in public shower areas.
- Water-resistant casting material: check with competition committee for requirements on size, materials, and acceptability.
- Special Olympics: additional staff needed to walk the length of the pool in the water or accompany participants swimming in a lane.

TREATMENT

- Awareness of banned substances in U.S. Swimming and FINA (American and international swimming governing bodies). Less problematic in NCAA participants.
- Shoulder (see Chap. 24) . Technique analysis by coach for proper form is most beneficial in rehabilitation and prevention. Prevention: rotator cuff strengthening regimen should be undertaken despite presence of signs or symptoms.
- Cervical spine (see Chap. 20). Down's syndrome population needs workup for atlantoaxial instability if diving activities are anticipated.
- Asthma (see Chap. 8).
- Eyes, ears, nose, and throat (see Chap. 10). Inner ear disturbances are problematic in divers due to their need to be in control of their spatial surroundings.
- Lacerations (see Chap. 16): in addition, several commercial products can be used to protect wounds. Some waterproof dressings include EnduraSPORTS tape, Johnson & Johnson Band-Aid Liquid Bandage, Conco Bulky Gauze Bandage, and OpSite Post-op waterproof dressing.
- Overtraining syndrome: rule out medical illness. Training break needed. Prevention is the key: allow rest and recovery, especially during heaviest training periods and postinjury return to activity.

RETURN TO PLAY

- Musculoskeletal injuries: see specific chapters above. As a general rule, most athletes can be released to controlled practices/sessions once range of motion and strength testing (functional testing) is adequate.

- Asthma (see Chap. 8).
- Inner ear disturbances: once symptoms resolve for divers. As tolerated for swimmers.
- Lacerations: protected wound and full range of motion of affected areas.
- Overtraining syndrome: as soon as athlete feels ready.

Bibliography

FINA Sports Medicine Reviews are located at www.fina.org.

Kammer CS, Young CC, Niedfeldt MW: Swimming injuries and illnesses. *Phys Sports Med* 27(4):51–54, 57–60, 1999.

Koehler SM, Thorson DC: Swimmer's shoulder: Targeting treatment. *Phys Sports Med* 24(11):39–50, 1996.

50

Tennis

Marc R. Safran

INTRODUCTION

- Most acute injuries are to the lower extremity.
- Most overuse injuries are to the upper extremity.
- Low back pain is usually due to overuse but may present as an acute injury.

THIGH

Common Injuries

- Strains—adductors, hamstrings, quadriceps (rectus femoris)

Treatment

- Strains—rest, ice, compression. Stretching and then strengthening. Non-steroidal anti-inflammatory drugs (NSAIDs).

Return to Play

- When full range of motion and adequate strength are achieved. Taping or wrapping when athlete first returns may help.

KNEE

Common Injuries (See Chap. 26)

- Medial or lateral meniscal tears—with joint line tenderness, swelling, decreased range of motion (ROM), locking, and giving way of the knee.
- Patellar tendinitis, or "jumper's knee," and Osgood-Schlatter disease in adolescents.

- Patellofemoral tracking problems (excessive lateral patellar compression)—more common in females.

Specialized Equipment Needs

- Patellar stabilizing brace or patellar tendon band may be beneficial.

Treatment

- Meniscus (see Chap. 26)
- Patellar tendinitis—activity limited by symptom, hamstring, and quadriceps stretching and strengthening. Relative rest, ice, ultrasound, NSAIDs, and patellar tendon taping.
- Patellofemoral—quadriceps strengthening leg press not to exceed 90 degrees of flexion), McConnell taping and patella-restraining brace.

Return to Play

- Meniscus—is treatment-specific. Average range is 6 weeks with partial meniscectomy to 6 months with a meniscal repair.
- Patellar tracking/overload or patellar tendinitis—activity is limited by symptoms.

LEG

Common Injuries

- Shin splints or medial tibial stress syndrome—leg pain—pain in shin, particularly lower inner leg.
- Tennis leg—tear of calf at the medial head of the gastrocnemius/distal muscle tendon junction.

Specialized Equipment Needs

- Shin splints associated with flat feet may benefit from cushioned arch supports.
- Tennis leg—prevent by stretching the calf and using a heel lift.

Treatment

- Shin splints—rest, arch supports, strengthen ankle (especially posterior tibialis muscle), ice, NSAIDs.
- Tennis leg—rest, occasionally crutch use, ice elevation, compression. Stretching and strengthening of calf.

Return to Play

- Shin splints—as tolerate symptoms, Use arch supports.
- Tennis leg—able to hop on affected leg without pain.

BACK

Common Injuries (See Chap. 21)

- Lumbosacral sprains, stress fractures to pars interarticularis, and disk injuries.

Treatment

- Rest, ice, compression, ROM exercises, strengthening of lumbosacral and abdominal musculature, rehabilitation of deficiencies in lower extremities, and bracing. Epidural injections and surgery may be considered with disk injuries.

Return to Play

- Sprains—activity limited by pain. Stress fracture—typically 3 to 6 months, occasionally back bracing. Back surgery—following 4–6 months of rehabilitation.

ABDOMEN

Common Injuries

- Abdominal strains—usually the rectus abdominis on the nondominant side.

Treatment

- Rest, ice, compression, stretching, strengthening of the abdominal musculature.

Return to Play

- Activity limited by pain.

UPPER EXTREMITY
Common Injuries

- Overuse injuries are common and may be exacerbated and require treatment during tournament.
  - Elbow—tennis elbow (lateral epicondylitis—recreational player; medial epicondylitis—high-level player (see Chap. 23).
  - Shoulder—rotator cuff inflammation (due to impingement or instability) (see Chap. 24).
  - Stress fracture of the ulna (uncommon but unique to tennis).
  - Wrist—fracture of hook of hamate; de Quervain's syndrome; tendinitis of the extensor carpi radialis brevis and longus and flexor carpi ulnaris; recurrent instability of the extensor carpi ulnaris; ulnocarpal impingement; triangular fibrocartilage tear.
  - Hand—radial digital nerve compression of index finger, ulnar artery thrombosis.

Specialized Equipment Needs

- Brace for medial and lateral epicondylitis

Treatment

- Inflammation and tendinitis—RICE, stretching, strengthening, NSAIDs, ultrasound, and taping of affected area.
- Tendon instability—requires surgical repair.
- Stress fractures—rest.
- Fractures—surgery or immobilization by casting. Hook of hamate fracture often treated by excision.
- Nerve compression—rest and NSAIDs.

Return to Play

- Inflammation and tendinitis—activity is limited by symptoms.
- Fractures—varies by degree and site of fracture.

OTHER COMMON INJURIES

- Bee stings (see Chap. 7)
- Muscle cramps
- Heat illness (see Chap. 17)

Bibliography

Safran MR: Injuries sustained in tennis and other racquet sports, in Fu FH, Stone DA (eds): *Sports Injuries: Mechanisms, Prevention, and Treatment,* 2d ed. Philadelphia: Lippincott, Williams & Wilkins, 2001, pp 617–656.

Safran MR, Stone DA: Tennis and other racquet sport injuries, in Safran MR, Van Camp SP, McKeag D (eds): *Spiral Manual of Sports Medicine.* Philadelphia: Lippincott-Raven, 1998, pp 613–614.

51

Track and Field

Evan Bass
Bernadette Pendergraph

COMMON INJURIES

Runners

- Sprinters/hurdlers <400 m
  - Acute hamstring strains: imbalance of quadriceps and hamstrings
  - Groin strains (see Chap. 25)
  - Achilles rupture: previous tendinosis or explosive push off (see Chap. 27)
  - Plantar fasciitis and plantar fascia injury (see Chap. 28)
- Distance runners >800 m, steeplechase
  - Patellofemoral syndrome (see Chap. 26)
  - Shin splints
  - Achilles/gastrocnemius rupture: previous tendinosis (see Chap. 27)
  - Plantar fasciitis: poor flexibility (see Chap. 28)
  - Spike lacerations: mass start of race
  - Heat illness: multiple events, inadequate hydration (see Chap. 17)
- Hurdlers, steeplechase
  - Groin strains (see Chap. 25)
  - Straddle injuries (see Chap. 15)
  - Knee sprains (see Chap. 26)
  - Trail leg contusions
  - Achilles/plantar fascial strain (see Chap. 28)

Throwers

- Javelin
  - Rotator cuff strains (see Chap. 24)
  - Medial epicondylitis and elbow ulnar collateral ligament injury (see Chap. 23)
  - Low back strain: rotational forces of throw with sudden deceleration (see Chap. 21)
  - Groin strains (see Chap. 25)

- • Patellar/quadriceps strain (see Chap. 26)
  - • Meniscus tear (see Chap. 26)
  - • Penetrating injuries: wayward throw at spectators and other competitors
- • Shot put
  - • Groin strain (see Chap. 25)
  - • Patellar tendon strain (see Chap. 26)
  - • Wrist/finger hyperextension (see Chap. 22)
- • Discus/hammer
  - • Rotator cuff strain (see Chap. 24)
  - • Groin strain (see Chap. 25)
  - • Blister of throwing hand

Jumpers

- • Long/triple jump
  - • Lumbar strain (see Chap. 21)
  - • Hamstring strain: occurs at takeoff
  - • Knee injury (see Chap. 26)
    - • Anterior cruciate ligament (ACL) tear: occurs on landing, especially at edge of pit.
    - • Meniscus tear.
    - • Patellar tendinitis.
  - • Achilles rupture: occurs on takeoff (see Chap. 27)
  - • Heel bruise: repetitive landings
- • High jump
  - • Cervical strain/spinal cord injury: especially with flop-style jump (see Chap. 20)
  - • Shoulder dislocation (see Chap. 24)
  - • Lumbar strain (see Chap. 21)
  - • Patellar tendinitis (see Chap. 26)
  - • Posterior tibial tendon strain: compression of medial ankle on takeoff (see Chap. 27)
  - • Ankle sprain (see Chap. 27)
  - • Heel bruise: repetitive landings
- • Pole vault
  - • Head injuries (see Chap. 6)
  - • Cervical strain/spinal cord injury (see Chap. 20)
  - • Shoulder strain: occurs with set of pole and push off (see Chap. 24)
  - • Lumbar strain (see Chap. 21)
  - • Fractures: landings outside of pit (see Chap. 18)
- • Lower extremity injuries in sprinters

SPECIALIZED EQUIPMENT NEEDS

- • Situate medical care near pole vault.
- • Most injuries can be treated with a first aid kit, ice, compression wraps.
- • Sport massage—multiple-event athletes.

- Stretching—quadriceps, hamstrings, Achilles.
- Cell phone for unexpected emergencies.

RETURN TO PLAY

- Individualized by athlete and event.
- Considering risk of further injury.

Bibliography

Otis CL: Track and field, in Sallis RE, Massimino F (eds): *Essentials of Sports Medicine.* St Louis: Mosby, 1997, pp 554–557.

Shaw D: Track and field, in Safran MR, McKeag DB VanCamp SP (eds): *Manual of Sports Medicine.* Philadelphia: Lippincott-Raven, 1998, pp 613–614.

Track and field, in Mellion MB, Walsh WM, Shelton GL (eds): *The Team Physician's Handbook.* Philadelphia: Hanley & Belfus, 1990, pp 585–598.

52

Triathlon and Duathlon

John Martinez

INTRODUCTION

- Multisport races that combine swimming, biking, and running (triathlons) or running and cycling (duathlons).

ORGANIZATIONS

- ITU—International Triathlon Union
- WTC—World Triathlon Corporation
- USTA—United States Triathlon Association

RACE SPECIFICS

- The lengths and distances of these races can vary greatly.

Sprint Distances

- Triathlons—¼- to ½-mi swim, 8- to 16-mi bike, 2- to 5-mi run
- Duathlons—2- to 3-mi run, 8- to 16-mi bike, 2- to 4-mi run

Olympic Distances

- 0.9 mi (1.5 km) swim, 24-mi (40-km) bike, 6.2-mi (10-km) run

Endurance (Ironman) Distances

- 2.4-mi (3.8 km) swim, 112-mi (180-km) bike, 26.2-mi run (full marathon)

EVENT SPECIFICS

- Swim
  - May be mass start or in waves separated by time intervals.
  - Traumatic injuries to face common in mass starts due to kicking of feet.
  - Wet suits allowed for age-group athletes if water temperature is less than 78°F.
  - Wet suits allowed for professional/elite athletes if water temperature is less than 72°F.
- Bike
  - Age-group racers; individual time trial.
  - Aerobars allowed, disk wheels per race director's policy (not allowed at Hawaii Ironman due to wind conditions on bike course).
  - Drafting not allowed—warning, time penalty, or disqualification.
  - Professional/elite athletes—some Olympic and Sprint distances are draft-legal.
- Run
  - No pacesetters or outside support allowed other than aid stations.

COMMON INJURIES

Head, Face, and Dental Injuries/ Trauma (See Chaps. 6, 10, 11)

- Swim—head and face injuries more common during mass swim starts. Result from close proximity of competitors and being kicked or struck during swim.
- Bike—severe head injuries from bike trauma
  - Includes concussion, skull fractures, and traumatic brain injuries such as subdural and epidural hematomas.
- Specialized equipment/prevention
  - Helmet required for bike portion. Helmet should meet ANSI or SNELL standards.
  - Helmet should be replaced after one hard impact even if no damage is evident.

Eye Injuries/Trauma

- Swim
  - Corneal abrasions and orbital/eye trauma from mass swim starts
  - Specialized equipment/prevention
    - Swim goggles
- Bike and run
  - Corneal abrasions and foreign bodies
  - Specialized equipment/prevention
    - Sunglasses

Hyponatremia

- Serum sodium level less than 135 mg/dL
- May be fatal. Can present with mental confusion and seizures or be relatively asymptomatic.
- Causes
  - Excessive free water intake during race.
  - Seen in slower athletes, who have more time to drink at aid stations and less fluid loss by sweating.
- Treatment
  - If altered mental status or seizures, transport!
    - If normovolemic or hypervolemic, do not give intravenous fluids!
    - If mild symptoms, allow body to eliminate excess fluid by diuresis.
    - No studies show quicker improvement by giving diuretics.

Dehydration

- Excessive fluid loss from sweating, vomiting, and diarrhea.
- Due to inadequate fluid intake before and during race.
- Prevention
  - Adequate access to liquids on race course (see below).

Exercise-Associated Collapse

- Athlete who collapses or requires assistance during or after an event.
- Usually vasovagal and hypotension due to loss of muscle pump action of legs while running.
- Be concerned and vigilant of athletes who collapse *before* finishing.
- Prevention
  - Encourage finishers to continue to walk after completing race.
  - Avoid massages or sitting for 30 min after end of race.
- Treatment
  - Supportive care, have athlete lie down and elevate legs.
  - Oral fluids as tolerated.
  - Intravenous fluids usually not indicated.

Hypothermia

- Most common during open-water swim, even with use of wet suit.

Hyperthermia

- Uncommon in longer endurance races due to slower pace.

- Swim—slightly increased risk of hyperthermia with use of wet suit.
- Bike—rare due to cooling effect of air-flow.
- Run—suspect in athletes who significantly increase pace in last miles of race (see Chap. 17).

Rhabdomyolysis

- Excessive muscle breakdown with potential for acute renal failure.
- Caused by excessive workout, heat stress and dehydration, sickle cell trait.
- Diagnostic tips
    - Agitation, nausea, vomiting, or confusion.
    - Moderate to severe muscle pain.
    - Anuria or decreased urine with dark or brown urine.
    - Elevated CK and urine myoglobin.
- Treatment
    - Intravenous hydration and rapid transport to hospital for definitive care.

Musculoskeletal Injuries

- See chapters for swimming, running, and cycling (Chaps. 32, 39, 49).

MEDICAL STAFF

- Proper medical coverage requires coordination between stationary and mobile medical staff.

Race Medical Director

- Physician in charge of organization

Physicians

- One physician per 200 athletes

Nurses and Midlevel Providers

- One nurse and mid-level per 100 athletes

Mobile Medical

- Vans—medical provider staff (physician or trained midlevel provider)
  - Two-way radio
  - Medical equipment bag
  - Backboard
  - C-collars

FLUID STATIONS

- Based on ITU guidelines for international–Olympic distance
  - Swim start
    - Two paper cups per athlete
    - 200 mL of water per athlete
    - 100 mL of electrolyte fluid replacement
  - Swim finish or swim-bike transition
    - same as above
  - Bike course—aid stations
    - Every 10–12 km for Olympic distance
      - One water bottle per person
      - 350–500 mL of fluid replacement
    - Every 10 mi for longer distance
  - Bike-run transition
    - Same as swim start and swim-bike transition
  - Run course aid stations every mile
    - Three paper cups per athlete
    - 200 mL of water
    - 100 mL of electrolyte fluid replacement
  - Finish line—recovery area
    - Fluids—same as above
    - Food—high carbohydrate content—(i.e. bagels, fruits, pretzels)

MEDICAL TENT EQUIPMENT

- Intravenous fluids
  - Lactated Ringer's solution
    - Has potassium. Avoid using unless serum potassium level of athlete is known.
  - D5½NS or D5NS
    - Event duration <4 h
      - D5 with ½NS—first liter.
      - ½NS subsequent liters.
      - Consider hospital transfer after second liter if not improved.
    - Event duration >4 h
      - D5NS—first liter.
      - NS subsequent liters.
      - Consider hospital transfer after third liter if not improved.

Medications and ACLS Equipment
(See Chaps. 2, 3, 4, and 61)

- Cardiac (ACLS) drugs, defibrillator, AED
- Intravenous benzodiazepam or other sedative
- Intravenous magnesium—cramping
- Intravenous antiemetics—intractable vomiting
- Albuterol (nebulizer or inhaler)—asthmatics
- Laboratory
    - Glucose, sodium, potassium, magnesium, and CBC most helpful.
- Medical records
    - Triathlon governing bodies require postrace report of medical treatment of all athletes.
    - Summary statistics are compiled by race director.
    - Prerace medical questionnaire
        - Completed before race by all athletes
        - Compiled list of all athletes with significant medical problems should be available to medical staff in the medical tent during race.
    - Medical treatment record
        - Include race number and name, time in and out of tent.
        - Brief history, examination, diagnosis, treatment, and names of medical providers.

EMERGENCY TRANSPORT

- Identify one designated hospital as receiving hospital if possible.
    - Direct communication between medical tent, hospital, and EMS.
    - Local EMS rules may have to be followed.

Bibliography

Roberts WO: Mass-participation events, in Lillegard WA, Butcher JD, Rucker KS (eds): *Handbook of Sports Medicine: A Symptom-Oriented Approach,* 2d ed. Burlington, MA: Butterworth Heinemann, Elsevier Science/Harcourt. 1999.

53

Volleyball

Kimberly G. Harmon

EPIDEMIOLOGY

- 800 million people worldwide play volleyball.
- 187,000 volleyball-related injuries are treated by physicians annually.
- 20–30 percent of all injuries are acute.
- Injury rate is similar in both practices (4.5 injuries per 1000 athlete exposures) and games (4.9 injuries per 1000 athlete exposures).
- Among college athletes, practice injury rate in volleyball is similar to that in other sports.
- Volleyball game injury rate among college athletes is the lowest among sports tracked by the NCAA Injury Surveillance System.

COMMON INJURIES

- Ankle sprains (see Chap. 27)
  - Represent 15–60 percent of acute injuries in volleyball (vs. 10–30 percent of all sport-related injuries).
- Most often occurs when landing from a jump.
  - Blocking or attacking.
  - Often occurs when foot goes underneath the net, over the center line in the "conflict zone."
  - Injuries can be decreased with a training program that teaches players to avoid the center line during play by jumping straight up rather than up and forward.
- Knee injuries—15 percent of acute injuries (see Chap. 26).
- Thumb—6 percent of acute injuries (see Chap. 22).
- Finger—4 percent of acute injuries.
- Muscle strains.
  - Account for 20–30 percent of all acute injuries.
  - Common in groin, hamstrings, quadriceps.
- Abrasions—"floor burns."
- Contusions.
  - From collisions with other players or the floor and when diving.

SPECIALIZED EQUIPMENT NEEDS

- Athletic equipment needs
  - Ankle braces
    - The value of prophylactic ankle bracing or taping is debated.
    - May decrease injuries by providing proprioceptive feedback.
    - In athletes with previous history of ankle injury, generally considered advisable, in addition to appropriate rehabilitation program.
  - Knee pads
    - Help prevent contusions, abrasions, and traumatic bursitis.
  - Defensive pants.
    - Padded from hip to knee and can prevent contusions and abrasions.
  - Volleyball equipment that is safe.
    - Stable nets and poles.
    - Padded supporting wires.
    - Adequate clear space surrounding court.
- No specialized medical equipment required (see Chaps. 59, 60, and 61).

RETURN TO PLAY

- Ankle sprain
  - When able to jump on one foot, land, cut, and run pain-free.
  - Tape or ankle brace recommended initially.
- Torn anterior cruciate ligament (ACL)
  - After surgery (6–12 months).
  - With demands of sport, conservative treatment is unlikely to be successful, and a failed trial of conservative treatment places the knee at risk for additional damage.
- Torn medial collateral ligament (MCL)
  - When knee has full range of motion, strength is 90 percent of opposite knee, there is no tenderness over the ligament and no pain with valgus stress testing or functional movements.
- Thumb/finger sprain
  - When no pain is felt while playing taped
- Muscle strains/contusions
  - When 90 percent strength of opposite leg with no pain with functional activities after adequate warmup.
- Floor burns
  - Immediately, after covering any bloody or weeping areas.
- Abrasions
  - Return to play after dirt and contaminants removed. This may be particularly difficult if playing in sand.
  - Wounds that are bleeding or seeping need to be covered.
- Muscle strains
  - For quadriceps strains, immobilize in flexion for first 48 h.
  - Crutches as needed to ambulate.

- Neoprene sleeve may provide comfort and help keep muscle warm when athlete returns to play.
- Return when player able to cut, jump, and run without pain.

Bibliography

Bhairo NH, Nijsten WWN, Van Dalen KC, Ten Duis HJ: Hand injuries in volleyball. *Int J Sports Med* 13:351–354, 1992.

Briner WW, Benjamin HJ: Volleyball injuries. *Phys Sports Med* 27(3):48–60, 1999.

Fandel D, Mellion MB: Volleyball, in Mellion MB, Walsh WM, Shelton GL (eds): *The Team Physician's Handbook,* 2d ed. Philadelphia: Hanley & Belfus, 1997.

Hirshman HP: Volleyball, in Safran MR, McKeag DB, Van Camp SP (eds): *Manual of Sports Medicine.* Philadelphia: Lippincott-Raven, 1998.

Schultz LK: Volleyball. *Phys Med Rehab Clin North Am* 10(1):19–34, 1999.

54

Wrestling

Ken Honsik

INTRODUCTION

Description

- Wrestling is one of the oldest and most demanding individual sports. Competitors wrestle in short periods, attempting to score points for take-downs, escapes, reversals, near falls, and ultimately pins. Wrestlers can also be penalized points for improper equipment, uniforms, and—most importantly—illegal holds and moves, which put the other wrestler at risk for injury.
- Two main forms
  - Freestyle (international/intercollegiate—*athletes may utilize or attack upper or lower body.*
  - Greco-Roman—*athletes may only attack and utilize upper body.*
- Role of medical personnel
  - Recognition and management of serious injuries such as c-spine and head trauma.
  - A *timely* on-mat evaluation to determine athlete's ability to continue safely within a strictly limited length of time.
  - Control bleeding and minimize blood exposure to other athletes.
  - Provide treatment for athlete's injuries after a tournament or match and education on rehabilitation, prevention, and return-to-play guide-lines.
- Injury time outs
  - Intercollegiate freestyle wrestling (high school/college) allows $1\frac{1}{2}$ minutes of cumulative injury time. The referee may call for an official time out if it is felt that the wrestler must be evaluated medically before continuing.
- Bleeding time
  - High school—cumulative time of 5 min.
  - College—two bleeding time outs are permitted, their length being at the discretion of the referee.
- Essential to have clear view of matches taking place to allow for ex-pedient evaluation and provide evidence for mechanism of injury.

COMMON INJURIES

Knee (See Chap. 26)

- Ligament sprains
  - MCL and LCL more common than ACL injuries.
  - Evaluate for significant laxity. If grade 1 (no laxity), athlete may continue match.
- Meniscal injuries
  - Very common in wrestlers secondary to increased torsion forces
  - Lateral more common than medial
  - Evaluate ROM and stability. If full ROM, no mechanical locking, and no new laxity, consider allowing athlete to continue if athlete so desires.
- Patellar subluxation/dislocation
  - Assess ROM and function.
- Prepatellar bursitis
  - RICE: consider aspiration, beware of possible septic bursitis.
  - Neoprene knee sleeve or brace (*do not* restrict ROM).

Shoulder (See Chap. 24)

- Acromioclavicular sprain
  - Very common: RICE, return to match if no significant displacement and full function of shoulder.
- Dislocation/subluxation
  - Primary dislocations should be reduced and athlete removed from competition.
  - If recurrent and immediately reduced, consider return to match if shoulder exhibits full ROM and strength. (This is controversial and situation-dependent.)
- Sternoclavicular sprain/dislocation
  - Assess for possible posterior displacement and cardiopulmonary complications.
  - If no displacement and wrestler able to take full breaths, consider return.

Back (See Chap. 21)

- Strains and spasm common, secondary to attempted lifts from poor leverage positions.
- Pain and level of function determines return to play.

Ribs

- Very common secondary to compression, torsion, and direct impact mechanisms.

- Muscle strain vs. fracture.
- Check for crepitus, step-off, and/or pulmonary complications (i.e., pneumothorax).
- Return to play is controversial and usually limited by athlete's ability to take full breaths.

Head and Neck

- Severe injuries rare because of rules preventing dangerous slams and maneuvers.
- Muscle strains common because head used for leverage in multiple moves.
- Brachial plexus injuries—burners or stingers common.
- If c-spine injury suspected, see Chap. 20.
- Concussions should be managed per accepted guidelines (see Chap. 6).

Face (See Chap. 10)

- Epistaxis
  - Extremely common because of direct blows such as the cross-face maneuver.
  - Have athlete blow nose to expel clot, tilt head forward, apply direct pressure to nares; application of ice may help.
  - Pledget or "nose rocket" may be used to stop bleeding and left in place until competition or activity is completed.
  - Wrestler may not be permitted to continue if bleeding is not controlled.
- Nasal fracture
  - May reduce deformity acutely.
  - Do not reduce once swollen.
  - Evaluate for septal hematoma.
  - Athlete may wear protective face mask to continue.
- Auricular hematoma ("cauliflower ear")
  - Common, especially at levels that do not require headgear.
  - Aspirate *once* at the end of a tournament (last match), using sterile technique with a 22- or 25-gauge needle (butterfly works best).
  - Place compression dressing after aspiration.
    - Aluminum finger splint compressed over gauze pressure dressing, collodion strips, dental molding (has been used with mixed success), suturing a button to compress the hematoma after draining (recommended for recurrent hematomas).
    - Inform parents of possible permanent deformity and to watch for infection.

Skin

- Herpes gladiatorum, ringworm, impetigo
    - These lesions disqualify an athlete from competition unless cleared by a physician and or adequately treated.
- Lacerations (see Chap. 16)
    - Suture, Steri-Strips, cyanoacrylate
    - Lacerations/abrasions must be completely covered. Semipermeable barrier products work very well for this purpose.

Pulmonary/Physiologic

- Rules are now allowing for athletes to be treated for preexisting conditions, such as asthma and diabetes, during the match.
- Emphasis has recently been placed discouraging the practice of "dropping weight" to compete in a lower weight class. This practice may result in profound dehydration.

TREATMENT/RETURN TO PLAY

- Treatment is either *temporary* (return athlete to match) or *definitive* (adequate time for healing, rehabilitation, and prevention of recurrent injury.
- Goal of team physician/athletic trainer is to prevent athlete from returning to match if unsafe or at risk of more serious injury *and* to make sure the athlete is in peak condition before he or she returns to the mat.

SPECIAL EQUIPMENT

- Suture pack (see Chap. 16)
- Cyanoacrylate
- Steri-Strips
- 10-mL syringes with 22- and 25-gauge butterfly needles
- Aluminum splints (cheap, "hind legs of frog" splint works best), collodion (messy/strong smell), dental molding material (expensive), compression dressings (always easy to find)
- Semipermeable membrane dressings
- Pledgets or cotton nose plugs
- Universal precaution blood cleanup kits
- Gloves!!!!!

ORGANIZATIONS

- USA Wrestling
- NFSHSA—National Federation of State High School Associations

- NCAA
- IOC—International Olympic Committee

Bibliography

Dienst WL, Dightman L, Dworkin MS, Thompson RK: Pinning down skin infections: Diagnosis, treatment, and prevention in wrestlers. *Phys Sports Med* 25(12):45, 1997.

Kelly TF: Wrestling, in Mellion M, Walsh M, Shelton G (eds): *The Team Physician's Handbook*, 2d ed. Philadelphia: Hanley & Belfus, 1997, p 700.

National Federation of State High School Associations: http://www.nfhs.org/sportsmed/procedure.htm

NCAA Wrestling Rules: www.NCAA.org/library/rules/2001/2001_wrestling_rules_book.pdf

Part 4

General Topics

55

Mass Gathering
Medical Care

Jeff T. Grange

BACKGROUND

- "Mass gathering medical care refers to organized emergency health care services provided for spectators and participants in which at least 1000 persons are gathered at a specific location for a defined period of time" (National Association of Emergency Medical Services Physicians).
- Common misconception: mass gathering medical care is analogous to standard emergency medical services.
- What makes mass gathering medicine unique?
  - Medical personnel must navigate large crowds often without clear landmarks.
  - Barriers to access often prevent utilization of motorized transport vehicles.
  - Environmental factors such as weather can produce large numbers of patients in a short period of time.
  - The working environment may be hostile/austere and/or dangerous (mosh pits, racetracks, etc.).
  - There may be specialized rescue/safety requirements.
  - Communication challenges due to distances and increased noise levels at some venues (rock concerts, motorsports, etc.).
  - Lack of sufficient resources.
  - VIP medical care.
  - Prolonged time and/or distance to hospitals.
  - Potential for terrorist activity or other disasters and multiple casualty incidents.
  - Increased potential for patients refusing necessary medical care due to desire to remain at event.
- Many smaller gatherings have many of the same characteristics (commercial airliners, passenger trains, offshore oil rigs. etc.).
- Goals of medical care at a mass gathering:
  - Provide basic first aid to promote an enjoyable atmosphere and prevent minor problems from becoming more serious.

- Provide advanced medical services to promote rapid and safe transfer of patient to an appropriate medical facility, thus reducing chances of death and disability.
- Reduce number of *unnecessary transfers* of patients to hospitals, thus diminishing the impact on the local EMS system and hospitals.
- Avoid impacting the EMS system in a way that dilutes its ability to respond to community residents or to provide backup medical assistance in the event of a multiple casualty incident (MCI) or disaster.
- Avoid incurring ongoing liability for promoter.
- Attempt to maintain good public relations for promoter.

- Bottom line: provide the same (or better) quality of medical care as could reasonably be expected by a normal citizen outside the venue.
- Very little in medical literature and few standards in mass gathering medicine.
- Medical literature describes incidence of medical care ranging from 0.12–6.00 per 1000 spectators with cardiac arrests ranging from 0.3–4.0 per 1 million spectators.
- A large mass gathering may present patients with complaints ranging from basic first aid to anything that you might see in a similar-size city (heart attacks, traffic accidents, childbirths, kidney stones, lacerations, sprains, abdominal pain, etc.).

BASIC MEDICAL ACTION PLAN

- A *basic medical action plan is the key* to medical care at any mass gathering. It should address the following components:

Physician Medical Oversight

- Medical literature clearly demonstrates that physicians can positively impact decision making in the field, especially regarding nontransports and triage decisions.
- A locally licensed physician/medical director should be appointed for every mass gathering.
  - Should be knowledgeable in out-of-hospital care/EMS/mass gatherings and have plan for both direct and indirect medical oversight. He or she should also be available to all personnel during event.
  - Medical director must participate in design and implementation of medical action plan.
  - Medical director should institute appropriate protocols for anticipated common chief complaints, allowing nurses and other medical personnel to provide appropriate care without requiring every individual to be seen by a physician. A physician does not need to become personally involved in the care of every individual patient.
  - Medical director should be easily identifiable (credentials, vest, uniform, etc.).

Medical Reconnaissance

- Check with local and state authorities regarding any requirements for medical care at mass gatherings.
- Do a risk assessment of venue (wooden grandstands—fire risk; low fences at racetrack—spectator injuries; access concerns—stampede risks, walkways—pedestrian capacity, pedestrian/vehicle intersections; etc.).
- What type and how many medical problems at last similar event? If possible, attend a similar event and evaluate elements contributing to successful or problematic EMS delivery.
- How will event impact the local EMS system?
- Will alcohol be served? If so, what is the estimated impact?
- Since every event is different, evaluate the following factors for your specific event:
  - Crowd composition, crowd volume, crowd density, crowd mood, crowd control, crowd mobility, physical barriers, time to access patients, entrance and exit locations for spectators and participants, outdoor vs. indoor, warm temperatures and potential for heat-related illnesses, cold temperatures and potential for cold-related illnesses, daytime vs. nighttime event, rain plan, threat of thunderstorms/lightning, wet/slippery vs. dry ground conditions, ingress and egress for emergency vehicles, VIPs, etc.
  - Consider availability of alcohol, illicit drugs, water, food, shelter.
  - Is there a plan to deal with threats against the venue (bombs, biochemical threats, etc.)?
- What are the local (non-event-related) medical resources?
  - Hospitals
    - Trauma centers, burn centers, community emergency departments, children's hospitals
  - Ambulances
  - Helicopters

Negotiations for Event Medical Services

- Both general and professional liability insurance should be provided by event promoter/manager.
  - Get "occurrence" coverage, *not* "claims made" coverage.
- Do not rely on Good Samaritan statutes!
- Compensation—may be monetary or nonmonetary, but in general "You get what you pay for!" Also discuss provisions for meals, parking, lodging, etc.

Level of Care

- Who will I treat? Participants only, spectators only, both?

- What level of care? EMT-A (basic), EMT-paramedic, nurse, nurse practitioner, athletic trainers, physicians?
- Although a minimum of ALS care is always preferred, *EMT-Basic* (including automatic external defibrillator, or AED) is considered by most to be the *minimum acceptable level of care* at any mass gathering.
- The level of care at a mass gathering should reflect that which is available in the surrounding community.
- Certain *high-risk events* (boxing, auto racing, motorcycle racing, etc.) *should have Advanced Life Support (ALS) such as EMT-paramedic as a minimum and preferably have physicians qualified to provide emergency airways and other emergency intervention. Should also be knowledgeable with prehospital resuscitation and the local EMS system.*
- Consider "comfort care" providers (chiropractors, massage therapists, etc.) when appropriate.

Human Resources

- All personnel should know their role, responsibilities, and chain of command.
- In general, the further away the event from higher levels of medical care, the higher the level of on-site care should be.
- In general, the higher-risk the event, the higher the level of on-site care should be available.
- Deployment—many strategies.
- Personnel should be fully oriented and trained and deployed prior to start of event.

Medical Equipment (See Below and Chaps. 59, 60, and 61)

- Consider check-in and check-out procedures.
- Have plan for restocking as equipment is used.

Treatment Facilities

- A medical care center is usually needed only for large mass gatherings, prolonged events, high-patient-volume events, or events with prolonged transport times.
- Usually keep highest medical authority here—it is more efficient to bring the sickest patients to a predesignated location rather than have highest medical authority go to each patient.
- Needs good access to on-site patients and off-site emergency transportation.

- Consider security—especially when dealing with high-profile patients.
- Consider helicopter landing zones near the medical care center.
- Private patient care areas desirable.
- Medical care areas must be clearly marked.

Transportation Resources

- Internal transportation:
  - Requires planning—stairs vs. ramps, mud vs. dirt. Create designated emergency access routes, etc.
  - Various modes depending on venue and distances—motorized carts, backboards, litters, cots, ambulances, helicopters, bicycles, boats, etc.
  - May need ambulances and/or helicopters dedicated to large events.
  - All medical response vehicles should be clearly marked and highly visible.
  - Reserve parking areas for emergency vehicles.
  - Lights and sirens may improve response times to patients but may not be visible or audible at some venues.
  - Consider medically equipped bicycles for large mass gatherings with difficult vehicular access.
  - Have a plan for nonemergency transports.
  - Deployment of internal transportation:
    - Minimize response time.
    - Create safe, relatively unimpeded routes.
- External transportation:
  - Have established emergency evacuation routes that are kept free of obstacles and people.
  - Consider need for law enforcement escort of emergency vehicles.
  - Many modes may be appropriate, depending on event and venue—ground ambulance, helicopter, airplane, snowmobile, boat, litters, etc.
  - Attempt to distribute the patients between hospitals to prevent "overload" of any one receiving facility.
  - Transport time may be prolonged (desert races, mountain expeditions, adventure racing, etc.)
  - Preplan if crossing county, state, and international borders may become necessary.
    - Medical license, certification issues
    - Passports
  - Communications.
  - Have plan for emergency resources returning to event/mass gathering.

Public Health Elements

- Food and water management and availability.
- Waste management concerns.
- Traffic management.
- Consider preventive medical needs:
  - Condoms at rock concerts.
  - Helmets, fire suits, fuel cells at motorsports events.
  - Hearing protection available at loud events.
  - Misters at potentially hot outdoor events/venues.
  - Consider restricting alcohol sales when appropriate.
  - Inspect spectator barriers (fences, walls, etc.) at high-risk events.
  - Consider metal detectors at certain high-risk events and political conventions.
  - Consider searching all spectators at high-risk events that may involve large numbers of gang members.
  - Consider "no colors" policy (clothing/items that represent gang membership must be removed prior to entering event/venue) for events that may involve gang members.

Access to Care

- Minimize time interval to provide care for patients.
- Educate all staff, participants, and spectators regarding how to access medical care.
- Ensure compliance with the Americans with Disabilities Act.
- First aid stations and/or care center locations should be in event programs/guides.
- Consider child ID bracelets at large mass gatherings.

Emergency Medical Operations

- Establish relationship and lines of communication with other venue disciplines and public safety services.
- Have an emergency action plan for each event, venue, or facility.
- Know what the emergency action plan says and what the roles and responsibilities of staffers are.
- Know your resources in case of a terrorist threat or incident:
  - Bomb squad
  - Hazardous materials team
  - Local lab to confirm or exclude suspicious materials as hazardous biological and/or chemical agents.

Communications

- Have plan with local *public safety answering point* (PSAP) for 911 calls during events.
- Have plan to communicate with local EMS system and hospitals.
- Have a backup plan.
- Have radio designations.
- Use "plainspeak" rather than codes.
- Test system prior to event!
- Review radio etiquette for those who may be unfamiliar with it.
- Consider head sets if noisy environment (concerts, auto races, etc.).

Command and Control

- Consider centralized hub [emergency operations center (EOC)] for command and control, communications, and dissemination of information.
  - Should be clearly marked.
  - Should be a fixed location.
  - Should have representatives from event administration, security, maintenance, public relations/public information, fire department, medical/EMS.
- Know lines of authority and responsibility for each medical position.
- Know where the medical team is integrated into the overall administrative structure.
- Be familiar with and use the Incident Command System (also known as the Incident Management System) (see Chap. 62).
- For large mass gatherings or events involving multiple agencies, consider invoking a "unified command" model.

Documentation

- All patient contacts should be documented in a standardized fashion.
- The medical record is not only a medical record but also a legal, risk-management, continuous quality improvement (CQI), and research document.
- Have an "against medical advice" (AMA) form for patients who refuse treatment that is deemed necessary to help reduce event/venue liability.

Continuous Quality Improvement

- Goal: constant improvement of medical care and system.
- Whenever possible, debriefings should be done in a positive light.
- Generate a list of recommendations and conclusions.

Dealing with a Death

- Whenever possible and appropriate, "Nobody dies at the venue."
- Pronounce en route to hospital or in emergency department.
  - Better control of situation.
  - Initiate resuscitation.
  - Prevent public spectacles (respect for patient and family members).
  - Coordinate public relations.
- Have a plan and coordinate with local coroner.
- Remember "It's not *if*, it's *when.*"
- Plan to secure site, vehicle, etc., until investigation is complete.

Dealing with the Media

- Danger! Beware! They can make you look really bad or really good!
- Remember to honor patient confidentiality.
- Check state regulations regarding what can be revealed about high-profile patients.
- Remember that if you do not "give them something . . . ," they'll go elsewhere and find something (whether it is accurate or not).
- Make sure that you have accurate facts before you speak to the media.
- Have a designated spokesperson.

COMMON INJURIES

- Motorsports (auto)—burns, head and neck injuries, blunt abdominal and chest trauma, cardiac events (see Chap. 41).
- Motorsports (motorcycle)—head and neck injuries, extremity fractures, blunt abdominal trauma, blunt chest trauma.
- Motorsports (boat)—drownings, head and neck injuries, blunt abdominal trauma, and blunt chest trauma.
- Concerts—cardiac (classical), overdoses (rock), extremity trauma (rock concerts with mosh pits, crowd surfing, and crowd diving).
- All mass gatherings—heat exhaustion, minor first aid, alcohol and drug intoxication.

SPECIALIZED EQUIPMENT

- Radios
- Head sets
- Vehicles
  - Ambulances
  - Miniambulances

- Golf carts
- Bicycles
- Motorcycles
- Helicopters
- Boats
- Uniforms
- Airway, breathing, circulation (ABCs) (see Chaps. 3, 4, and 5)
  - Combitube
  - Defibrillators
  - Medications
  - Intravenous supplies and fluids
- Rescue/extrication
  - Stair chair
  - Reeves sleeve (consider for insulation for defibrillation in metal grandstands)
  - Kendrick or similar extrication device
  - Splinting supplies
  - Wheelchairs
  - Bandages
- Medical bags (see Chaps. 59, 60, and 61).
- Standardization of all medical equipment is desirable (i.e., all defibrillators same make and model, all ambulances, medical bags, and first aid stations stocked the same, etc.).
- Miscellaneous
  - Map with all stationary medical stations, mobile medical resources, staging areas, predesignated treatment areas for MCIs, and landmarks should be available.
  - Some medications may require refrigeration (succinylcholine, tetanus toxoid, etc.).
  - Flashlights.
  - Sheets, blankets, pillows, when appropriate, for first aid stations.
  - Sunglasses, sunscreen, hats, etc., for protection from environment.
  - Personal protective equipment—gloves, eye protection, universal precautions.
  - Consider x-ray capability for large mass gatherings with large numbers of extremity fractures (i.e., motorcycle races).

TREATMENT

- *Have a medical action plan prior to event—most important.*
- Notification of medical problem:
  - May come from ushers, volunteers, security/law enforcement, public address system, 911 calls, walk-ins, television during live broadcast events, etc.
  - Maintain contact with the reporting party until you make patient contact.
  - Information is often secondhand, inaccurate, and vague.
- Dispatch appropriate medical personnel/resources
  - Consider certified emergency medical dispatchers (EMD).

- Must be familiar with facility!
- Have plan for 911 calls that may arise from the stands via pay phones or mobile phones.
- Locate patient(s):
  - May be very difficult (especially in general-admission areas).
  - Be as specific as possible—use common landmarks, section numbers, row numbers, seat numbers, gate numbers, etc.
  - Always know *your* location! You may need to request backup medical resources and/or security.
- Rescue/extrication may be required.
  - Scene safety—#1 priority.
    - Never turn your back on race traffic/mosh pit/etc.
    - Stop the event if necessary.
    - Consider parking rescue vehicles/ambulance to help protect scene.
    - Crowd control/security may be necessary.
  - Specialized equipment may be needed ("jaws of life," fire trucks, four-wheel-drive ambulances, backboards, extrication devices, etc.).
  - Have a plan for rescue/extrication of patient and practice it.
  - Consider using other spectators as appropriate for security/crowd control/etc.
- Triage—many incidents involve more than one person (especially in motorsports crashes).
  - Could there be other injured patients?
- Stabilization
  - Mass gathering medicine is show-business medicine, so remember, whenever possible, that "The show must go on!"
    - High visibility with high expectations!
      - Have a sense of urgency.
      - It is not only whether or not you did the right thing, it is also how it appears.
      - You will be "Monday-morning quarterbacked."
  - Only do what needs to be done, but *do what needs to be done!* (In the middle of a mass gathering/grandstand/concert/racetrack, etc.)
    - *Airway with c-spine* immobilization, breathing, circulation (ABCs) (see Chaps. 3, 4, and 5).
    - Consider risks and benefits when using defibrillator in occupied metal grandstands.
- Internal transportation (see above)
- Triage area/first aid station
  - Remember that some patients belong in a hospital (acute MIs, major trauma, etc.). In general, these patients should bypass any first aid stations or care centers to prevent delay in definitive care and be transported to closest appropriate medical facility as soon as possible.
- External transportation (see above)
- Definitive care
  - Know your local medical facilities (trauma centers, burn centers, closest emergency departments, hyperbaric chambers, etc.).

RETURN TO PLAY

- See appropriate chapters related to corresponding injuries.

Bibliography

Grange JT, Green SM, Downs W: Concert medicine: Spectrum of medical problems encountered at 405 major concerts. *Acad Emerg Med* 6(2):202–207, 1999.

Jaslow D, Drake M, Lewis J: Characteristics of state legislation governing mass gathering medical care. *Prehosp Emerg Care* 3(3):316–320, 1999.

Jaslow D, Yancey A, Milsten A: *Mass Gathering Medical Care: The Medical Director's Checklist for the NAEMSP Standards and Clinical Practice Committee.* Lenexa, KS: National Association of Emergency Medical Services Physicians, 2000.

Parillo SJ: Medical care at mass gatherings: Considerations for physician involvement. *Prehosp Disast Med* 10(4):273–275, 1995.

The Incident Command System, Student Manual. Washington DC: Federal Emergency Management Agency (FEMA), National Emergency Training Center, National Fire Academy, 1989.

56

Ethics and Sports Medicine

Rob Johnson

DEFINITION

- From Merriam-Webster's Collegiate Dictionary:
  - Ethics: The discipline dealing with what is good and bad and with moral duty and obligation.
  - A set of moral principles or values; a theory or system of moral values; principles of conduct governing an individual or group; a guiding philosophy.
- Intimately intertwined with medicolegal aspects of medicine.
  - Ethics = moral values.
  - Law = enforceable social rules (most notably in their definitions of confidentiality and informed consent).

GUIDING PRINCIPLES

- Adapted from the Fédération Internationale de Médicine du Sports (FIMS) Code of Ethics.
- Sports medicine physicians:
  - Have an ethical obligation to understand the demands (mental, physical, and emotional) of exercise, training, and competition.
  - Must support the autonomy of the athlete.
    - The principle of informed consent developed from autonomy.
    - Failure of informed consent weakens the athlete's autonomy.
    - Failure to give the athlete appropriate information diminishes his or her ability to make autonomous decisions.
  - Must avoid allowing the profit motive to influence the conduct of their sports medicine function.
  - Must cautiously determine the information that is suitable for public disclosure in the context of physician-athlete confidentiality.
  - Must disclose to the athlete his or her allegiance (agent of the athlete or agent of the team/management).
  - Should oppose training, practices, and competition that could be injurious to the health of the athlete.
  - Should maintain a high level of sports medicine knowledge and share this information with others.

- Should consult other experts appropriately.
- Must insist on professional autonomy, acting independently of coaches and management on behalf of the athlete.
- Must oppose the use or promotion of illegal performance-enhancing substances.

ETHICAL CHALLENGES TO THE TEAM PHYSICIAN

- Common causes of "breach of duty":
  - Pressure from the injured player
  - Pressure from management
  - Peer pressure
  - Threat of replacement
  - Economic considerations
- Pressure from coaches and management
  - Threat of replacement
  - Participant in deception ("injured reserve")
- Self-pressure
  - Desire to be a part of the "team"
  - Efforts to please coaches and management
  - Public relations/practice building

TYPICAL PHYSICIAN– PATIENT RELATIONSHIP

- Physician works exclusively on the patient's (athlete's) behalf.
- Patient (athlete) and physician work toward common goal of return to play.
- The relationship is confidential.

TEAM PHYSICIAN– ATHLETE RELATIONSHIP

- If the physician is the agent for the team, athlete confidentiality extends to the team, not just the athlete. The physician must remind the athlete of this relationship.
- The physician must carefully balance the welfare of the athlete with the welfare of the team.

SPECIFIC ETHICAL ISSUES

- Confidentiality
  - Key precept of medical ethics.
  - If the athlete retains the physician, the usual confidentiality issues prevail.

- If the physician interacts with the athlete in the role as team physician, the results of the encounter may be shared with coaches or other agents of the team.
- If acting in the role as a team physician, the physician should remind the athlete of his or her role as a representative of the team and the possibility of sharing medical information with team officials.
- If the athlete requests complete confidentiality, the physician may have to disqualify himself or herself from the encounter or refuse to accept these conditions and encourage the athlete to seek private consultation outside the team setting.
- Athlete confidentiality does not permit the use of misleading or incomplete information on examinations or medical clearance forms.
- Privacy in the training room is nearly impossible. The physician must not permit the training room setting to alter his or her recommendations or treatment because of these outside influences. Maintain and encourage as much privacy as the training room setting permits.

- Balancing return to play with general health.
  - A conflict often exists between an athlete's desire to return to play and sound medical decision making. The athlete may be motivated by competition, peer pressure, coach pressure, the fans, or potential wealth. The physician should be motivated by athlete welfare.
  - When two different but appropriate medical or surgical interventions conflict, the athlete must be fully informed of the options, including long- and short-term risks.
  - Athlete preference (as long as the athlete is informed) takes precedence over physician preference.
  - The physician's role is to fully inform the athlete about therapeutic options.
  - Beware of pressure from coaches and teammates.

- Informed consent
  - Discuss risks and benefits of therapies.
  - Make sure that the athlete fully understands information disclosed by the physician.
  - Special concerns exist for the pediatric athlete in the context of parent involvement.

- Advertising
  - Inform patients; do not mislead.
  - Avoid advertising that encourages inappropriate use of medical resources.
  - Advertising of associations with teams (professional and college, in particular) must be honest and not exploited. The label of excellence is to be earned, not purchased.
  - Financial sponsorships/relationships between team organizations and team physicians establish serious conflicts of interest, jeopardizing athlete and physician autonomy.

- Performance enhancement
  - The physician's role in discouraging illegal performance enhancement practices or substances need not be emphasized.
  - The physician's role regarding legal performance enhancement is a more difficult issue.

- Each physician must decide on his or her own philosophy regarding legal performance enhancers. Encourage? Educate? Support?

QUESTIONS TO GUIDE PHYSICIANS THROUGH THE MAZE OF ETHICAL CHALLENGES

- Will the medical decision or therapeutic intervention be of benefit to the athlete?
- Will the medical decision or therapeutic intervention be of benefit to the sport?
- Will the medical decision or therapeutic intervention be of benefit or credit to the medical profession?
- All the answers must be yes if the sports medicine physician is to act in an ethical, professional manner.

Bibliography

Attarian DE: The team physician: Ethics and enterprise. *J Bone Joint Surg* 83A(2):203, 2001.

Bernstein J, Perlis C, Bartolozzi AE: Ethics in sports medicine. *Clin Orthop Rel Res* 378:50–60, 2000.

British Medical Association, Board of Science and Education: Doctors' assistance to sports clubs and sporting events. *Prehosp Immed Care* 5:53–56, 2001.

Brown DW: Presidential address of the American Orthopaedic Society for Sports Medicine: Some thoughts on perspective and the business of medicine. *Am J Sports Med* 27(6):694–698, 1999.

Capozzi JD, Rhodes R: Ethics in practice: Advertising and marketing. *J Bone Joint Surg* 82A(11):1668–1669, 2000.

International Federation of Sports Medicine: FIMS code of ethics in sports medicine, 1997.

Leach RE: Editorial: Job auction. *Am J Sports Med* 23(4):379, 1995.

Levine BD, Stray-Gunderson J: The medical care of competitive athletes: The role of the physician and individual assumption of risk. *Med Sci Sports Exerc* 26(10):1190–1192, 1994.

Maron BJ, Brown RW, McGrew CA, et al: Ethical, legal, and practical considerations impacting medical decision-making in competitive athletes. *Med Sci Sports Exerc* 26(10 Suppl):S230–S237, 1994.

McCrory P: No pain, no gain. The dilemma of a team physician. *Br J Sports Med* 35(3):141–142, 2001.

Pipe AL: JB Wolffe Memorial Lecture. Sport, science, and society: Ethics in sports medicine. *Med Sci Sports Exerc* 25(8):888–900, 1993.

Stevens SR: Winning medicine: Professional sports team doctors' conflicts of interest. *J Contemp Health Law Policy* 14(2):503–529, 1998.

57

Legal Issues for the Team Physician

Brian Birnie

APPLICATIONS

- Includes breadth of sporting world, from community-based youth soccer teams to the highly paid professional athlete.
- This advice comes in the form of a brief look at some of the legal concepts to consider, not as a game plan to put into place.
- Differing levels of athletes have different training considerations; similarly, physicians working with different levels of sporting teams may have different levels of legal concerns.

BEFORE YOU SAY YES TO THE TEAM, SOME THINGS TO CONSIDER

- Team physicians come from many different medical backgrounds, from family practitioners to internists to orthopedic specialists. Feel confident in your abilities before agreeing to the position.
- In many community settings, the physician may have some personal relationship to the team. Be careful to not let that relationship color your advice to the players or the team.
- Look to the history of the team in deciding if this team has been well taken care of in the past and to see what would be realistically expected of the person in the role of team physician.

TRY TO GET IT IN WRITING

- If you decide to participate as a team physician, a good means of avoiding pitfalls later is to have a written contract with your duties spelled out. The contract may be with a school district, a community based group (think AYSO), a club team (growing in popularity), or a professional sports team.
- Your contract should discuss your duties, compensation, responsibilities for providing supplies, travel requirements, etc. If you are to be

compensated, determine if your duties are for the season or per game, whether follow-up care is to be provided at your office also paid for, etc. Employing legal counsel to review and negotiate a fair contract is money well spent.

PREPARTICIPATION PHYSICALS

- Often the starting point for a patient-doctor relationship.
- Duty of care is to the patient—in this case, the athlete—and *not* to the third-party payer or team management.
- Decisions regarding fitness to participate are shared with the patient; the player enjoys a confidential relationship with the physician. Do not share your medical opinions with the media or others unless you have permission to do so from the athlete. Get this permission in writing in order to avoid legal problems.
- The team physical may be performed by the athlete's primary care physician. Some suggest providing specialists for these physicals—use of multistation physicals with specialists examining each athlete. The standard of care for specialists may be higher than for nonspecialists. Use caution in having a specialist render an opinion outside his or her specialty.
- A physician must fully disclose to the athlete any information that the physician finds to be pertinent to the athlete's ability to perform. An athlete has every right to rely on the opinion of the team physician as to whether he or she is fit to play. Physicians should not be "bullied" by management (or media or parents) to allow an athlete to participate if it is not in the athlete's best interest.

RETURN-TO-PLAY DECISIONS

- There are different scenarios for different levels of athletes. The physician's duty at all times is to the athlete, not to those who might put pressure on him or her. Liability may arise if the athlete returns prematurely to the field/arena/court and suffers further injury.
- Use of painkillers to enable an athlete to return to play may cause more problems in the long term. Keep records of prescriptions and document discussions with the player regarding return-to-play status.
- Long-term health damage caused by narcotic usage, steroids, etc., may be the basis of a lawsuit against both the physician and the team if it can be proven that the physician and team management sacrificed the health of the athlete for the good of the team.

INFORMED CONSENT

- Medical treatment by a physician relies on the theory that the patient is given all the information needed to make an "informed" consent for medical care.

- Team physicians dealing with minors must make certain they know the jurisdiction's legal requirements for treating minors. Consent-to-treat forms should be signed by parents and kept current and with the team at all times. Some jurisdictions may allow a minor to agree to some incidental types of treatment, depending on the minor's age. Each jurisdiction may be different; consult local counsel if there is a question.

"GOOD SAMARITAN" ISSUES

- By rushing on to the field to aid an injured player, is the doctor playing the role of a good Samaritan?
- Some aspects of the theory to consider: Does the physician have a pre-existing relationship with the player, making it his or her "duty" to render aid, or is the physician merely expected to act as team doctor and being paid to do only this?
- "Good Samaritan" statutes were enacted because the public wanted physicians to render aid in emergency situations; these statutes differ from state to state.
- Some legislatures have enacted specialty statutes dealing with the issue of physicians who act as team doctors at sporting events.
- Essentially, if you are acting as a team physician and your player is injured, you probably are outside the realm of being a good Samaritan, since the relationship you have with the team is to render aid in just these types of circumstances. A primary idea behind most good Samaritan statutes is that you are not being compensated for rendering this type of aid. If a team physician is being paid for his or her services, then this too would not make the actions subject to good Samaritan coverage.
- Good Samaritan status is a defense and still must be argued in the event of a lawsuit. Even if this is a true defense, it will cost the physician money. It does not replace good liability insurance.

LICENSURE ISSUES

- If you travel with the team outside the jurisdiction in which you are licensed to practice, will you be practicing medicine without a license?
- Prevalent philosophy is that "practicing" medicine is more than just acting as a team physician.
- Ideas to consider: Are you only on occasion, temporarily, sporadically rendering medical aid while traveling with the team? Most jurisdictions will not consider this to be a problem unless you set up an office, start charging fees, and in essence take on a more permanent look. Team physicians who are under paid contract for rendering aid to the team are not considered to be "charging" for their services for these types of questions. They are under contract whereever they go; physicians donating their time are obviously not charging fees.
- Will you be able to admit athletes to a local hospital? Probably not, only because you would likely not have staff privileges at a hospital outside your licensed jurisdiction.

- Each licensing jurisdiction does have different standards in this regard, and advice from these licensing boards should be sought.
- The American Medical Association may also be able to provide an overview of the different licensing requirements in various jurisdictions.
- Insurance may not be in effect if you are practicing outside of area in which you are licensed.

LIABILITY INSURANCE FOR THE TEAM PHYSICIAN

- Prior to undertaking the duties as team physician, carefully review your malpractice insurance policy, particularly if it is held as part of a group or partnership. Supplemental insurance to cover you while you are acting as the team physician will help to protect other physicians you might be in practice with.
- Who will pay for your insurance coverage while you are acting as the team physician? This is one of the issues to be addressed in your contract with the management (remember to get it in writing).
- Coverage should include all the same areas that you would want to have covered in an insurance policy for your private practice.
- Outside counsel with expertise in the language of insurance contracts should be consulted regarding any specific questions a team physician might have; the team's lawyer may prove to be less than a candid advisor on such issues.

SIDELINE PREPAREDNESS: WHOSE RESPONSIBILITY, WHAT TO BRING, WHO PAYS?

- The team physician must be able to provide the team with a well stocked "black bag"—actually, most teams have things that look more like small portable supply cabinets.
- Team physicians should require teams to have at each practice, game, tournament, etc., all the supplies stipulated to by the physician. Transportation of these items should be the responsibility of the team, but the physician must make sure they are on location before play begins.
- Teams should bear the financial burden for the costs of these items, and they should be considered the property of the team. The physician should undertake to make sure that all supplies are in good condition.
- Supplies should be stocked that would be needed for a particular sport and the injuries most likely to occur in that sport (tennis would be different than football).
- For specific lists of items that would be needed on a sport-specific basis look at websites for organizations such as American Academy of Family Physicians and the American Medical Society of Sports Medicine (also see Chaps. 59, 60, and 61).

RECORD KEEPING

- Keeping good records is the secret of avoiding a lot of trouble down the road.
- These records should be kept in the same serious manner as if care and treatment were being rendered in your office.
- Consent-to-treat forms should be updated and should always travel with the team! Dealings with minors must be handled carefully; check local statutes for what you can or cannot do without a parental consent.
- Reduce to writing all decisions regarding treatments, prescriptions, options, etc. Be aware of statutory requirements on length of time for keeping these records. You may need to warehouse your records after you have stopped acting as team physician.
- Keep a log of phone calls, referrals to experts, follow-up concerns, etc.
- An ounce of prevention is worth all the pounds of trouble that the lack of good documentation can cause you later.
- If you dictate your notes, read the final transcript before signing; once you have signed it as being what you said, it is very hard to argue later that you meant something else.
- Remember medical records are confidential; do not share what you know with anyone without the express written permission of your patient, the athlete. If your patient is a minor, be aware that he or she may have the right of confidentiality in some circumstances. When in doubt consult an attorney.

FINALLY

- Most team physicians find their experience to be enjoyable.
- Try to get a written agreement/contract regarding your services.
- Check on licensure issues if you will be traveling outside your licensed area.
- Keep good records—for everything.
- Have a good liability insurance policy.
- Make friends with an attorney who can help with the legal stuff.

Bibliography

Gallup EM: *Law and the Team Physician.* Champaign, IL: Human Kinetics, 1995.

58

The Psychology of Injury

Robert Corb

PREDICTING SPORTS INJURIES

- Personality factors potentially increase the risk of injuries for athletes who:
  - Have an external locus of control meaning they feel less in control and may take more risks.
  - Are very low or very high in self-confidence. Injury may serve as an excuse or athlete may feel invulnerable.
  - Are high in trait and competitive-state anxiety. This results in:
    - Increased muscle tension
    - Fatigue
    - Reduced flexibility
    - Decreased attentional focus
- Stress levels—direct relationship between overall stress level and risk of injury
  - Life events, especially negative stressors, increase likelihood of injury.
  - History of previous injury is predictive of reinjury or new injury.
  - Probability of injury increases with lack of adequate coping mechanisms, such as:
    - Social support
    - Psychological skills training (i.e., relaxation skills)
    - Tendency to self-medicate

ATHLETES' RESPONSES TO INJURIES

- Stress response—injury is a stressor that triggers a three-part response.
  - Cognitive appraisal—an effort to intellectualize and understand the experience.
    - Seeks to answer the question "Why me?"
    - May involve denial, negotiation, rationalization.
  - Emotional response—generally more difficult to assess, especially in male athletes.
    - Described as the "grief" response (see below).
    - Corresponds to a call for help.

- Behavioral response—athletes tend to minimize extent of injury.
  - Play in pain
  - Fail to notify medical staff of extent of injury
  - Artificially increase activity level to hide injury
  - Responding to question "What now?"
- Acute response must focus on all three domains:
  - Athlete needs accurate information regarding extent of injury in order to make cognitive appraisal.
  - Athlete needs emotional connection with medical staff to begin to accept reality of injury.
  - Medical staff and athlete must share expertise: athlete knows his or her body but medical staff understands injuries.
- Grief response—three phases, focus on phase one for acute injury treatment.
  - Athletes and nonathletes experience injuries differently.
    - Athletes tend to view themselves as invulnerable.
    - Physical ability is central to athlete's identity.
    - Loss of mobility translates into loss to be grieved over through emotional responses.
  - Phase one—shock-like state involving:
    - Denial of seriousness of injury
    - Anger toward self/others, especially those perceived to have caused the injury
    - Attempts to negotiate (i.e., minimize) extent of injury
  - Phase two—as immediate shock wears off, an intense preoccupation with injury begins.
    - Depressive symptoms, including changes in appetite and/or sleeping patterns, loss of motivation, sadness, anhedonia, possibility of self-medication
    - Increased anxiety, resulting in loss of concentration, obsessive thoughts, increased nervousness, angry outbursts, and interpersonal difficulties
    - Feelings of guilt, resulting in crying, troubled dreams, difficulty being involved in team activities
  - Phase three—acceptance of injury and reorganization of life after injury
    - View of injury as a challenge to be overcome, an opportunity
    - Increased commitment to rehabilitation and return to competition

PATIENT VARIABLES AND THE DOCTOR-PATIENT RELATIONSHIP

- Patient's need for control
  - Injury represents loss of control for athlete
  - May result in increased need for control in doctor-patient relationship, or
  - Desire to cede all control to medical personnel.

- Self-confidence
  - Athletes high in self-confidence may have trouble listening to and trusting their physician (athlete knows his or her body best).
  - Athletes low in self-confidence may want to have physician take complete responsibility for diagnosis and treatment.
- Speed of decision making—interacts with patient s (and doctor's) need for control
  - Patient with slow decision-making style and high need for control can be difficult to work with.
- Introversion-extroversion—tendency in either direction exacerbated by stress related to injury.
  - Introverted athlete:
    - May require additional probing to gather all information relevant to extent of injury.
    - More prone to social isolation and depression.
  - Extroverted athlete:
    - More likely to use denial and social involvement to cope with injury.
    - May seek to minimize seriousness of injury and need for treatment.
- Interpersonal expressiveness
  - Intellectual expressiveness:
    - Characterized by a need to be logical and structured in decision making related to treatment options
    - Difficulty in expressing emotions
  - Affective expression:
    - Tendency to be negative (critical, confrontative).
    - Exacerbated as a result of injury.
    - Respond to cry for help by injured athlete with patience.
- Acute response must recognize athlete's individual differences:
  - Assess athlete's need for control and speed of decision making—provide athlete with control over situation where medically appropriate.
  - Extent of previous relationship between medical staff and athlete (i.e., trust level) will influence athlete's willingness to provide information about extent of injury.

SPORTS PSYCHOLOGY AS ADJUNCTIVE THERAPY

- Sports psychologist can provide consultation for physicians and/or adjunctive therapy for patients.
- Psychologist focuses on three domains:
  - Cognitive response related to meaning of injury for athlete:
    - Athlete's use of positive (accurate) and negative (inaccurate) self-talk
    - Cognitive restructuring (injury as opportunity or challenge)
    - Rehabilitation as new competitive environment

- Affective response:
  - Responding to grief process and loss of identity with normalization
  - Possible individual and/or group therapy
- Behavioral responses—enhancing coping skills such as:
  - Social support
  - Stress management
- Psychological skills training to aid rehabilitation process:
  - Relaxation training
  - Mental imagery
  - Goal setting
- Pain management—athletes tend to have higher pain tolerance.
  - Use psychological skills training to address pain.
  - Focus on secondary gain associated with "pain behavior" (return-to-play decisions).
  - Be aware of addictive tendencies with pain medication.
  - Athlete may self-medicate with nonprescription drugs.

RETURN TO COMPETITION—ASSESSING PSYCHOLOGICAL READINESS

- Psychological readiness means understanding the meaning of the injury and of being recovered:
  - Affective readiness—fears about:
    - Reinjury
    - Physical limitations
    - Performance issues
    - Role on team
    - Expectations of self and others (coaches, teammates, etc.)
  - Behavioral readiness:
    - Ability to perform at same level as prior to injury
    - Revisiting the site or action associated with the injury
  - Cognitive readiness:
    - Self-talk associated with playing again
    - Appraisal of coping mechanisms
- Importance of multidisciplinary assessment including:
  - Medical staff
  - Trainer
  - Physical therapist
  - Sports psychologist
  - Coaches
  - (Fully informed) athlete
- Career-ending injuries—special attention paid to identity concerns of athlete ending his or her career:
  - Sudden loss of identity
  - Lack of control over situation
  - Additional grief process without usual social support system (teammates and coach)
  - Need for referral to sports psychologist

Bibliography

Heil J: *Psychology of Sports Injury.* Champaign, IL: Human Kinetics, 1993.

Heil J: The injured athlete, in Hanin YL (ed): *Emotions in Sport.* Champaign, IL: Human Kinetics, 2000.

Nideffer R M: The injured athlete: Psychological factors in treatment. *Orthop Clin North Am* 44(2):373–385.

Williams J, Roepke N: Psychology of injury and injury rehabilitation, in Singer RN, Murphey M, Tennant LK (eds): *Handbook of Research on Sports Psychology.* New York: Macmillian, 1993.

Part 5

Appendixes

59

The Team Physician's Bag

Aaron Rubin

The team physician may carry a variety of materials to games and the training room. The contents will vary from sport to sport, home or away, training room visit or game, and by the number of participants. This list will help the team physician design his or her own bag and create a checklist that can be updated to fit the situations encountered. In Table 59.1 below, some space is provided for individualization of the list.

Some supplies and medications are restricted by state medical and pharmacy laws. This may create special problems if the team physician is traveling across state or national borders. Controlled substances have not been included in this list.

There is some redundancy in the team physician's bag, the trainer's kit (see Chap. 60), and EMS supplies (see Chap. 61). Some items listed will not be necessary if a paramedic ambulance is present—also depending on the supplies carried by the athletic trainer. Items often carried by the trainer are indicated in the table with "T" and by EMS with "E." The athlete or facility may be charged for products supplied by the paramedic squad or ambulance.

Table 59.1 Items Carried by the Team Physician and/or EMS/Athletic Trainer

Item	EMS/ Trainer	Event 1	Event 2	Event 3	Inventory
Pocket gear					
Bandage shears		1			
Exam gloves		2			
Pocket mask		1			
Penlight		1			
Knife/multitool		1			
4 × 4 sponges		2			
Pen and paper		1			
Airway		1			
Cellular phone		1			
Sideline instruments					
BP cuffs (various sizes)	E, T*	1			
Oto/ophthalmoscope		1			

(continued)

Table 59.1 (*Continued*)

Item	EMS/ Trainer	Event 1	Event 2	Event 3	Inventory
Sideline instruments (*Continued*)					
Thermometer	E, T	1			
Glucose monitor	E	1			
Pulse oximeter	E	1			
Needle forceps		1			
Hemostat		2			
Scissors		1			
Disposable cautery		1			
Headlamp		1			
Batteries (to fit above)					
Eye tray					
Cobalt blue light		1			
Flourescein strips		1			
Irrigating solution		1			
Tetracaine, 0.5% unit dose		2			
Topical ophthalmic antibiotic ointment		1			
Neurologic/orthopedic					
Air splints	E, T	1 set			
"Sam" splint	T	1			
Cast padding		1 roll			
Readi splints (fiberglass)					
4 × 35 in.		1			
3 × 15 in.		1			
3 × 12 in.		1			
Knee immobilizer	T	1			
Elastic bandages (3 4, and 6 in.)	E, T	1 each			
Finger splints (aluminum)	T	2			
Crutches	T	1 pair			
Triangular bandages	E, T	2			
Tape	E, T	1 roll			
Rigid backboard	E, T				
Cervical collars (sizes)	E, T				
Face-mask removal device	T	1			
Wound care					
Gauze pads	E, T	12			
Bandages	E, T	Assorted			
Saline irrigation	E, T	1			
Povidone-iodine swabs	E, T	12			
Lidocaine 1% injection plain		1			
Lidocaine 1% injection with epinephrine		1			
Disposable suture tray		2			
Suture (4-0 nylon, 6-0 nylon, 4-0 absorbable)		2 each			
Sterile gloves		4 pair			
Sterile fields		1			
Steri-Strips, assorted		3			
Tincture of benzoin ampules	T	3			
Topical antibiotic unit dose	T	3			
Syringes, assorted needles	E	2 each			
Sharps disposal container	E	1			

Table 59.1 (*Continued*)

Item	EMS/ Trainer	Event 1	Event 2	Event 3	Inventory
Wound care (*Continued*)					
Biohazard bag	E, T	1			
Roll gauze (3, 4, and 6 in.)		2 each			
Nonadherent bandages		4			
Bioocclusive dressing		4			
Exam gloves		12			
Medications (non-ACLS)					
Albuterol inhaler with aerochamber	E	1			
Epinephrine 1:1000 (Epi-pen)	E	2			
Diphenhydramine, 25-mg injection	E	1			
Diphenhydramine, 25-mg capsules		30			
Antacid tablets		30			
Antinausea tablets/injection		12			
Antidiarrheal tablets (loperamide 2 mg)		12			
Ibuprofen 200 mg		50			
Acetaminophen 325 mg		50			
Anesthetic ear drops		1			
Aspirin 81 mg	E	50			
Aspirin 325 mg		50			
Nitroglycerin 0.4 mg	E	25			
Travel medications					
Penicillin 250 mg		12			
Cephalexin 250 mg		12			
Ciprofloxacin 250 mg		12			
Azithromycin 250 mg		6			
Miscellaneous					
Bag or case		1			
Blanket or space blanket		1			
Prescription pad		1			
Information sheets for injured (head injury, ankle sprain, knee injury, wound, etc)		Set			
Injury recording system		1			
Micro–tape recorder		1			
Rain jacket/poncho					
Appropriate clothing					
Protective goggles/mask/ gown/gloves	E	1			
ACLS					
See Chaps. 61 and 64					
Consider automated external defibrillator	E	1			
Oxygen	E	1			
Bag-valve-mask device	E	1			
Combitube	E	1			
Cricothyrotomy kit	E	1			
Medications (see Chaps. 61 and 64)	E				

*Key: T, athletic trainer; E, EMS.

60

Athletic Trainer's Kit

Julie Max

ATHLETIC TRAINER'S KIT AND SIDELINE SUPPLIES

The equipment and supplies needed on the sidelines can vary depending on individual needs, budget, and personal preferences. However, there are some items and supplies that are considered "standard" sideline equipment. What follows is a suggested list of emergency and general supplies used to meet the needs of 40–50 athletes on the sidelines of a sporting event.

This does not include the Physician's Kit (see Chap. 59) or what is carried by most EMS units (see Chap. 61).

Most certified athletic trainers will have their own personal kits in which some of these items will be found, but they will also use large duffelbags or trunks in which to store and transport the remaining items. This list does not include items (such as preventive taping) kept in the training room to prepare the team before a game or practice.

Using the following table, create your own supply list for various sports. Once you have set your personal levels for these sports, use this as an inventory against which to check your supplies before your events (Table 60.1).

Table 60.1 The Athletic Trainer's Kit and Sideline Supplies

Item	Sport— Football	Sport	Sport	Sport	Sport	Inventory
Air or cardboard splints	Assorted					
Hard cervical collar	1					
Oropharyngeal airway	1					
Blanket	1					
Crutches	2 pair					
Ice chest and ice	20 lb					
Plastic bags	50					
6-in. Ace wraps	10					
4-in. Ace wraps	10					
Face-mask removal device	1					
Adhesive tape, 1½-in.	12					
Underwrap	6					
Elastikon, 3-in.	4					
Lightplast 2- and 3-in.	4					
Heel and lace pads	12					
Plastic ice wrap	1					
Bandages—various sizes	box					
Tape adherent (Tuf-skin)	bottle					
Steri-Strips 1/8-in.	12					
Cotton-tipped applicators	12					
Tongue Blades	12					
Skin Lube	1 tube					
Hydrogen peroxide	1 bottle					
Antibiotic ointment	1 tube					
3 × 3-in. gauze pads	50					
4 × 4-in. gauze pads	20					
Telfa pads	12					
Heat balm	1 tube					
Bandage scissors	2					
Tape cutter ("Shark")	2					
Forceps or tweezers	1					
Nail clipper	1					
Triangular bandage	12					
Penlight	2					
Mirror	1					
Blood pressure cuff	1					
Stethoscope	1					
Multifunction tool	1					
Pen	5					
Eyewash	2					
Contact lens care kit	1					
Thermometer	1					
Lip balm	1					
Foam and felt	Assorted					
Moleskin	Assorted					
Mouthpieces	6					
Ibuprofen	50					
Acetaminophen	50					
Antacid tablets	50					

61

Emergency
Medical Supplies

Jim Schiller

The sideline or event physician should be aware of the supplies and capabilities of the local EMS unit in his or her area. Supplies in an individual ambulance or rescue squad will vary from location to location.

When the 911 system is activated, the responding units will be carrying a preestablished list of drugs and equipment. This approved list is developed from the state-approved standard drug and equipment list, which will vary from state to state as well as county to county. The governing authority of each state will allow counties and regions to deviate from this as long as they can show sufficient justification. Some areas have longer transport times, which may require a greater degree of intervention than would apply in a metropolitan setting.

Another example would be event-specific. One local fire agency implemented a bicycle-based EMS delivery system during the holiday season at a local shopping mall that could have over 100,000 people present at one time. In this instance, the local governing agency had to be petitioned for permission to deviate from the standard drug and equipment list. The requested list still included all the first-line cardiac medications, including analgesics, but there was neither need nor space to carry all the usual equipment. These bike patrols can be extremely useful in crowded venues with limited access to traditional ambulances and EMS squads.

Table 61.1 Emergency Medical Supplies—Advanced Life Support, Bike Units, and Inventory

Item	ALS Squad	Bike	Inventory
Medications			
Activated charcoal	50 g	25 g	
Adenosine	30 mg	18 mg	
Epinephrine 1:1000, 10 mL	6	1	
Epinephrine 1:1000, 1 mL	2	1	
Epinephrine 1:10,000, 10 mL	3	2	
Albuterol inhalation 2.5 mg	4	2	
Aspirin, chewable, 81 mg	1 bottle	1 bottle	
Atropine 0.4 mg/mL	2	0	
Atropine 1 mg/mL	4	2	
Calcium chloride	1 g	0	
Dextrose 50%	50 g	1	
Diphenhydramine injection	50 mg	50 mg	
Furosemide injection	100 mg		
Glucagon	1 mg	1 mg	
Dopamine	400 mg		
Magnesium sulfate	10 g		
Naloxone	10 mg	2 mg	
Nitroglycerine tablets or spray	2 bottles	1 bottle	
Normal saline injection, 10 mL	2	1	
Pitocin	20 units		
Phenylephrine HCl	1 bottle	1 bottle	
Procainamide	1 gm		
Terbutaline	2 mg		
Verapamil injection	15 mg		
Lidocaine	300 mg	200 mg	
Lidocaine	2 g		
Viscous lidocaine	2 oz	2 oz	
Controlled substances			
Midazolam 5mg/mL	40 mg	40 mg	
Morphine sulfate	60 mg	60 mg	
IV Fluids			
Normal saline 250 mL	3	2	
Normal saline 1000 ml	6	2	
Solutions			
Normal saline irrigation 1000 mL	3		
Equipment			
Antiseptic swabs	box	box	
Syringes TB, 3, 5, 10, 20, 60 mL	2 each	1 each	
Hypodermic needles 18, 20, 22, 25 gauge	2 each	1 each	
IV catheters 14, 16, 18, 20, 22, 24 gauge	2 each	2 each	
Intraosseous needles	2	2	
Three-way stopcock	1		
Solution administration set	5		
Buretrol administration set	1		
IV extension tube	2		

(*continued*)

Table 61.1 (*Continued*)

Item	ALS Squad	Bike	Inventory
Equipment (*continued*)			
Conductive defibrillator pads	2	2	
ECG Pads			
Rigid cervical collars, pediatric/adult	2 each		
Sterile burn sheets	2		
Meconium aspirator	2	2	
OB kit	1		
Endotracheal tubes, cuffed, 6.0, 7.0, 8.0	2 each	2 each	
Endotracheal tubes, uncuffed, 2.0, 3.0, 4.0, 5.0	2 each	2 each	
Adult pertrach device	1		
Pediatric pertrach device	1		
Naso/orogastric tubes, 10, 12, 14, 16, 18	1 each		
Suction catheters, 6, 8, 12 Fr	1 each	1 each	
Yankauers tonsil tip	1	1	
Small-volume nebulizer	2	1	
Malleable stylet, adult and pediatric	1 each	1 each	
Water-soluble lubricating jelly	1	1	
Oropharyngeal airways (infant, child, adult)	1 each	1 each	
Nasopharyngeal airways (infant, child, adult)	1 each	1 each	
Vaseline gauze	2	2	
Nasal cannulas (adult and pediatric)	2 each	2	
Adult non-O_2 rebreather mask	2	1	
Adult simple O_2 mask	1	1	
Pediatric O_2 mask	2	1	
Saline locks	2	2	
One-way flutter valve	1	1	
Ankle and wrist restraints	1	0	
Pneumatic or rigid splints	4		
Sterile compression bandages	12	2	
Gauze pads (4×4)	12	6	
Roller bandage 2, 3, 4, 6 in.	6		
Bandage shears	1	1	
10×30 universal dressing	2	2	
Emesis basin	1		
Bedpan or fracture pan	1	0	
Urinal	1	0	
Equipment			
Ambulance cot and collapsible stretcher	1	0	
Straps to secure patient to cot	1	0	
Sheets, pillows, pillowcases, blankets	2 each	0	
Portable O_2 with regulator	1	1	
Glucose monitoring device	1	1	
Communications radios 800 MHz	2	1	

Table 61.1 (*Continued*)

Item	ALS Squad	Bike	Inventory
Equipment (*continued*)			
Defibrillator/monitor/pacemaker	1	1	
Head immobilization devices	2	0	
Long backboard with straps	1	0	
Pediatric immobilization board	1	0	
Short extrication device	1	0	
Traction splint	1	0	
Triage tags (START system)	30	0	
Suction device	1 battery	1 manual	
Suction device (wall-mounted)	1		
Laryngoscope handle with batteries	1	1	
Laryngeal blades #1, 2, 3, 4, curved and straight	1 each	1 each	
Magill forceps, pediatric and adult	1 each	1 each	
In-ambulance O$_2$ source	1	0	
Ventilation bags (ambu bags) with connections, adult and pediatric	1 each	1 each	
End-tidal CO$_2$ device	1	–	
Stethoscope	1	–	
Blood pressure cuffs (infant, pediatric, adult, large, thigh)	1 each	1 each	
Pressure infusion bag	1	1	
Flashlight	1	1	
Pulse oximeter	1	1	
Thermometer	1	1	
Gallon or more of potable H$_2$O	1		
Nonporous gloves	1 box	20	
Goggles, face masks, gowns	3 each	2 each	
Optional equipment			
Antishock trousers (adult and pediatric)			
Automatic ventilator			
Combitube			
Esophageal obturator airway			
IV infusion device			
IV warming device			
Manual suction device			
Chemistry profile tubes			
Vacutainer and needles			

62

Incident Command System

Jim Schiller

INCIDENT COMMAND SYSTEM (ICS)

- Organizational system used by many emergency systems.
- Designed to provide chain of command for an upper-level leader to control the actions of three to seven subordinates.
- This allows the "boss" to share the responsibility and success of the organization.
- Team physician may become involved if a mass casualty incident (MCI) occurs at a forum or event. An MCI is defined as one involving casualties that overload the initial response. For example, if the stands collapsed at a sports venue with more injuries than the medical staff can initially care for, an MCI exists.
- With the threat of terrorists, weapons of mass destruction, biological threats, natural disasters, structural failure or fire, there is the possibility for a large number of casualties at sporting venues.
  - The physician may be the incident commander (IC) or may serve under the IC and provide direct patient care. The physician may act as IC until more help is available and resources are brought to the scene.
- The ICS is broken into two groups: the command staff and the general staff.
  - Command staff
    - Incident commander (IC)
      - Takes charge of the overall incident.
      - Should be familiar with the local agencies responding to the incident.
    - Safety officer
      - Responsible for the overall safety for members involved in the incident.
    - Liaison officer
      - Works between agencies involved in the incident.
    - Public information officer (PIO)
      - Keeps media and public informed.
      - Team physician should not discuss incident with the media unless directed by the PIO. This provides consistent information to the public.

- The team physician also carries the added responsibility of maintaining patient confidentiality.
- General staff
  - Operations
    - Responsible for mitigating and dealing with the physical incident.
      - Medical—this is the likely area for the team physician.
      - Rescue.
      - Fire suppression.
      - Hazardous material.
      - Security.
  - Planning
    - Collects, evaluates, disseminates, and uses information concerning the incident.
    - Records status of incident, resources available, technical specialist, and demobilization.
  - Logistics
    - Provides facilities, services and materials.
  - Finance
    - Tracks costs and cost recovery.

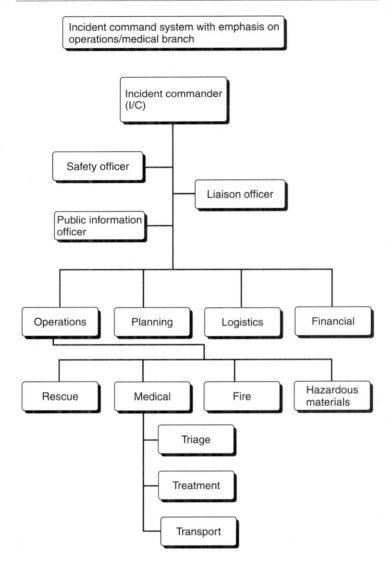

63

Emergency Action Plan

Aaron Rubin

- The Emergency Action Plan should be filled out for every venue and event. Copies should be distributed to all key personnel as well as local emergency services.
- The nearest intersection and directions to the venue should be recorded.
- Cell phones and radios should be checked in advance of the event as well as at the event.
- *Call 911 for emergencies at most locations in the United States.*
- Knowing direct number for ambulance service for nonemergent transports can prevent unneeded activation of EMS system. Check with local jurisdictions for how to obtain nonemergent ambulance service.
- Direct number for Rescue/Fire and Police/Sheriff as backup in case of failure of local EMS system.
- Number for local ER and trauma system useful in discussing management directly with ER staff.
- Personnel names and contact information should be provided.
- The team physician or athletic trainer will act as the incident commander and care for athlete until EMS responds (see Chap. 62).
- Have a designated person to organize parents and have them meet the medical team after emergency care has been completed. Parents are often present in the stands, and this will help keep them from interfering with care while still being present for medical history and transport questions.
- Someone must direct EMS personnel and make sure gates and doors are open and not blocked.
- An action plan should be filled out for times when the team physician is not available, such as practice, conditioning, and times other than game time.

Emergency Action Plan

Venue_____

Address_____

Nearest major intersection_____

Communications: Cell phone check_____

                  Radio check_____

Phone locations_____

Map

EMS 911

Rescue fire agency_____Phone_____

Police/sheriff:_____Phone_____

Nonemergent ambulance_____Phone_____

Nearest hospitals: General ER_____ER phone_____

                     Trauma center_____ER phone_____

Personnel

Incident commander_____Cell/radio_____

Attend athlete_____Cell/radio_____

Communication (call 911)_____Cell/radio_____

Security_____Cell/radio

Direct EMS/assure access_____Cell/radio_____

Direct/call parents_____Cell/radio_____

Other key personnel_____Cell/radio_____

_____Cell/radio_____

_____Cell/radio_____

64

Emergency Cardiac Care: Algorithm/AHA*

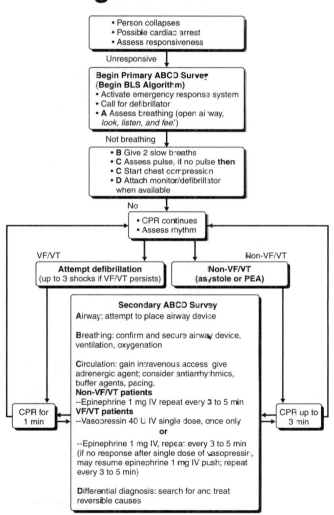

65

Out-of-Hospital Use of AEDs: Algorithm/AHA*

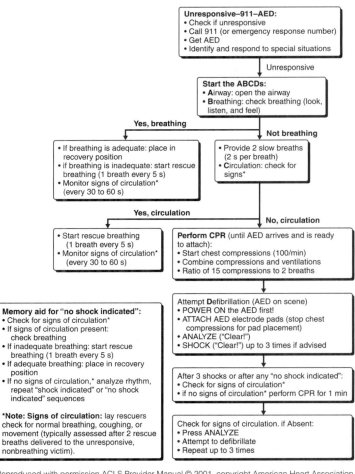

Unresponsive–911–AED:
- Check if unresponsive
- Call 911 (or emergency response number)
- Get AED
- Identify and respond to special situations

Unresponsive

Start the ABCDs:
- **A**irway: open the airway
- **B**reathing: check breathing (look, listen, and feel)

Yes, breathing

- If breathing is adequate: place in recovery position
- if breathing is inadequate: start rescue breathing (1 breath every 5 s)
- Monitor signs of circulation* (every 30 to 60 s)

Not breathing

- Provide 2 slow breaths (2 s per breath)
- **C**irculation: check for signs*

Yes, circulation

- Start rescue breathing (1 breath every 5 s)
- Monitor signs of circulation* (every 30 to 60 s)

No, circulation

Perform CPR (until AED arrives and is ready to attach):
- Start chest compressions (100/min)
- Combine compressions and ventilations
- Ratio of 15 compressions to 2 breaths

Memory aid for "no shock indicated":
- Check for signs of circulation*
- If signs of circulation present: check breathing
- If inadequate breathing: start rescue breathing (1 breath every 5 s)
- If adequate breathing: place in recovery position
- If no signs of circulation,* analyze rhythm, repeat "shock indicated" or "no shock indicated" sequences

***Note: Signs of circulation:** lay rescuers check for normal breathing, coughing, or movement (typically assessed after 2 rescue breaths delivered to the unresponsive, nonbreathing victim).

Attempt **D**efibrillation (AED on scene)
- POWER ON the AED first!
- ATTACH AED electrode pads (stop chest compressions for pad placement)
- ANALYZE ("Clear!")
- SHOCK ("Clear!") up to 3 times if advised

After 3 shocks or after any "no shock indicated":
- Check for signs of circulation*
- if no signs of circulation* perform CPR for 1 min

Check for signs of circulation. if Absent:
- Press ANALYZE
- Attempt to defibrillate
- Repeat up to 3 times

Glossary

AAN	American Academy of Neurology
ABCs	airway, breathing, and circulation
ABCDEs	airway, breathing, circulation disability, environment examination
ABGs	arterial blood gases
AC	acromioclavicular
ACE	angiotensin converting enzyme
ACL	anterior cruciate ligament
ACLS	advanced cardiac life support
ACSM	American College of Sports Medicine
AED	automated external defibrillator
AGE	air gas embolism
AHA	American Heart Association
AIIS	anteroinferior iliac spine
AITFL	interosseous membrane of the anterior talofibular ligament
ALS	advanced life support
AMA	against medical advice
AMS	acute mountain sickness
ANSI	American National Standards Institute
APL	abductor pollicis longus
ASA	acetylsalicylic acid (aspirin)
ASIS	anterosuperior iliac spine
ASTM	American Society for Testing and Materials
ATFL	anterior talofibular ligament
AVN	avascular necrosis
AYSO	American Youth Soccer Organization
BLS	basic life support
BP	blood pressure
BURP	backward, upward, and rightward pressure
CDC	Centers for Disease Control and Prevention
CFL	calcaneofibular ligament
CNS	central nervous system
COX-2	cyclooxygenase-2
CPK	creatine phosphokinase
CPR	cardiopulmonary resuscitation
CQI	continuous quality improvement
CT	computed tomography
CTM	cricothyroid membrane
DAN	Divers Alert Network
DCS	decompression sickness
DIPJ	distal interphalangeal joint
DVT	deep venous thrombosis
EAC	exercise-associated collapse
ECC	emergency cardiac care
ECG	electrocardiogram

ECRB	extensor carpi radialis brevis
ECRL	extensor carpi radialis longus
EDC	extensor digitorum communis
EDL	extensor digitorum longus
EEG	electroencephalogram
EIB	exercise-induced bronchospasm
EMD	emergency medical dispatcher
EMS	emergency medical service
ENT	ear/nose/throat
EOC	emergency operations center
EPB	extensor pollicis brevis
ER	emergency room
ETC	esophageal-tracheal combitube
ETT	endotracheal tube
FCR	flexor carpi radialis
FDA	U.S. Food and Drug Administration
FDP	flexor digitorum profundis
FDS	flexor digitorum superficialis
FHL	flexor hallucis longus
FIFA	Federation Internationale de Football Association
FIMS	Fédération Internationale de Médicine du Sports
FOOSH	fall on outstretched hand
GU	genitourinary
HACE	high-altitude cerebral edema
HANS	head and neck safety
HAPE	high-altitude pulmonary edema
IC	incident commander
ICS	incident command system
ICU	intensive care unit
IOC	International Olympic Committee
IPV	infantile paralysis (poliomyelitis) vaccine
IVP	intravenous pyelogram
LCL	lateral collateral ligament
LCPD	Legg-Calvé-Perthes disease
LE	lateral epicondylitis
LFTs	liver function tests
LMA	laryngeal mask airway
LOC	loss of consciousness
LUQ	left upper quadrant
MAST	medical antishock trousers
MCI	mass/multiple casualty incident
MCL	medial collateral ligament
MMR	measles/mumps/rubella vaccine
MO	myositis ossificans
MPJ	metacarpophalangeal joint
MRI	magnetic resonance imaging
NAEMSP	National Association of Emergency Medical Services Physicians
NCAA	National Collegiate Athletic Association
NFSHSA	National Federation of State High School Associations

NFPA	National Fire Protection Agency
NG	nasogastric
NSAID	nonsteroidal anti-inflammatory drug
NTG	nitroglycerin
OPA	oropharyngeal airway
OR	operating room
ORIF	open reduction and internal fixation
PAF	plasminogen activating factor
PCL	posterior collateral ligament
PEA	pulseless electrical activity
PIO	public information officer
PIPJ	proximal interphalangeal joint
PLRI	posterolateral rotatory instability
PNC	percutaneous needle cricothyrotomy
PSAP	public safety answering point
PT	physical therapy
PTA	posttraumatic amnesia
PTFL	posterior talofibular ligament
RAST	radioallergosorbent test
RGA	retrograde amnesia
RICE	rest, ice, compression, and elevation
ROM	range of motion
RSI	rapid sequence induction
RTP	return to play
RUQ	right upper quadrant
SAR	search and rescue
SC	sternoclavicular
SCFE	slipped capital femoral epiphysis
SITS	supraspinatus, infraspinatus, teres minor, subscapularis
SNELL	Snell Memorial Foundation
SPECT	single-photon-emission computed tomography
TAI	traumatic aortic injury
Td	tetanus and diphtheria vaccine
TENS	transcutaneous electrical nerve stimulation
TFCC	triangular fibrocartilage complex
TLSO	thoracolumbar spinal orthosis
TM	tympanic membrane
TMJ	temporomandibular joint
UCL	ulnar collateral ligament
URI	upper respiratory infection
USSF	United States Soccer Federation
UTI	urinary tract infection
VF	ventricular fibrillation
VT	ventricular tachycardia
WBGT	wet-bulb globe temperature
WHO	World Health Organization

Index

NOTE: Page numbers followed by *f* indicate figures; those followed by *t* indicate tables.

Hold chart 14 inches from eye in good light.
Record each eye separately with and without glasses.

S P O	48 pt	
R T S	36 pt	
I N J U R	26 pt	20/200
I E S A N D	14 pt	20/100
E M E R G E N C I E S	10 pt	20/70
A Q U I C K -	6 pt	20/40
RESPONSE	4 pt	20/25
MANUAL	3 pt	20/20

Pupil Gauge (mm)

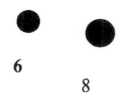

2   3   5   6   8   9